$24.95

NUTRITION MANAGEMENT FOR FOODSERVICES

NUTRITION MANAGEMENT FOR FOODSERVICES

Leslie E. Cummings
College of Hotel Administration
University of Nevada, Las Vegas

Lendal H. Kotschevar
School of Hospitality Management
Florida International University

DELMAR PUBLISHERS INC.®

NOTICE TO THE READER

Delmar Staff
  Associate Editor: Cynthia Haller
  Editing Manager: Gerry East
  Production Coordinator: Larry Main
  Design Coordinator: Susan Mathews

Cover photo by Phil Haggerty, Saratoga NY.

For information, address Delmar Publishers Inc.
Two Computer Drive West, Box 15-015
Albany, New York 12212

COPYRIGHT ©1989
BY DELMAR PUBLISHERS INC.

Printed in the United States of America
Published simultaneously in Canada
by Nelson Canada,
A division of International Thomson Limited

10 9 8 7 6 5 4 3 2 1

Library of Congress Cataloging-in-Publication Data

Cummings, Leslie E.
  Nutrition management for foodservices.

  Includes index.
  1. Nutrition. 2. Food service. I. Kotschevar, Lendal
Henry, 1908–   II. Title.
TX353.C86   613.2   89-1219
ISBN 0-8273-3522-9
ISBN 0-8273-3523-7 (instructor's guide)

Contents

PREFACE

PART 1 Introduction: The Need for a Healthful Foods Program   1

Chapter 1   Foodservices and Healthful Foods / 2
        Chapter Goals / 2
        The Search for Health and Quality Foods / / 3
        The Foodservice Industry Acts / 5
        The Government and Nutrition / 6
        The Government and The Foodservice Industry / 9
        How Much Responsibility? / 12
        Discharging The Responsibility / 15
        Summary / 17
        Chapter Review / 18

Chapter 2   Fables, Foibles, Fraud, and Fact / 19
        Chapter Goals / 19
        Why People Eat As They Do / 20
        Misinformation / 24
        How Reliable Is Nutrition Information? / 26
        Sources Of Reliable Information / 31
        Government Information and Regulation / 33
        What Is Nutritious? / 38
        Things to Come / 38
        Summary / 39
        Chapter Review / 40
        Some Federal Publications On Nutrition: / 41

PART 2 Nutrition   43

Chapter 3   Eating for Optimal Health / 44
        Chapter Goals / 44
        Why Eat? / 44
        Kinds Of Nutrients / 45
        The Six Nutrient Categories / 46
        How Food Is Reduced to Nutrients / 47
        The Digestive System / 48
        Human Nutrient Needs / 50
        Is An Ideal Diet Possible? / 59
        Summary / 60
        Chapter Review / 61

Chapter 4   Carbohydrates / 63
        Chapter Goals / 63
        Recommendations for Carbohydrate Intake / 68
        Using Carbohydrates / 68

Carbohydrate Issues / 71
Managing Carbohydrate Intake / 75
Alcohol / 77
Summary / 78
Chapter Review / 80

Chapter 5   Proteins / 81
Chapter Goals / 81
What Is Protein? / 81
Protein Value / 82
How Much Protein? / 86
The Cost of Protein / 87
Functions of Protein / 87
Misconceptions About Protein / 87
Protein Metabolism / 89
Summary / 89
Chapter Review / 90

Chapter 6   Fats and Oils: The Lipid Family / 92
Chapter Goals / 92
Fat: Good Or Bad? / 92
The Roles Of Lipids / 100
Lipid Metabolism / 101
How Much Fat and Cholesterol? / 103
What to Do About It / 105
Cardiovascular Disease (cvd) / 111
Summary / 115
Chapter Review / 116

Chapter 7   Controlling Calories / 119
Chapter Goals / 119
Calorie Concerns / 119
Heredity Or Environment? / 121
Body Composition / 123
Ideal Weight and Energy Needs / 124
Estimating Calorie Need / 127
Panaceas for Weight Loss / 129
Adding Weight / 132
Maintaining Weight / 134
Steps to A Successful Program / 135
Chapter Review / 138

Chapter 8   Vitamins / 139
Chapter Goals / 139
Fat-soluble Vitamins / 141
Water-soluble Vitamins / 146
Summary / 155

Chapter Review / 158

Chapter 9 Water and Minerals / 160
Chapter Goals / 160
Water / 160
Minerals / 164
Macrominerals / 168
Trace Elements / 179
Summary / 188
Chapter Review / 192

PART 3 The Healthful-foods Program 193

Chapter 10 Managing Nutrients in Food Purchasing and Production / 194
Chapter Goals / 194
Nutrition In The Kitchen / 194
Purchasing to Secure Nutrients / 199
Storage Considerations to Protect and Preserve Nutrients / 203
Preserving Nutrients In Pre-preparing Food / 207
Preserving Nutrients In Cookery / 208
Policing Nutrients In Purchasing and Cookery / 213
Flavor Favors / 214
Summary / 215
Chapter Review / 216

Chapter 11 Marketing the Healthful-foods Program / 218
Chapter Goals / 218
The Nutrition-oriented Foods Program—What and Why? / 218
Bringing The Nutrition-oriented Foods Program to Life / 221
Getting to Know The Market / 225
The Nra's Four Segments: Opportunities Abound / 229
An Industry Perspective:
    Who Serves Nutrition-minded Guests? / 234
Summary / 238
Chapter Review / 239

Chapter 12 Bringing the Menu to Life / 241
Chapter Goals / 241
The Menu Opportunity / 241
Menu Management for Nutrition Programs / 243
General Menu Considerations / 243
General Menu Decisions about the Scope and Shape
    of the Menu and Program / 245
Specific Needs: Planning Notes By Foodservice Type / 246
Recipes and Menus: Special Programs for Foodservices / 250
Selecting and Developing Healthful Recipes / 252
Summary / 265

Chapter Review / 267
An Industry Perspective:
    Who Serves Nutrition-minded Guests? / 268

Chapter 13   Nutrition-oriented Programs: Telling and Selling / 269
Chapter Goals / 269
Telling About The Healthful Foods Program / 269
Menu Item Communication / 270
Menus: Married Or Separate? / 270
Guidelines for Operations / 270
Managing The Marketing Mix for Nutrition-conscious Guests / 281
Program Roll-out: Before, During, and Ongoing / 292
Summary / 294
Chapter Review / 295

Chapter 14   Preparing Employees for Program Success / 298
Chapter Goals / 298
Management's Responsibility / 299
The Communication Loop A Training Imperative / 300
Training Formats: Types Of Training Programs. / 303
Training Preparation / 305
Instruction / 307
Training Program Evaluation / 308
When to Begin Training / 308
Who to Train and Topics for Training / 308
Summary / 319
Chapter Review / 320

Chapter 15   Serving Special Dietary Needs of Guests / 322
Chapter Goals / 322
Diets and Foodservices / 322
Health Care Prescription: Nutrition Management / 323
Diets Significant to Commercial Foodservice Patrons / 324
Misunderstood Conditions,
    With Dietary Notes and Clarification / 330
Catering to Vegetarian Diets and Orders / 334
Summary / 338
Chapter Review / 339

Appendices   A / 340
              B / 354
              C / 362

Index   / 396

PREFACE

Within the last few years the relationship between food and health has moved into sharp focus. People are aware that how and what they eat are related to health. Eating right for health while eating for enjoyment is important to many people today. This will be emphasized even more in the future.

A change in dietary patterns has been noted by the foodservice industry. Many units make sure they have some foods that are fitness fare. Some have changed to new menu selections and/or different modes of food preparation. The trend today is toward light but good food and patrons are showing approval. Operators, however, have also learned that they can't sell nutrition without quality, and that quality has to come first.

The foodservice industry has made progress even though many in the industry have little knowledge of nutrients and what foods meet specific standards for good nutrient content. They have lacked the knowledge of how to merchandise programs that meet patrons' needs and desires. Dietitians, nutritionists, physicians, and health-promotion associations have helped them understand what must be done to meet the demand for fitness fare. Many programs have been based on trial and error. The National Restaurant Association has been helpful in supplying information, but many foodservice operators would like more. Educational institutions have recognized that eating patterns and patron's requirements have changed. They are including courses that provide information about food and health and how healthful food programs can be successful.

There is a need today for a text that can meet the needs of both operators and educators in developing adequate healthful food programs. This book has been written to answer that need. It gives some background on the change in eating attitudes, and defines what the various segments of the foodservices industry may have as a responsibility in meeting it. It also summarizes information needed to understand some of the rudiments of nutrition and diets, and how to obtain highly nutritious foods and how to preserve nutrients.

It ends with a discussion of how to identify whether a market exists for a healthful food program and how such a program is planned and managed. A final chapter gives information about some common diets.

The foodservice industry plays a significant role in our national health. About 42% of food dollars are spent for food consumed away from home. After deducting labor and other costs, this represents about 25% of the food consumed. This means that 25% of our nutrition is the industry's responsibility and it must be discharged in a creditable manner. The authors hope that this text will make meeting this challenge easier and more successful.

No book ever becomes a reality solely through the effort of the author or authors. Many others make valued contributions. Reviewers, editors, publishers, and others lend their assistance. Deans and colleagues also deserve credit for their support and counsel. Without such help this book could never have been brought to fruition and the authors would like to express their sincere thanks. Special thanks are due the following reviewers, whose excellent suggestions helped refine and shape the final text:

Nancy S. Graves, M.S., R.D.
Department of Restaurant, Hotel and Institutional Management
Purdue University
West Lafayette, IN

Evelyn B. Enrione, Ph.D., R.D.
School of Health Sciences, Dietetics, & Nutrition
Florida International University
Miami, FL

Ethel M. Fowler, M.S., R.D.
Dietary Technician Program
Palm Beach Junior College
Lake Worth, FL

Catharine H. Powers, M.S., R.D.
The Culinary Institute of America
Hyde Park, NY

Barbara VanFossen, M.S., C.H.E.
Program Director
Hospitality/Food Service Management
Jefferson Technical College
Steubenville, OH

Sue Larkin
Department of Hotel Technology
Schenectady County Community College
Schenectady, NY

ABOUT THE AUTHORS

Leslie Edwards Cummings, a registered dietitian, is Associate Professor in Food and Beverage Management with the top-rated hospitality program at the University of Nevada, Las Vegas. Ms. Cummings' Bachelor's, Master's, and current doctoral studies share as their focus Food Delivery Systems and Nutrition. Cummings' food-service industry experience includes health care, education and commercial fine dining, and management of operations from large scale catering to fast food.

An active author and speaker, Cummings' articles on nutrition and management appear in journals around the world. Distinctions include: Institute of Food Technologists Outstanding Scholar; study Fellowships in Australia and in the General Mills test kitchens; Phi Beta Kappa membership; and Article of the Year from the *Cornell HRA Quarterly Journal,* (1988).

Lendal H. Kotschevar, Ph.D. is currently distinguished professor at the top-rated School of Hospitality Management, Florida International University, Miami, Florida. He has had extensive experience in both the foodservice industry and hospitality education. He has published widely, including many popular textbooks in the area of foodservice management. In addition, Dr. Kotschevar has presented numerous papers for the National Restaurant Association, Club Manager's Association, Foodservice Executives Association, the American Hotel and Motel Association, and other organizations devoted to hospitality management.

Dr. Kotschevar has taught and lectured widely over the world and served for a number of years as consultant in Mass Feeding for the United Nations. He also had the distinction of serving as consultant to His Holiness Pope Paul in the preparation of the Pope's talk before the Congress for World Hunger in Rome in 1963.

Part **1**

Introduction: The Need for a Healthful Foods Program

Chapter 1
Foodservices and Healthful Foods

Chapter Goals

- To explain why we need nutritious food to be healthy.
- To describe briefly the desire of patrons for healthful foods and how foodservices have responded.
- To identify nutritional gaps in our national food consumption pattern.
- To discuss activities of the federal government that promote adequate nutrition.
- To list the recommendations of the Dietary Goals for the United States.
- To show how the National Restaurant Association (NRA) and the foodservice industry have addressed the challenge of providing nutritious foods.
- To examine the responsibility of foodservice units in providing nutrition.
- To provide a basis for discussing how the foodservice industry can develop healthful food programs.

Food is vital to life. It keeps us alive and makes us grow. Mild deprivation brings on hunger pangs; prolonged malnourishment can cause serious health problems, even death. Throughout most of history, much of man's time has been spent getting enough food. There was rarely a surplus. Even today many people are near starvation. As food grows scarcer, people drop everything else, because they want to survive.

Even when there is no food shortage, eating can be a concern, because food is closely linked with health and well-being. We must eat the right foods in the right amounts to be healthy. It is possible to eat far more than enough to avoid hunger pangs, and yet to be undernourished. In fact, overeating can be a form of malnutrition: frequently it produces obesity, a condition with undeniable health risks.

Foods contain substances vital to the body's functioning. Just because there is plenty to eat does not necessarily mean the diet is adequate. Unfortunately, our appestats are geared only to relieve hunger pangs. There are no sensors to tell us that we have had enough of certain nutrients and not enough of others. Nearly forty nutrients are necessary for health. Soothing hunger pangs is not enough. We have to eat right to function properly.

THE SEARCH FOR HEALTH AND QUALITY FOODS

When people eat away from home today, they want foods they like; foods that are healthful and affordable. The foodservice operation must be clean and provide pleasant surroundings, and service must be good. They want convenience—not only in location but in how they dine. It is more than just a filling station stop. It should be a pleasurable experience in which good food, pleasant surroundings, courteous service, and healthful food contribute to a gratifying experience.

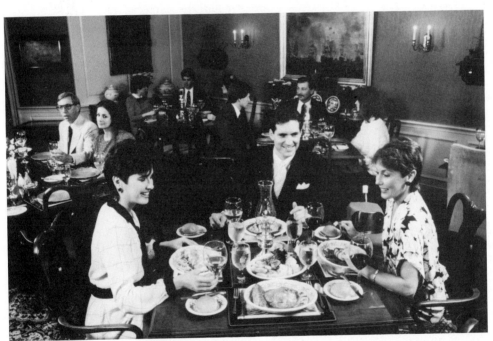

Figure 1-1 Pleasant clean, adequately furnished surroundings make for pleasurable good eating.

An emphasis on eating healthful foods was not always characteristic of Americans. Not so long ago we were a meat-and-potatoes people. In the early 1900s, when the population was largely rural, we did eat better, but with more urbanization we began to eat more fats and sugars, and to reduce our intake of fruits and vegetables. At the same time some of our health statistics changed. High blood pressure, heart diseases, and cancer became more prevalent. Table 1-1 shows heart diseases, malignancies, cerebrovascular disorders (largely strokes), and arteriosclerosis (hardening of the arteries) are, respectively the first, second, third and fifth leading causes of death of persons 55 years old and over. In many cases all four conditions are diet related. The death rate from heart disease was even higher 15 to 20 years ago. It is dropping now—some say because many people are exercising and eating better.

Though the U.S. has one of the highest living standards in the world, it ranks only 17th in health. In 1955 and 1965 extensive studies examined how American families ate. In 1955 approximately 60% of our households had "fairly good diets," and about 15% had what would be called "poor diets. According to the 1965 study, during a time when our standard of living was rising, the standard of nutrition was dropping. Only 50% of households had fairly good diets and 21% had poor diets. Since that time no mass studies such as these have been conducted, but smaller ones and other data indicate that there has been a turnaround. More households now have fairly good diets and fewer poor diets, but there is still much room for improvement.

TABLE 1-1
Leading Causes of Death of Persons 55 Years and Older, 1984

All Causes	Percent
1 Diseases of the heart*	45
2 Malignant neoplasms*	15
3 Cerebrovascular diseases*	15
4 Influenza and pneumonia*	4
5 Arteriosclerosis*	3
6 Accidents	2
Motor vehicle	1
All other	2
7 Diabetes mellitus*	2
8 Bronchitis, emphysema, and asthma	2
9 Cirrhosis of liver*	1
10 Infections of kidney*	1
All other causes	11

* Could be nutrition related. Adapted from National Center for Health Statistics.

Today poor nutrition is common among elderly persons, children and women; and a high income is no guarantee of good nutrition. Many who have plenty of money to spend for food spend it unwisely as far as nutrition is concerned.

For the most part, people are motivated to eat healthfully not out of a desire for a balanced diet but because they want to avoid extra calories (to maintain their weight) and to avoid foods high in fats and cholesterol (because they are associated with heart and blood vessel diseases). Salt is used sparingly, because it can elevate blood pressure. Eating properly is not just a matter of selecting the right nutrients but of getting them in the right foods. People are also interested in how safe food is in terms of additives and byproducts of processing. They often want a minimum of processing, believing that foods in the natural state contain more nutrients.

This desire for healthful and quality foods was engendered by the recent public awareness of the relationship between food and health. Excess calories, fat, cholesterol, junk food, and sodium have no place in today's "fit food," to use popular nutrition jargon; many say they should be avoided. "Lean n'Light" is the catch phrase that denotes optimal menu fare today.

This awareness of the relationship between food and health has been brought about by the patrons' expectations of what healthful food is. Patrons who are better informed about diet and how to stay fit want foodservices to provide such a diet for them when they eat out.

At the same time, this healthful food must be served in a way that does not detract from the enjoyment of eating. To some, the words "diet" and "nutrition" suggest self-denial—eating foods that are not particularly tasty but are "good for you."

Foodservices, realizing this, have gone out of their way to offer not only healthful foods, but those that are of high quality and as appealing in every way as anything else offered on the menu.

THE FOODSERVICE INDUSTRY ACTS

Interest in meeting this increasing desire for high quality and healthful foods is pervasive throughout the industry. Many restaurants, hotel dining operations, fast food units, worker feeding facilities, schools, and other foodservices have incorporated into their menus what patrons feel are healthful foods, and patrons have responded favorably. One of the first restaurants to feature health-oriented foods was La Patisse, in Berkeley, California. Today its success is being duplicated in many other fine, gourmet-type dining establishments, but family restaurants and others also saw a demand and moved to satisfy it.

A number of hotels, many of them chains such as the Hiltons and Marriotts, have established healthful-foods programs. An article titled "Hotel Meals: How Nutritious?" (February 1981 *Cornell Hotel and Restaurant Quarterly Journal*) by Barry Goldstein and Mary Tabacchi, examined the nutritional value of 83 menus from a cross-section of hotels. They made three significant assumptions: (1) the traveler understands nutrition, his or her requirements, and daily dietary goals and guidelines; (2) he or she would choose appropriate foods and not others; and (3) the hotel restaurants surveyed actually serve the portion sizes and precise recipes reported. Given these optimistic qualifiers, the authors reported that most nutritional needs could be met. The main nutrient problems were a shortage of vitamin B_6 and too much protein (twice the recommended 12% in the Dietary Goals). The authors concluded that sound nutritional choices are available in many hotel foodservices.

Fast food operations also have made changes. More vegetables are available, and salad bars have been introduced. The variety of offerings has been increased, some of which are intended to appeal to people interested in healthful eating. Buffet bars are featured. The nutritional value of some favorite menu items has been enhanced, as by adding lettuce and tomatoes to hamburgers. Many fast food operations are now publishing nutrition information about their foods. This change has been well received by the public.

Operations that feature ethnic foods have joined the march. The Hunan Restaurant in Philadelphia, Pennsylvania and Madame Wu's Garden in Santa Monica, California are good examples of the Chinese way of serving healthful foods. Chi-Chi's Mexican restaurants also have added health fare to the menu.

In the effort to meet public demand, foodservices have sought the assistance of many professionals and organizations that can advise on programs in eating for health, such as the American Cancer Society, the American Dietetic Association, the American Diabetes Association, and the American Heart Association (AHA). Their assistance created more confidence in the commitment of foodservices offering healthful foods. The AHA's "Creative Cuisine" and the ACS's programs have enjoyed considerable acceptance from patrons and from foodservices which have seen increased patronage, customer satisfaction, and profits. It is note-worthy that among those using the AHA's programs are fine dining establishments that serve gourmet food. In the Los Angeles area, over 40% of the establishments using the AHA's programs are of this type. Even supermarkets are trying to cash in on the ACS's slogan, "It's good for you" (Fig. 1-2).

THE GOVERNMENT AND NUTRITION

The U.S. government has shown concern for the state of nutrition of its citizens. Through agencies such as the Department of Agriculture (USDA), Health and Human Services (HHS), and others, it has gathered information on our nutritional status and has established educational programs. The government has also established a processed food enrichment program that requires the addition of certain vitamins

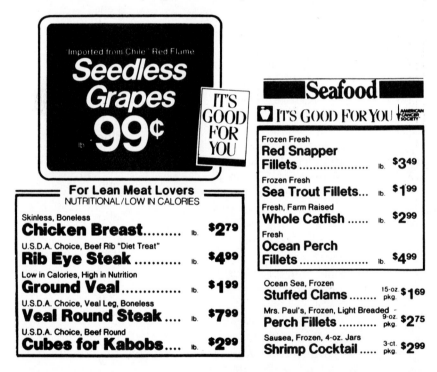

Figure 1-2—Note how even supermarket advertisements are attempting to capitalize on nutritional factors in selling certain foods. The slogan "It's good for you" is being popularized by the American Cancer Society.

and minerals to refined grains and cereals. It allows the addition of vitamins to fluid milk and margarine and of iodine to table salt. The National School Lunch Program was established to provide children with a better balanced diet. Later, breakfast and a feeding program for young children were added. The Food Stamp Program was designed to help the needy get food at less cost. The government also distributes surplus food to the poor and to charitable institutions. The Women, Infants, and Children (WIC) program was directed toward providing high quality foods to groups particularly vulnerable to becoming undernourished. Meals-on-Wheels, or Title VII Elderly Feeding Program, enables many senior citizens to get at least one balanced meal a day. Often this meal is delivered to their residence.

The government has in other ways encouraged better nutrition. The Food and Drug Administration (FDA) has set up a program called Nutrition Labeling (Fig. 1-3), which requires that processed foods in the retail market have certain nutritional information on the label if any nutritional claim is made about the food inside. Food processors can also voluntarily place on the label nutritional information per serving of the food. If a manufacturer makes a false or misleading claim in such labeling, the FDA can take action to stop it. Federal and state agencies are also charged with establishing and enforcing standards for quality and sanitation, (Fig. 1-4).

NUTRITION INFORMATION		
SERVING SIZE: ½ CUP		SERVINGS PER PACKAGE: 4
	MIX TO MAKE 1 SERVING	1 SERVING PREPARED AS PUDDING USING WHOLE MILK
CALORIES	90	160*
PROTEIN	1 g	5 g
CARBOHYDRATE	22 g	28 g
FAT	0	4 g
SODIUM	110 mg	170 mg
PERCENTAGES OF U.S. RECOMMENDED DAILY ALLOWANCES (U.S. RDA)		
PROTEIN	**	10%
VITAMIN A	**	2%
VITAMIN C	**	**
THIAMINE	**	4%
RIBOFLAVIN	**	10%
NIACIN	**	**
CALCIUM	**	15%
IRON	**	**
PHOSPHORUS	2%	15%

*SAVE 30 CALORIES/SERVING — USE SKIM MILK
**CONTAINS LESS THAN 2% OF THE U.S. RDA OF THESE NUTRIENTS.

FOR PUDDING: Mix contents with 2 cups milk. Cook and stir over medium heat until mixture comes to a full boil. Pudding thickens as it cools. Serve warm or cold.
For creamier pudding, place plastic wrap on surface of pudding while cooling; stir before serving. Top with COOL WHIP® Whipped Topping, if desired. Makes four (½-cup) servings.

FOR PIE: Cool cooked pudding 5 minutes, stirring twice. Pour into cooled, baked 8-inch pie shell. Chill 3 hours.

INGREDIENTS: SUGAR, DEXTROSE (CORN SUGAR), CORNSTARCH, COCOA PROCESSED WITH ALKALI, MODIFIED CORNSTARCH, SALT, POLYSORBATE 60 (FOR UNIFORM DISPERSION IN MILK), CALCIUM CARRAGEENAN (VEGETABLE GUM – THICKENER), FUMARIC ACID (STABILIZER), ARTIFICIAL AND NATURAL FLAVORS. 99 g

Figure 1-3 Nutrition labeling on a package of chocolate pudding; note the list of ingredients appears under this information.

The White House Conference on Food, Nutrition, and Health held in 1969 brought together leading scientists, nutritionists, dietitians, physicians, and others to evaluate the state of nutrition of the populace and to formulate a basis for a national nutrition policy. One of the outgrowths of this conference was the publication in 1977 by the U. S. Senate Select Committee on Nutrition and Human Needs (now defunct) of the *Dietary Goals for the United States*. These were revised in 1985 (Table 1-2).

The Dietary Goals proved to be controversial: some opponents claimed that we should not try to cover everyone just because some few need such guidance. In some cases the Goals were thought to be too specific. Other critics called for even stricter recommendations; still others wanted them relaxed. Undoubtedly they will be revised again in the future, but for the time being they remain a pillar around which we can center nutritional attention, and in this book we consistently refer to them as goals.

These 1985 revised Goals are less specific, and do not indicate various levels or amounts of food. Thus, the 1977 Goals indicated that complex carbohydrates constitute 48% of total calories and simple carbohydrates (sugars), 10%. These percentages were dropped from the revised Goals. They also recommended that fat intake be divided equally between saturated fats, monounsaturated fats, and polyunsaturated fats. Alcoholic beverages were not mentioned in the first Goals. In the

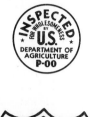

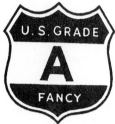
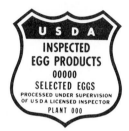
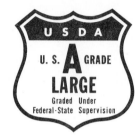

Figure 1-4 The three stamps on the top indicate the food has been inspected and passed and is fit for human consumption. The three grade stamps on the bottom are stamps indicating quality.

discussion below on following through on some of these recommendations, we consider both the 1977 Goals and the 1985 ones.

The Goals can help ensure proper intake of nutrients. Providing good nutrition is a balancing act: we must consume foods with enough protein, vitamins, minerals, and complex carbohydrates, and only enough fat, sodium, sugar, and alcohol to provide a satisfactory diet that does not contribute to health problems. Energy intake (calories) must also be tailored to energy expenditure for weight control.

TABLE 1-2
Percentage of Calories from Various Nutrient
Groups Recommended by U.S. Dietary Goals
and Actually Consumed.

Nutrient	Daily Calories		Recommendations
	Actually Consumed (%)	Recommended (%)	
Fat	42	30	Avoid too much total fat
			Avoid too much saturated fat
Protein	12	12	Eat adequate vegetable protein
Complex carbohydrates	22	48	Eat adequate "whole" plant foods
Sugar or simple carbohydrates	24	10	Avoid too much refined sugar, syrup, etc.

To assist in promoting the Goals, the 1977 Senate Committee recommended that the following steps be taken:

1. Establish a large scale public nutrition education program utilizing schools, food assistance programs, extension services, and the mass media.
2. Expand mandatory food and nutrition labeling.
3. Develop improved food processing methods to improve the nutritional value and safety of our foods.
4. Increase governmental support for research in human nutrition.

To meet these goals the following recommendations were made for selection and preparation of foods:

1. Increase consumption of vegetables, fruits, and whole grains.
2. Reduce intake of sugars and foods that contain large amounts of all types of sugars. Limit refined sugars to 10% of calories, and complex carbohydrates and naturally occurring sugars to 48% (total carbohydrate 58% of calories).
3. Limit intake of foods high in fat and substitute polyunsaturated fats for saturated fats. Consume the 30% of calories recommended for fat in the diet as 10% monounsaturated fat, 10% polyunsaturated fat, and 10% saturated fat.
4. Increase the consumption of poultry and fish while reducing consumption of meats, which contain fairly large amounts of saturated fats in their fatty components.
5. Obtain about 12% of calories from protein foods.
6. Consume nonfat milk and low-fat milk products, but allow whole milk and whole milk products for children.
7. Reduce the consumption of butterfat, eggs, and other high cholesterol sources. Those in good health may eat as many as three eggs a week, if intake of other cholesterol is controlled.
8. Try not to salt food and avoid processed foods with high salt content. Use spices and other seasonings to take the place of salt.

Our discussion in the chapters that follow will include many examples of how we can implement these recommendations.

THE GOVERNMENT AND THE FOODSERVICE INDUSTRY

The government also has attempted to stimulate attention toward nutrition in the foodservice industry. In 1975 the Federal Trade Commission (FTC) proposed a food advertising trade regulation that would consider menus as advertising media and require them to conform to its regulations on advertisements. Any claims made in a menu about nutritional value would have to be substantiated by giving the amounts of nutrients in foods sold. After many hearings a step-by-step plan of implementation was proposed:

Phase I: Require menus to carry information on calories and other nutrient- and health-related terms. Restrict the use of terms such as "natural" and "organic."

Phase II: Require nutritional information to support claims. Thus, statements such as "wholesome," "nutritious," "good for you," "low in calories," and "high in energy" would have to be substantiated.

Phase I was to start January 1, 1979.

The NRA and others in the industry opposed to the regulation attended the FTC hearings. During these FTC hearings the NRA made a statement articulating its stand on the proposal and its views on the difficulty foodservices would have in meeting some of the FTC's proposals. "We share the Commission's view that many Americans fail to apply nutritional principles in their eating habits. Whether this failure stems from ignorance of nutrition or from a conscious rejection of good principles in favor of personal tastes and desires, we do not know. Considering the broad dissemination of the elements of sound nutritional dietary components in our schools and in the press, it is possible we are faced with a widespread rejection of known dietary principles in favor of personal taste, preference and convenience. We may be confronted with an affirmation of the old adage that 'you can lead a horse to water, but you can't make him drink.' The proposed rule, however, is based on the assumption that ignorance is the prime cause and that the disclosure requirement will provide the needed education."

The NRA further pointed out that ethical standards of the Association already required truthful and accurate representation of menu statements and offerings. They agreed that patrons lacked the necessary knowledge of what foods to select and needed to be more knowledgeable, but the NRA argued that patrons might not understand the nutrition information even if it were given to them. And if patrons could not understand it or how it fit into their needs, they would not be in a position to use the information to make proper selections. Such information might be confusing and cause patrons to make improper selections.

The NRA also said the regulation could unfairly restrict foodservices from making legitimate claims about nutrition or health and that, if they did make such statements, they would leave themselves open to attack without recourse to any defense. Small foodservices would be hardest hit, because they could not afford the expense of ongoing legal fees and laboratory analyses of menu items to substantiate their claims.

Because of the strong arguments presented against the FTC proposal by the NRA and others, the FTC tabled the plan. However, the experience was a sobering one for the foodservice industry. It saw in such government regulation possible requirements that would be very difficult to meet, might not serve the intended purpose, and might harm the industry.

Labeling on food packages is the responsibility of the USDA's FDA, which in 1979 proposed that menus meet the same requirements as food packaging (i.e., if a menu made a nutritional claim, the claim must be substantiated). Also, basic information required on *all* labeling of packaged food would be required on *all* menus.

The NRA and the foodservice industry again opposed the regulation, and in January 1979 the NRA published a nutrition policy statement that "reaffirmed the tradition of concern for the health and well-being of restaurant customers." It said it was "fully aware of the increased interest by government, the scientific community, and members of the public in nutrition, and encouraged scientific research in nutrition." The NRA agreed that the foodservice industry should play a role in communicating nutrition information and should assist patrons in selecting a better diet. Finally, the NRA committed its membership to cooperating with the government, scientific agencies, the media, and the general public in promoting good nutrition to the extent they could.

Again the NRA and the industry were able to forestall action. The FDA decided to recommend that the individual states take up the matter and pass appropriate legislation. However, the NRA went a long way in committing the industry to good nutritional efforts, saying it had concern for the health and well-being of patrons; encouraged scientific research in nutrition; and it should play a role in communicating nutrition information and to help patrons select better diets. This was a big step forward from its 1975 statement.

After the 1982 elections, government interest in nutrition and the foodservice industry waned; however, in 1986 some U. S. Congressional leaders became dissatisfied with the states' lack of progress in passing legislation regarding labeling regulations. Only one state, New York, had done anything about it. A bill was introduced in Congress that would require all food chains with at least 10 outlets to provide patrons with ingredient lists for the products sold. The bill was backed by the AHA, the Center for Science in the Public Interest, and other groups. In reaction to this movement, McDonald's, Burger King, and other chains now publish pamphlets containing ingredient information. In the end, the 1986 proposal died in committee owing to an overall lack of support. The position of the NRA at the time when this book is being completed is to strongly back nutrition support by the industry within limits of its ability to provide it and to staunchly oppose government interference.

Many feel that progress is being made and that if the foodservice industry is allowed to develop programs voluntarily, a more sound and practical policy will be the result. The fact that selling nutrition produces profits and patron satisfaction is bringing about a greater attempt by foodservices to offer foods desired by patrons. Progress in the last 10 years has been significant.

However, those pushing for governmental regulation ask, "Why is it that action is taken only when federal or state authorities or agencies pick up the cudgels?" The task cannot be done overnight; there is danger that it would miss the mark, do little good, and harm the industry. Foodservices are moving to promote better nutrition on a broad front, and this text is one evidence of this progress.

The desire of patrons for foods they regard as healthful is increasing. As we have seen, government interest in seeing that certain labeling requirements be added to those we have has not abated. The government has decided, at least for the time, to drop the issue of making menus conform to labeling laws.

Whether more government regulation would or would not be in the public interest is arguable. Many feel we are overregulated today, that much of the regulation we have is not beneficial (and in some cases actually harmful). In a competitive society there are usually enough pressures to bring about a compromise that suits the majority's wishes. A *laissez faire* (let things be) approach may be the safest and surest way to reach desirable goals.

HOW MUCH RESPONSIBILITY?

It is estimated that about 25% of the total food consumed in this country is produced in foodservice operations (Fig. 1-5 and 1-6). The proportion of food dollars spent for dining away from home is 42%. Subtracting nonfood items such as labor, rent, and other costs from this 42%, we estimate that 25% is spent then for food itself. If so, the foodservice industry bears the responsibility for providing 25% of the nutrition for the U.S.

How much responsibility should the foodservice industry have in providing good nutrition to the public? Some would go so far as to have us remove certain foods from the menu, furnish nutrition information, provide dietary needs, and attend to a host of other matters. Others say that the industry has no responsibility whatever. People are capable of selecting where and what they eat; those are their choices. The authors feel that the foodservice industry's proper responsibility lies midway between these two points of view.

It seems reasonable that responsibility would vary with how much freedom of choice a patron has in where and what to eat; with the type of foodservice operation and its goals; and with the amount of food a patron consistently consumes in one operation, among other considerations. Certainly a restaurant does not have the same responsibility as a hospital, or a college or prison foodservice, where people must eat what is offered because selection is limited or nonexistent. We will examine some of the factors and see whether we can define boundaries within which various types of foodservice operators might feel they properly have a responsibility for serving healthful foods. There has long been a need for such a definition.

It should be obvious that different foodservices have different goals, perform different services, serve different patrons who have varying needs, and operate under vastly different conditions to mention just a few of the variables in the problem. These differences presuppose different levels of responsibility vis-á-vis nutrition. A drive-in offering only a few items cannot be expected to serve a complete, nutritionally balanced meal. A restaurant cannot be expected to provide nutrition advice. A diabetic eating in a restaurant should know which foods are permitted and which are not. For diabetics choice of foods can be a matter of life and death, and restaurants should not have to participate in decision making. There are many analogous situations, but let us examine the variables and how they may influence responsibility.

For the purpose of analyzing these varying responsibilities, let us divide foodservices into three categories: free-choice operations, partially "captive" operations, and captive ones. The dividing lines are not always sharp. A dining facility in a factory may be free choice but also be partially captive. Workers can eat there or not, can select what they want, but since it is the only eating facility available to them, they are partly captive. Unless they carry their own food or don't eat, they have to eat there.

Free-choice operations are those where patrons have free choice to select the operation, and to select what they want, and to eat what they want. In some, the menu is extensive enough to provide a nutritionally complete meal; in others such as a drive-in, the offerings are limited and a complete meal is not available. Many

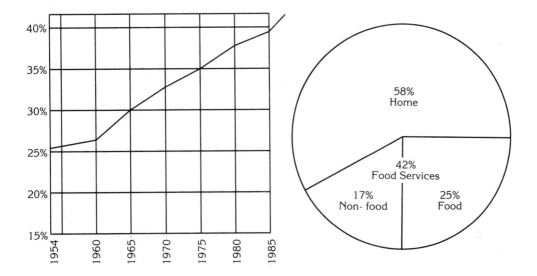

Figure 1-5 This graph shows how the percentage of food dollars spent for food away from home has increased in the last 30 years in the United States. (Adapted from NRA data)

Figure 1-6 How the American food dollar is spent.

restaurants, cafeterias, hotel foodservices, fast food operations, and others comprise this group. For the most part, they can be regarded as profit oriented.

The partially captive group varies considerably. School foodservices, college dormitory systems, airlines, cruise ships, trains, worker feeding units, and many others fall into this category. The distinguishing feature is that only a part of all food consumed is consumed by a person in the operation. Often, but not necessarily, a substantial part of the diet is obtained elsewhere.

The captive group has two kinds of foodservices. One kind serves most or all the food patrons get but is not principally health related. Examples are prisons, boarding schools, and other services whose purpose is to provide good, healthful food to basically healthy patrons. The other kind serve persons who have special health-related nutritional needs such as the people in hospitals, nursing homes, extended care centers, and even health spas.

How do the nutritional responsibilities of each of these three groups differ? It must be remembered that the responsibility can vary as the nature of the operation varies from one group to another.

Free-Choice Group

When a patron is free to select the place and the food and to eat it or not, a facility has little responsibility for seeing that the patron has adequate nutrition. In such operations, the patron has almost total responsibility for what he or she eats. The facility has only a general, broad responsibility that is common to all three groups in the foodservice industry.

Partial-Choice Group

Some in this group serve given individuals so briefly or so sporadically that inadequate nutrition could be tolerated (although the operation, certainly, should meet its obligation); for example an airplane service that serves only one or two meals or a cruise ship that serves patrons for only a week or so. A child eating in elementary school eats five of 21 meals per week there, so a greater proportion of the total nutrition is provided by the cafeteria than by some other operations. When an operation serves even more of the food, the responsibility increases. The degree of freedom one has in selecting food and in eating what is taken also is a factor. In elementary and secondary schools, the Type A lunch now is often of the offer-serve type: five foods from representative nutritional groups must be offered, but the child only has to take three. Thus, some responsibility resides with the patron to make good nutritional choices. In the same way, other patrons share responsibility to the extent that choices are available to them. In some cases, it is possible that a facility will or should promote good nutritional choices. School feeding programs may be one of these. Also, a cafeteria may be asked by management to do some nutritional promotion and prepare some special foods to tie in with the operation's wellness program.

Captive Group

Operations that serve captive diners have a clear responsibility to provide adequate nutrition. Too much of the diner's food is consumed there for it to be otherwise. In some institutions, such as prisons and boarding schools, it may even be desirable for the facility to provide for some special dietary needs. The facility also must bear some responsibility for trying to promote good nutrition in order to maintain the health and well-being of those it feeds. In the case of a hospital or other health-related unit, there is an even greater responsibility to see that the food is nutritionally adequate, even to the extent of limiting or dictating a patron's selections; but, even in this group, patrons often have a choice of food within a prescribed range and, so, still retain some limited responsibility. A health-related unit bears responsibility for seeing that a patron eats what should be eaten, even to the extent of offering some other permitted food so as to encourage consumption. Often records must be kept of how well a patron is eating what is served so that, if the right kind or amount is not being eaten, steps can be taken to correct the situation. Note in Figure 1-7 how the greater share of nutritional responsibility falls to the facility and only a little falls to the patron.

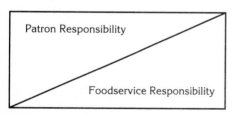

Figure 1-7 As patrons lose more and more freedom of choice in where, when, and what they will eat, the responsibility of foodservices for nutrition usually increases.

General Industry Responsibility

A significant part of the nutrition in the U.S. is provided by foodservices, and our national health, productivity, and well-being are clearly affected by this circumstance. Foodservices have a clear duty to the national interest as well as to individual patrons to discharge this overall responsibility in a creditable manner. There are limits to what can be done that are partly functions of the nature of the facility and the type of patron. A fast food unit that serves light snacks cannot be charged with the responsibility of serving a nutritionally complete meal, but a facility with a menu that makes it possible to select a complete meal might assist the patron in selecting foods that are adequate and nutritionally balanced. Then it is up to the patron to make the proper selection.

Every foodservice should make a conscious effort to see that the foods offered contain all the nutrients they should. Food of adequate nutritional quality should be purchased within the limits of the food itself, and nutrients should not be lost by mishandling or poor preparation. (Of course, if the item is a cola syrup which is mixed with a carbonated water to make a soft drink, the operator has little choice. The sugar, at least, provides energy!) Figure 1-8 illustrates facility responsibility in a step-by-step rise in responsibility.

DISCHARGING THE RESPONSIBILITY

The responsibilities for nutrition presented above may be somewhat greater than some believe they should be. Others may think they are not enough. However, if the foodservice industry is to provide a significant share of the population's nourishment, the responsibilities as outlined are a constructive and timely first step. Informed by knowledge, with skill and commitment, continuing progress should culminate in

A Drive-ins, such as hamburger, chicken, pizza, snack bars, vending machines, or others serving partial meals.
B White-tablecloth restaurants, family restaurants, or cafeteria, coffee shops, etc.
C Any of those in A or B, above, that feature healthful foods; they may or may not make nutritional claims for them or they may try to give helpful nutritional information.
D Elementary and secondary schools, college dormitories, transportation, business and industry feeding units, prisons, etc.
E Hospitals, nursing homes, some retirement homes, etc.

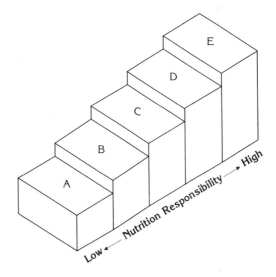

Figure 1-8 Degrees of nutritional responsibility in different foodservices. Kinds of establishments in each category.

providing patrons with what they want today. Certainly, they are not out of line with previously cited stands taken by the NRA.

Is the industry prepared to discharge these responsibilities? Certainly health-care foodservices have been doing so for a long time, because high nutrition standards are among their goals. As public operations are pressed to meet these responsibilities, even as outlined, follow-through may be more difficult. Traditionally, nutritional responsibility has not been a prominent factor in their operation and was not included in their goals. This need and opportunity is something that has come about in the past few years.

Any discussion of responsibility must also address the primary need to present food of good quality. If the quality of the food is poor, the patron usually does not eat it, and the food and the effort are wasted. Implementing a healthful-foods program is not an onerous, unpleasant task: rather, it means capitalizing on skillful, palatable preparation of nutritious fare, and it is a program that can pay off.

In a free economy, a public foodservice has the right to serve what it wants. If it fails to serve what appeals, the business will not survive. This is the way our economic structure has of eliminating those who cannot meet the market's demands. Too often critics have assumed that menu offerings should be dictated by nutritional considerations alone, or by the health beliefs of various public interest groups rather than by regular patrons and by what is best for the business of the foodservice. While public-spirited decision-makers may wish to "push nutrition," if this offends patrons or denies them certain food items they come for, it might be business suicide for a foodservice to move too far. This should be recognized. The law of supply-and-demand works both ways. Foodservices that supply items that patrons demand will, in turn, be in demand. They will be more likely to prosper. Failure to perceive and supply those demands means patrons will not patronize the operation.

Public foodservices are not in business to teach patrons how to eat to maintain health. Patrons must take charge of their own nutritional information needs. If we know what we want to eat and it is not available at one facility, we can patronize one that meets our demands or prepare our own food.

We also have to recognize that patrons are not experts in nutrition. There is a lot of misinformation about, and foodservices are often badgered by patrons who believe it. Nutrition and diet are complex subjects, and most people, though they may have plenty of "information," are not very knowledgeable. What the majority know about nutrition and health is what they hear or read in popular sources. Most lack complete and accurate information on what constitutes a good diet and what sound nutritional principles are. Henry J. Heinz II discussed this lack in an article in *The New York Times* in 1981, calling us a "nation of nutritional illiterates."

There are many indications that we need to establish better education programs on nutrition and diet in order to dispel a tremendous amount of misinformation that is rampant throughout the populace. Through education, we can bring about changes in our own behavior and in others that will result in more healthful food choices being made at home and away from home. Better informed patrons would make it easier for foodservices to discharge their responsibility.

In the chapters that follow we will be discussing briefly some of the current misinformation about health and foods and presenting some basic facts about healthful foods and human needs. We also will see how foodservices can deliver healthful foods and turn it into an asset.

SUMMARY

The foodservice industry can take great pride and satisfaction in the service it provides the nation. It is an extremely important service that allows the economy and society to function freely. It is a massive industry in terms of business dollar volume and in the enormous number of employees. Another important factor is that this industry is vital to our long-term health through nutrition since about one fourth to one third of the food consumed is purchased this way.

The foodservice industry has been criticized for failing to execute its responsibility to provide healthful foods by some patrons, by nutrition and health authorities, and by the government. Because of this, as early as 1979 the NRA published a position paper on nutrition, affirming its interest in nutrition and healthful food and in meeting its obligations in seeing that adequate standards are maintained in these areas. It also indicated it would be active in providing nutrition information.

Operations that serve the general public for profit (commercial establishments) have a lower level of nutritional responsibility than those that serve patrons with few choice alternatives, such as those in prisons, live-in schools, and hospitals. A balanced diet should not be expected by patrons when operations, such as fast food services, serve only partial meals. When menus are extensive enough to provide a variety of foods and where complete meals are served, the operation's responsibility for nutrition is greater. Patrons should be offered a range of foods from which they can select a balanced meal. Patrons who freely choose where and what they eat have more responsibility for selecting a proper diet than persons who have less choice of where and what to eat. The patron who must eat in a specific operation and must eat what is offered, has less responsibility and the operation, more. Health-care facilities have the greatest responsibility, since one of their goals is to provide adequate nutrition, which often is a part of the medical treatment.

Discharging these various levels of responsibility may require that some foodservice personnel and managers become more knowledgeable in nutrition than they now are. The necessary level of knowledge will vary with the responsibility carried by the facility. Hospitals and some institutional foodservices may now have personnel who are knowledgeable about nutrition, but some commercial and institutional foodservices may have to educate some of their personnel.

Foodservice professionals are beginning to recognize that more emphasis must be put on nutrition. They realize that they face a new challenge in discharging the responsibility of their operations vis-á-vis nutrition. However, there are clear opportunities to advance business objectives on the whole, and foodservices can look positively on these and take advantage of them. Later chapters in this text explore how this might be done.

Chapter Review

1. List and briefly describe 10 reasons why the foodservice industry should pay more attention to nutrition and 10 reasons why it should not.
2. If a patron complains about the nutritional quality of a meal and management feels it is following good nutritional practices, how should the manager handle the problem? Describe a situation and present ideas on how management should respond to such criticism and how it might be prevented.
3. Briefly summarize the nutrition-related responsibilities of various kinds of foodservices serving (a) free-choice (b) partial-choice and (c) "captive" patrons.

Chapter 2
Fables, Foibles, Fraud, and Fact

Chapter Goals

- *To point out types and sources of information and misinformation on how to eat to be healthy.*
- *To discuss why people eat the way they do.*
- *To show how those who wish to profit from nutrition fraud sometimes misuse facts to gain their ends.*
- *To discuss fad diets.*
- *To present the position of natural and organic food advocates and describe how some nutrition authorities agree and disagree.*
- *To list sources of good information on healthful eating.*
- *To show how the government provides information on nutrition and tries to regulate to assure healthful and safe eating.*
- *To cover briefly how this text will move in subsequent chapters to show what the nutrients are and to present a way of assuring that such nutrients are present in foods served in foodservices.*

Is there truly a pot of gold at the end of the rainbow? Does garlic lower blood pressure? Is raw sugar more healthful than refined? Does consuming a lot of meat make people aggressive? Are grapefruit and fat so antagonistic in the body that grapefruit burns up fat? Why are lobster and milk taken together said to make a poison? Is sexual performance enhanced by eating oysters? Would drinking a tonic of jellyfish ashes cure goiter?

Perhaps you don't believe *all* these things, but do you believe one or more? As far as we know, "yes" is the right answer to only one. Just as no one has ever been known to find gold at the end of the rainbow, no one has ever lowered blood pressure by eating garlic. It lowers only one's chances for a kiss. Raw sugar has some calcium, iron, impurities, and coloring matter that refined sugar lacks, but these extras are not enough to make raw sugar significantly better than ordinary refined white sugar. Eating meat does not cause aggression. Peaceful Eskimos eat a lot of it, whereas vegetarian tribes in the South Seas are ferocious warriors. Grapefruit and fat are compatible, and neither particularly eliminates the other from the body. Lobster bisque and lobster Newburg are delicious milk and lobster combinations that many eat without coming to harm. Whoever invented the idea that fish, especially oysters, stimulate libido, no one knows. Some hypothesize that the phosphorus in fish and shellfish acts as a sexual stimulant, but lots of other foods that contain phosphorus do not have this reputation. The only true statement could be that jellyfish cures goiter. Jellyfish contains iodine and iodine cures goiter.

WHY PEOPLE EAT AS THEY DO

How people eat is deeply tied to identity and environment. Both factors influence basic eating patterns that, once established, are extremely difficult, if not impossible, to change. It is often said that it is easier to change a person's religion than the way he or she eats.

If we understand how deeply ingrained eating habits are, we have a much better understanding of how to influence eating patterns. Often, the way to effect such changes lies in finding some way to move into one of these deeply set patterns and work from there.

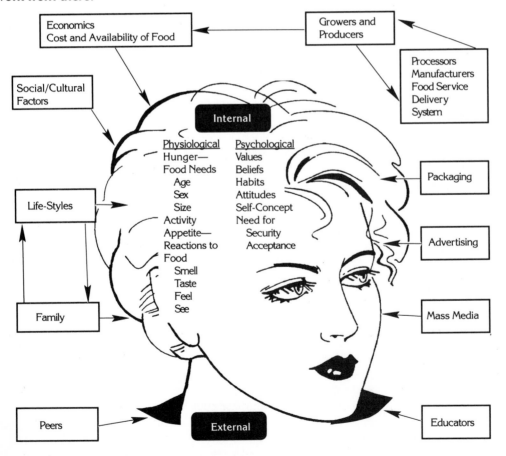

Figure 2-1 Influences on Our Food Habits—External and Internal

Many factors influence eating habits. (Fig. 2-1). There are outside factors such as mass media, education, advertising and packaging, sociocultural influences, family, and peers, but, internal factors also influence us—values, beliefs, attitudes, and habits. Eating habits are a function of physiological and psychological needs and natural, ethnic, social, religious, economic, and individual influences; some people even approach eating as an art.

Physiological Factors

One of the most compelling reasons why we eat is a built-in physiological mechanism, hunger. This basic instinct is necessary to our survival. When we have eaten enough, the hunger mechanism shuts off. It is such a strong instinct that at times it can over-ride other powerful instincts such as love and fear. We may eat out of habit, choosing to eat because we are stimulated by the sight, smell, flavor, or texture of food. Children love sweet things because their mouths and tongues have so many taste buds for sweetness. Most older persons crave sweets less because they have lost a lot of those taste buds.

We need more food in infancy and adolescence, when we are growing fast. Pregnant and nursing mothers also have increased needs. After about age 45 the need for calories drops though the need for other nutrients does not. Females usually eat less than males: persons with greater body mass must eat more to maintain their weight. Activity level also affects eating patterns. It takes extra energy to play a couple of sets of tennis. Environment can be an influence: in cold weather we need more calories to maintain body heat, and we may increase our consumption of food to that end.

Psychological Factors

Eating is tied deeply to the psyche. Food is so important—so satisfying and so closely tied to emotions—that sometimes the emotions dictate how we eat. Many people overeat when they are upset. A person may have some unpleasantness at the office and that night be upset with dinner. There is nothing wrong with the food. It is a psychological response to the stress. Directors of college foodservices know that the conjunction of the stress of examinations and the boredom of the long academic year come together in the spring and prompt student food riots. In this period smart directors "beef up" their menus with steaks, strawberry shortcakes, and other treats to forestall boredom and food criticism. Some pregnant women crave certain kinds of foods. While such craving may be based on some physiological factor, the real cause is often a psychological one.

Natural Factors

Some people eat certain foods because they are readily available. South Americans eat a lot of plantain, a cousin of the banana, because they can grow it more easily than other starch sources. Many peoples build their eating habits around fish because it is plentiful in their area. Eskimos eat a lot of blubber, because it is in good supply in their food sources. If we ate as much, the high concentrations of vitamins A and D would make us ill. China has two main carbohydrate sources; in the south the main carbohydrate is rice, and in the north, where only wheat can be grown, it is noodles and dumplings. Millions of Chinese have never tasted rice, because they cannot grow it. We could go around the world noting that natives of each country or area eat what they do because it is what they have: whatever prospers locally is what they eat.

Ethnic Factors

Often ethnic or national or regional eating patterns are bound up with what a culture has—its indigenous food, but separate cultures that have similar food resources nevertheless develop peculiar cooking styles. Germans eat a lot of sausage, partly because of the foods that are available but also because they have developed a liking for this kind of food. Irish and Polish people both eat a lot of potatoes, but they prepare them in quite different ways.

When a region, nation, or culture develops a distinct way of preparing food, we call it a *cuisine.* Within a given cuisine we often find *styles* of cooking. Thus, France has one cuisine but three styles of cooking: in the north butter is the main fat; in the south olive oil is the main fat; and in the west the main fats are goose grease and lard. In each of these three areas the food is quite distinctive, but there are many common patterns characteristic of French cuisine.

In Italy there are two styles. Italy's cuisine is built around pasta, but in the south the tomato is much more prominent than in the north. A given dish can appear at tables dressed in red sauce or in white, or cream sauce. Thus, clam sauce with pasta can be either red, with a tomato base, or white, without tomatoes. China has at least seven distinct styles of cooking but basic cooking methods and foods are so similar that they belong to one cuisine. It is said that the United States has no cuisine, only styles of cooking: Southern, Cajun, Creole, Pennsylvania Dutch, etc. (One wag disputes this, saying the national cuisine is the hamburger, fries, and a milkshake or carbonated beverage.)

Social Factors

Social customs also dictate how people eat. Particular foods are considered appropriate—even integral—to certain occasions: Wedding or birthday cake, tiny hors d'oeuvres at a reception. Soup, followed by fish, chicken, the main course, salad, cheese, and finally dessert is one socially accepted pattern for a very formal meal. At a Fourth of July picnic it would be unthinkable not to serve hot dogs.

Some cultures, the Chinese for example, build their social system around food. Food was a part of everything the Chinese did—weddings, ancestral worship, social meetings, large gatherings. The food and the manner in which it was served had great symbolic meaning. The standard Chinese greeting was not "How are you?" but, "Have you eaten today?" This was a paramount consideration in a race that built its culture around its food. When someone lost a job, the lament was, "My rice bowl is broken!"

To a lesser extent, the Jewish people built many of their social patterns around food, and we know this is true to some degree, in every culture.

Religious Factors

Patterns of eating and choices of food often are deeply affected by religious beliefs. Seventh Day Adventists do not eat meat, nor do Buddhists. In some countries where people of different religious groups live side by side there can be deep, bitter conflict because of eating habits. In one city in Bangladesh a terrible riot broke out, because some daring Moslems killed a cow and dragged it into the Hindu section, where the cow is worshiped. The Hindus retaliated by killing a hog—which Moslems abhor—and dragging it into the Moslem area.

A number of Christian faiths use food in communion ceremonies to remember Jesus Christ. Breaking bread and sharing wine at the first communion, Jesus said, "Do this in memory of me." And in one of the most ancient Christian prayers is the phrase, "Give us this day our daily bread." At special times of the year people of certain faiths eat or forego certain foods. Jews eat unleavened bread and other special foods during Passover; Moslems fast daily from dawn to sunset during the ninth month, Ramadan. Until recently Roman Catholics ate no meat on Fridays. Even now they may fast or eat no meat on certain days.

Economic Factors

Some people eat as they do because they cannot afford to eat any other way. For those who must live at subsistence level, including many in the United States, although other food is available, it is not within their reach. Their eating patterns are determined by their income. It is often such people who suffer malnutrition and poor health because of inadequate diet. Eating patterns developed from economic necessity are not deeply ingrained, they are dictated by circumstances.

Personal Factors

Every person is unique, so even among those of one religion, region, culture, or economic level, patterns of eating vary. This is because people have individual likes and dislikes. Their tastes differ. Individuals' or groups' specific ways of eating sometimes make it difficult to serve the public. There are so many variations that those serving the public find it difficult to find a common ground of acceptance. This is always a challenge to the foodservice industry.

Attitudes and Beliefs

Some of us eat a certain way because we believe we ought to. Such a belief does not arise from religious or cultural customs, we just "learn" it. People who are knowledgeable about nutrition tend to follow a pattern of eating that conforms to what they have learned. A distance runner may also eat a particular way because he or she has learned that such a diet confers endurance. Other people modify their diets in response to a physician's advice, to improve their health. The number of people who are making informed choices about diet has increased in recent years.

Eating As an Art

Finally, some people eat a certain way for the pure enjoyment of it. They make an art of eating. It is a sensuous and emotional experience. For them, enjoying a fine meal can have the qualities of seeing a fine play, hearing a great symphony, or reading a beautiful poem. Such a meal, properly planned, begins with foods that develop, or whet, the appetite, then continues with different courses that variously stimulate the palate until finally, at the *pièce de rèsistance* (usually the entree), there is a gustatory crescendo. The palate is fully aroused, and the food is consumed with relish and satisfaction. The subsequent courses are planned to sustain a subsiding appetite and finally a sweet closes the meal and the appetite tapers off.

MISINFORMATION

If people eat as they do because they believe it is the right way, it is extremely important that they be given accurate information that does promote healthful eating. Today there is a lot of misinformation abroad on how we should eat. Often it is based on old wives' tales or popular misconceptions. Some foodservice patrons attempt to foist their misguided opinions onto operations personnel, who can correct these misconceptions more effectively if they understand something of their origins.

Charlatans and Quacks

No stranger things are done than in the name of nutrition. P.T. Barnum said there was a sucker born every minute, and those who prey on the nutritionally gullible prove it every day. The cost without benefit of buying so-called health foods, vitamins, drugs and related items runs into the billions each year; Americans' vitamin bill alone is over $2.2 billion; over $100 million a year, it is estimated, is spent by people who hope extra vitamin E will do them some good. Diet products are second to pain relievers in drug sales. People buy not only drugs but amulets, girdles, belts, charms, clothing, machines, incantations, even deities in bottles, hoping to realize some utopian dream of good health. Mail-order dietary assistance is available. One company claims to be able to give you a complete analysis of your dietary status just by analyzing the vitamin and mineral makeup of one hair. Another company promises to evaluate your health status by analyzing a list of what you say you eat. They claim that the results are as accurate as a blood test.

The limits of human gullibility are boundless. Imagine this: An enterprising person started to market blue-shelled eggs from South American Aruncana chickens, claiming they contained more protein and iron and less cholesterol than regular eggs. The public took the bait and new henneries sprouted all over the country. Things were going well until someone at the University of California at Davis analyzed the eggs and found they were no different than regular eggs. The market collapsed, and all the promoter had was egg on his face.

Marketers of many questionable nostrums prey on the emotions of fear, pride, vanity, insecurity, shame, or fantasy. Many people want desperately to lose weight, and they are prime targets for those selling "surefire" weight-loss programs. Almost any claim interests them. Likewise, almost everyone is tired at some time or other during the day but this "normal" feeling is played upon to sell a tonic that cures "iron-poor blood."

Many sales pitches rely on testimonials. They appeal not to logic but to emotion. The customer identifies with some cultural, ethnic, or personal attribute of the spokesperson and is more likely to buy what is being pitched. The claim is usually elaborate, subjective, and unsubstantiated. Weight-reducing advertisements often feature "before" and "after" pictures. The emotional impact of the now-svelte successful dieter who was once obese confounds reason: people who should know better give in to hope and desire and order the product that will "change their lives" (Fig. 2-2).

Burn fat, get lean with a new, scientific workout.

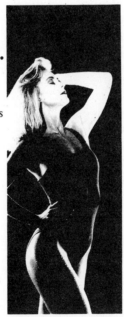

Most workout videos fall into one of two categories: glamorous, and flashy. They feature great-looking celebrities who put on a great show, but know very little about the conditioning you really need. These programs can leave you feeling sore, tired, and hopelessly inadequate.

We think you'll find our *Lean Body Workout* model glamorous too, but there is a lot more substance to our program and its model, Cynthia Kereluk. Cynthia was Miss Canada in 1984 and is an exercise physiologist who has the top-rated exercise show on Canadian network television.

By combining her abilities with those of Dr. Ladislav Pataki, who was a chief architect of the Soviet Bloc's athletic training systems before he defected to the United States in 1985, we have been able to produce the most effective exercise video ever conceived. This program is perfect for you, whether your goal is losing weight, toning up or gaining flexibility.

Figure 2-2 In the past Americans got more exercise because we worked harder. Today a far greater proportion of the population have sedentary jobs, and many fewer do heavy physical labor that burns a lot of calories. People have to exercise to maintain weight and remain fit. This clipping advertises an exercise videotape for home use. It is somewhat different from some ads for exercise videos that make sensational claims. *(Courtesy Sybervision)*

A common approach is to take a well-known scientific fact and apply it inappropriately, twisting the facts to enhance the product. Or, a number of solid scientific principles are stated and a false one is slipped in. Or, a scientific fact may apply in one case but not in others. Vitamin E helps fertility in rats but not in humans, but this does not stop a promoter of vitamin E from claiming that it does. Pantothentic acid does change gray hair to a darker color on a rat, but we can't make it work this way on human beings. Still people buy it for this purpose. Sometimes marketers coin pseudo-scientific terms to mislead people.

Why do people fall for these shams and come-ons? Trust, gullibility, ignorance, faith, conceit, desperation, hope, delusion, and other factors lead people astray when they should know better. Until we can change human nature, some people will be misled—not all by clever manipulation, some because they *want* to believe. Barnum's observation will probably be true for a long, long time.

HOW RELIABLE IS NUTRITION INFORMATION?

The author of the book or article says, "Eat my way and you'll gain everything anyone desires. You'll have better health, be more active, and have more fun; you'll think better and be free of the danger of some of our biggest killers." Every year hundreds of articles and books on diet and nutrition are published, and some sell millions of copies. They make popular reading. Some are downright good. Others may give information that is absolutely worthless, and what is worse, some of these diets can be dangerous to your health.

It is difficult to know whether something is reliable or not. Often the author's credentials are telling. The author should be a well-respected authority and a member of reputable scientific organizations and should have proper education credentials. One popular book that had a lot of converts on a particular diet but was severely criticized by nutrition experts was written by a man who had a doctorate from an unaccredited California college. It is good to be suspicious of mail-order academic degrees.

Often one can apply a test. Are the claims based on scientific tests or on anecdotal claims? In other words, are the results clearly proven? It is often desirable for tests to use an experimental group and a control group in order to prove that a significant difference exists. Also, if a number of variable factors are allowed to operate simultaneously it may be impossible to know which factor caused the results or whether a combination of the factors did so. An eating regimen that stipulates the dieter must eliminate stress and get a lot of exercise may reduce weight because the dieter exercised more, or the result could be a complementary result of the three combined factors. It is wise to see what other reliable people think of the work. If a respected authority says it is not in keeping with present scientific thought, that is a caution that one should be somewhat skeptical.

Some diet books recommend a regime that is plainly inadequate. Some needed nutrients are missing, and if the regimen is followed too long malnutrition or other serious problems could result. Other publications make claims that are false. A recent book prescribed a diet to end pain. While there was not much wrong with the diet nutritionally, it provided no pain relief.

Watch out for extravagant claims such as an extraordinary loss of weight, adding years to your life, or even getting rid of pimples. Find out whether the claims are valid. Sometimes a diet that purports to solve a problem is not specific to the problem. Others publish results that were never proven. One authority has said, "Be careful of claims that a specific food does a specific job. Foods just don't go to a special place and go to work doing the job we want."

Some programs produce a result, which is, however, meaningless. A program for an athlete may raise the level of blood sugar without improving his or her performance. The information in some commercial publications on health problems of current interest, such as hypertension, cancer, and heart disease may be reliable but is also available at less cost from a source such as the American Dietetic Association, American Diabetes Association, the American Heart Association (AHA), or the American Cancer Society.

A prominent physician, Dr. Victor Herbert of Mount Sinai School of Medicine, New York City, said, "People want to believe in magic. They see nutrition as a religion, not a science." He is right, and the religion has many converts.

Fad Diets

Following a fad diet can give variety to life; it gets us away from the humdrum of everyday living and leads us to expect something wonderful to happen. We are a nation of fad dieters. We go from one fad diet to the next. A new diet appears and catches on. Adherents multiply and the diet becomes the "in" thing. Many claim the diet works wonders; extravagant claims of pounds lost in short periods are made, spreading the diet like prairie fire. Within a few weeks there are millions on the diet; it has reached epidemic proportions. As with other fads, the rise is rapid. Then, similarly, there is a sudden backlash, and adherents fall away almost as fast as they built up.

The number of people in this country on medically prescribed diets is substantial (around 20% among elderly persons), but, the number on self-prescribed diets is tremendous. Most such diets do no harm; frequently they do little good; but some diets can be very harmful. The "Zen diet", which restricts food intake to some vegetables, cereals, legumes, and Oriental foods, killed some people and harmed a lot of others' health. Many users of a popular weight-loss diet wound up with nausea, vomiting, diarrhea, irregular heartbeat, and liver damage and maintained no weight reduction. In any diet proper balance of nutrients is important. A weight-reduction diet needs some carbohydrate, some protein, but only a bit of fat. If carbohydrate isn't there, ketosis can develop that can result in death. Few if any weight-reduction diets should go below 900 to 1200 calories a day, depending on the individual. Some liquid protein diets that hold calories to about 600 a day have been shown to be dangerous unless closely medically supervised.

Meganutrient diets (diets high in one or more vitamins or minerals) have been recommended for almost every problem from mental disorders to athlete's foot.

Massive doses of vitamins can be harmful, especially if the vitamins are the fat-soluble ones such as A and D. The popular "rainbow pill" that contains vitamins and other substances has been the cause of serious health problems among those who took it.

Natural or Organic Foods

A significant portion of our population are devotees of "natural" and "organic" foods. While they are sometimes regarded as being outside the main stream of nutrition, they have been a force in promoting good nutrition and have been aggressive enough to gain the public's attention for their views. Some nutrition authorities feel that the claims of natural food enthusiasts cannot be substantiated and often are downright erroneous. Others recognize that some health food promoters advocate principles that are questionable but that others do some good. In the discussion that follows, we shall first look at the negatives and then at facts that can be considered positive. It is important to remember that the views of extremists often get lumped with those of moderates, and all are then identified unfairly as being of one mind.

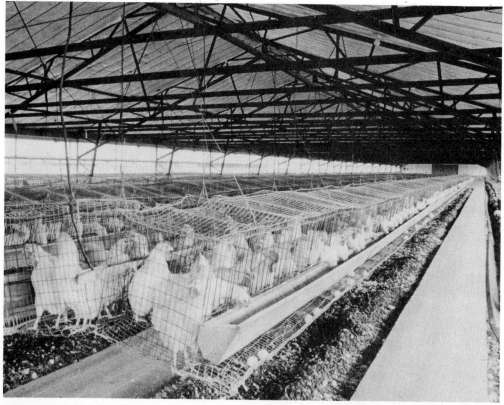

Figure 2-3 Some natural food advocates say eggs produced under the controlled conditions shown here are not as nutritious as eggs produced in a barnyard environment. Others argue that eggs produced under these sanitary conditions, with a controlled atmosphere and a high nutrient diet, are of better quality and higher nutrient value than eggs produced under uncontrolled conditions. *(Courtesy USDA)*

Natural food advocates say they want their food to be much like that that came to markets around 1900, when there were no pesticides, bactericides, hormone stimulants, or other chemicals that today are used to promote food crops. They inveigh against making foods different from products of the old days. They are against synthetics: "egg custards" that have no eggs, "pecan meats" made of soy, "beef broth" that never saw beef.

Devotees of organic foods share many of these beliefs, and they want their food to be grown in soil fertilized with manure and other organic matter without benefit of chemical fertilizers, pesticides, etc. They also want eggs produced by hens that run free. They claim the eggs produced in highly mechanized henneries by specially bred chickens are not as nutritious (Fig. 2-3).

Organic and natural food advocates often grow their own food. They also tend to purchase the rest from health food stores or from health food sections in supermarkets. Both groups eschew processed foods and food additives. They prefer fresh foods, whole-grain foods, and products such as fruits dried without sulfur or other additives.

Tests to identify differences in the nutritional quality and safety of foods grown in soil fertilized organically and with chemicals have shown no differences. Plants cannot differentiate between an organic and a synthetic nutrient. Nor can the human body distinguish between the minerals and other substances in organically grown foods and others. As far as we can tell, there may be no benefit in eating organically grown foods. The nutrient value is often the same, provided that the soil is adequately fertilized by whatever substances.

Most of the chemicals used to protect growing plants are washed off by rain or in preparing the products for market. Tests have shown some to be harmless. Herbicides and pesticides reduce costs of production and produce greater yields, and quality is often improved. Potatoes come from the ground without scab. Apples have a smooth skin and bright color without insect damage. Keeping qualities of many foods are also enhanced. Actually, if we stopped using all substances that help us produce our foods, there might not be enough food (Fig. 2-4).

Growing foods under natural or organic conditions does not guarantee that the food will not be harmful. In fact, some respected medical and nutrition authorities have said that a number of the products sold in health food stores may be more harmful than other foods. A recent article in the *Medical Letter on Drugs and Therapeutics*, a nonprofit, physician-edited journal, warned that many items in health food stores can be harmful. At one point it stated, "Many who patronize health food stores do so out of concern over the possible harmful effects of food additives, yet some of the plant materials and other foods sold there may be more harmful" than regular foods. Table 2-1 lists some foods known to be harmful. There are many others and all could be described as "natural."

Some nutrition authorities are critical of natural or organic diets that are extreme or bizarre. Claims that natural or organic foods are the only right ones and condemnation of the kind of diet recommended by nutrition authorities also draws their fire. These authorities see a lot of "snake-oil promotion" in the program and point out that natural foods can be a waste of money, and do little good or even do harm. They feel it would be better if organic food enthusiasts followed a diet that includes more standard food patterns rather than extremes. Some authorities say a natural or organic food program *that follows good nutritional standards* will do no harm and may even be more healthful than the ordinary one most Americans eat.

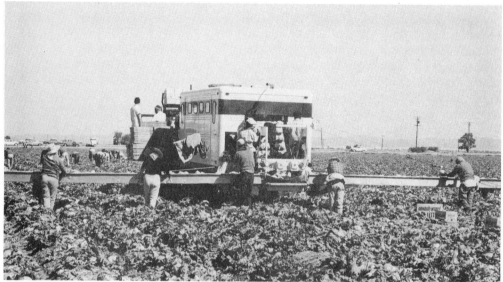

Figure 2-4 Advocates of modern farming methods say that such methods not only improve crop yields but also produce foods of higher quality and nutrient value. (*Courtesy USDA*)

Some natural food buffs condemn the use of antioxidants (sodium benzoate, butylated hydroxyanisole [BHA]) to keep fats and oils from turning rancid and then embrace a popular health potion like Life Extension Formula, which contains some of these same antioxidants. It is said that some foods available in special food stores at special prices are identical to those found in supermarkets at much lower prices and come from the same distributors. Assays turned up the same amounts of additives, pesticides, bactericides, and other substances considered harmful. Sanitation has also been questioned because of the custom of repackaging in the store from bulk stocks. Some "health" foods do not stack up to claims made for them. Granola is highly regarded by natural and organic food advocates, yet lacks vitamin A, riboflavin, niacin, vitamin D, vitamins thiamine, pyridoxine, and folacin, nutrients contained in many dry breakfast cereals. About 30% of granola's calories come from fat, and it contains a lot more sugar than cornflakes. It does, however, contain calcium, which cornflakes lack.

The criticism of harmful substances being added to our foods has been helpful. The finding of polychlorinated biphenyls (PCB) in flour and other foods caused the government to lower the amount that can be used, and eventually it will be banned entirely. The use of DDT has been considerably restricted since it was found to persist in milk. The use of stilbesterol and some other suspected cancer-causing agents has been stopped. Natural and organic food enthusiasts have been quite vocal in all of this and have stimulated public awareness and governmental action.

The government tries to keep harmful substances out of foods. It has set up what is called the GRAS list (generally recognized as safe), a list of additives that may be used in processing foods. Many permitted substances are chemicals or compounds such as sorbitol and monosodium glutamate (MSG). The government constantly reviews the list and revises it. There are natural and organic food advocates who say that some things on the list are harmful and should be removed. MSG is one. Others say that some things not allowed should be on the list. For the most part, such substances are used to improve quality, improve nutrient value, make food easier to work with, give it color or flavor, or preserve it; they are not considered harmful, and serve to improve the food.

TABLE 2-1
Some Foods Known To Be Harmful

Food Item	Harmful Effect
Licorice root	Heart failure or cardiac arrest
Pennyroyal oil	Kidney and liver toxicity
Horsetail	Nerve dysfunction as that associated with beri-beri
Burdock root tea	As little as one half cup can cause blurred vision, slurred speech, bizarre behavior, inability to urinate, and hallucinations
Chamomile tea	Severe allergic reactions
Sassafras root bark tea	Liver toxicity; has been found to cause cancer in animals
Radishes, turnips and cabbages	Can interfere with iodine absorption, causing goiter
Solanine*	The greenish spots found in potatoes that have been exposed to sunlight are poisonous, but only in large quantities (17 pounds of potatoes)
Olive oil*	Suspected of containing a carcinogen
Carrots*	Suspected of containing a hallucinogen
Shrimp*	Some contain high levels of arsenic, which if consumed over a long period, could be very harmful

* Either the quantity must be very great or only some samples may be harmful at times.

The diets promoted by healthfood enthusiasts are often very nutritious. They contain a lot of raw vegetables and fruits, and whole-grain products, and very little fat, sugar, and empty calories. There is nothing wrong with wanting foods in the forms that nourished the human race for millennia. These groups have been aggressive and effective in pushing their claims against some additives, pesticides, and other substances—to our benefit. The government has been forced to give the GRAS list closer scrutiny and to test some additives far more rigorously to determine safe levels.

SOURCES OF RELIABLE INFORMATION

The AHA and other public interest groups work with foodservices planning menus, providing recipes, and helping in other ways to see that good programs are set up. Most state and local health boards have people on staff who can provide reliable nutritional and diet information. Much good information is also published by trade associations such as the Cereal Council and the National Restaurant Association (NRA). The National Dairy Council and the National Livestock and Meat Board do much in this area. Even publications of large corporations give helpful facts. Our news media do a good job; columnists and food editors have large audiences. (Fig. 2-5).

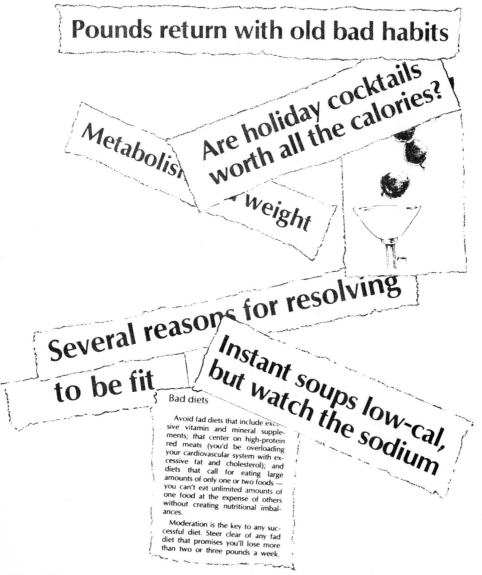

Pounds return with old bad habits

Are holiday cocktails worth all the calories?

Metabolis~ ~weight

Several reasons for resolving to be fit

Instant soups low-cal, but watch the sodium

Bad diets

Avoid fad diets that include excessive vitamin and mineral supplements; that center on high-protein red meats (you'd be overloading your cardiovascular system with excessive fat and cholesterol); and diets that call for eating large amounts of only one or two foods — you can't eat unlimited amounts of one food at the expense of others without creating nutritional imbalances.

Moderation is the key to any successful diet. Steer clear of any fad diet that promises you'll lose more than two or three pounds a week.

Figure 2-5 Daily newspapers often contain considerable information on health and fitness. The clippings came from just one issue of a Midwestern daily.

It is paramount that the information we use come from reliable sources. Most professional journals are fairly reliable; association information might be slanted in favor of those the association represents, but the best ones are highly reliable. The news media are conscientious, but sometimes material is put together hastily without adequate documentation or the writer is not conversant with the problem and inadvertently gives incorrect information. Some publications are not scientific journals, but because the articles are well researched, the information often can be depended upon.

Many hospitals are now extending their services and dietary staff may be available to work with persons outside the hospital in food and health programs. Hospitals are even giving courses to provide better information. Local groups of American Dietetic Association members often set up a Dial-a-Dietitian program: members take turns answering questions phoned in.

Elementary and secondary schools have instituted programs in health and nutrition. Junior, community, and four-year college programs also have courses in diet and nutrition. Some offer programs leading to certification as a registered dietitian. Many hotel and restaurant management programs have courses aimed at giving nutrition information and content on how to set up and implement programs for good nutritional planning.

GOVERNMENT INFORMATION AND REGULATION

The Food and Drug Administration (FDA), Public Health Services (PHS), Federal Trade Commission (FTC), Environmental Protection Agency (EPA), U.S. Postal Service (USPS), the Department of Agriculture (USDA), and other federal agencies either provide good information or assist the foodservice industry through regulation. Every foodservice worker should be familiar with these services so as to serve the public better. These agencies and others help us to protect our patrons, protect the safety of our food supply, and obtain good nutrition information. State and local laws and regulations contribute as well. At the end of this chapter, a few of the publications available at no charge from government agencies are listed. One need only write requesting them. The bibliography at the end of this text lists some of the best information sources available today.

FDA

The Department of Health and Human Services (HHS) has under it a number of agencies that work to benefit the foodservice industry. The most important of these is the FDA, which administers the Pure Food, Drug, and Cosmetic Act of 1938 and its many amendments. It is charged with seeing that food on the market is "fit for human consumption," preventing false labeling, and requiring that foods meet certain Standards of Identity. If a label makes any nutritional claim, the claim must be supported. It administers the GRAS list of over 3000 substances. The FDA also establishes sanitary standards for food manufacturing plants. It is also charged with the administration of the 1976 Ordinance and Code used by states and local communities for inspection of the sanitation and operational standards of foodser-vices.

Labeling

Under the provisions of the Food, Drug, and Cosmetic Act, the FDA is charged with seeing that labels on food packages conform to certain standards. The following information *must* appear:
1. Product name
2. Product form (i.e., diced, sliced, dried, etc.)
3. Net weight of contents
4. Name and place of business of the manufacturer, packer, or distributor
5. Ingredient contents, in descending order of predominance by weight

The requirement "ingredient contents, in descending order of predominance by weight" is not required of what are called "common foods,"—foods whose composition is supposedly well known, such as catsup. Non-common foods must list the ingredients they contain in this descending manner. Some ingredients in non-com-mon foods, like spices, flavors or colors, can be named by general category rather than by name. If any artificial or imitation product is used, the word "imitation" or "artificial" must be used before the ingredient. Specific kinds of dyes, if used, must be named. Thus on a label on a package for flan (Spanish style custard) the ingredients are listed as "sugar, calcium carrageenan, locust bean gum, salt, artificial flavor and color; contains FD&C yellow dye No. 5; contains no eggs."

In 1971 an additional labeling requirement was introduced. A label must contain required nutrition information when a nutrient has been added to a food, such as vitamin A or D in milk, or when a nutritional claim is made on the label or in advertising. The information that must then be on the label is:
1. Serving size and number of servings per container
2. Calories per serving
3. Protein, fat, carbohydrate, and sodium content in grams per serving
4. Percent of U.S. Recommended Daily Allowance (USRDA) of each serving for protein, vitamins A and C, thiamin, riboflavin, niacin, calcium, and iron. (In 1985 sodium and potassium amounts were added.)
5. When claims are made for a specific nutrient or nutrients (i.e., saturated or polyunsaturated fatty acids or cholesterol), the amount must be provided. In the list of nutrients an asterisk (*) or a zero (0) can be used to indicate a nutrient that is less than 2% of the USRDA per serving.

The FDA requires that if the protein in a food is better than or equal to the protein in milk (casein), its percent of protein can be stated on the basis of a USRDA of 45 grams, but, if the protein has a value less than milk protein, the need percent must be based on 65 grams a day. Thus, if the product is Swiss steak in gravy, where the protein in the steak is equal in value to that of milk protein, the protein value can be based on 45 grams, but if it is string beans, that have a protein of lower value than milk protein, the value has to be based on 65 grams. The proportion of protein food in the product is also considered. Thus, if a volume of corned beef contains more corned beef than potatoes and onions, the standard can be 45 grams, but if it is mostly potatoes and onions and little meat, the standard is 65 grams. Some manufacturers voluntarily list the amounts of cholesterol, fiber, and other substances.

Nutritional labeling has provided consumers with valuable information on some nutrients in food. Many consumers do not use it; some do not know how, though, with the growing interest in health and nutrition more and more are learning. The 1977 *Dietary Goals for the United States* urged Congress to require nutrition labeling on all packaged foods. Many packagers today give this information voluntarily, even though they are not required to do so. Some federal regulatory agencies have asked for additional information on food labels:

1. Ingredients by percent of total weight
2. Spices and coloring ingredients named individually
3. If oil content exceeds 10%, the kind of oil must be named.

There has also been some feeling that, whenever cholesterol content is declared, ingredients such as sugar (in addition to total carbohydrate), potassium, and fatty acids should be identified.

The FDA sets up and administers what are called Standards of Identity. They state exactly what a non-common food must contain. (A non-common food is one whose ingredients are not generally known.) Catsup is a common food but mayonnaise is not. There are 275 standards. If a food does not meet the standard, it cannot bear the name of the standard. Thus, for a product to be called "cheese" it must contain 51% or more milkfat on a dry basis; if it does not, it may not be called cheese. Sometimes the words "cheese food" are used for products that do not meet the standard for cheese. Standards of Identity also cover shape or form of a product. Thus, if the label says "cubed," the product must be of a specific size and cube-shaped. If it says "peach halves," the product must be of a specific variety of *Prunus* and be in halves, not broken pieces. The standards have been helpful in giving consumers what they expect when they buy a product.

FTC

The FTC was established to see that fair business practices are followed and that advertising is truthful and not misleading. It also regulates marketing for ethical practices. It acts as a deterrent against spreading misinformation about nutrition. The USPS has the right to stop misrepresentation of products distributed through the mails.

One may wonder how publishers of newspapers, magazines, and books can legally publish misinformation about nutrition. The United States Constitution guarantees the freedom of the press and publications do not have to conform to FTC or postal regulations. Such publications are not considered advertisements, and the FDA can get into the act only when food labels make health claims.

Other Government Information Agencies

A number of agencies in the federal government provide information about food and health that is of help to food service industry representatives. Both the USDA

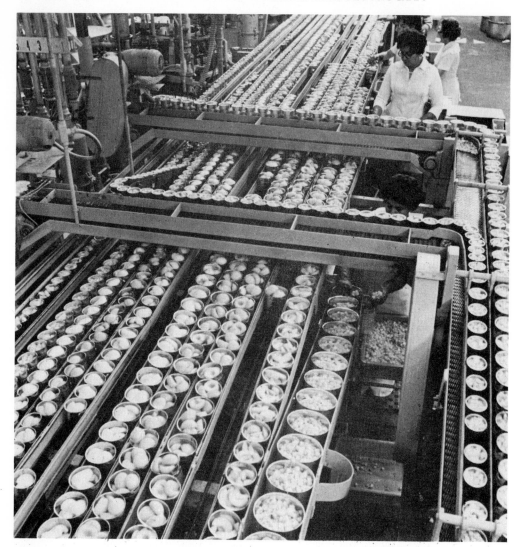

Figure 2-6 A modern cannery like the one shown here meets the high sanitary standars required by the FDA for food processing plants. (*Courtesy National Food Processors Association*)

and HHS devote considerable staff and money to provide good information. The PHS can be helpful. The USDA, by establishing standards for grading food and then supervising such grading, helps assure consumers that they are getting the quality they are promised.

Food safety is also a concern of the government, and a number of agencies work to that end. The USDA administers the "Inspected and Passed" program, which sees that meat and poultry and their products are fit for human consumption. It also is charged with seeing that processing plants meet specific operational and sanitary standards (Fig. 2-6). The FDA under the Pure Food, Drug, and Cosmetic Act, is empowered to maintain high standards of sanitation in food processing. The PHS is

```
                NUTRITION INFORMATION
                         PER SERVING
                   SERVING SIZE: 1/2 CUP
                  SERVINGS PER CONTAINER: 3
      CALORIES ..................... 170
      PROTEIN ................. 8 GRAMS
      CARBOHYDRATE .......... 12 GRAMS
      FAT ..................... 10 GRAMS
      SODIUM ................... 140 MG
      PERCENTAGE OF U.S. RECOMMENDED
      DAILY ALLOWANCES (U.S. RDA):
      PROTEIN .... 20    NIACIN ........*
      VITAMIN A .... 4   CALCIUM .... 30
      VITAMIN C ....*    IRON ........*

      THIAMINE .... 2    VITAMIN D ... 25
      RIBOFLAVIN . 20    PHOSPOROUS 25
      *CONTAINS LESS THAN 2% OF THE U.S.
      RDA OF THESE NUTRIENTS.

      INGREDIENTS: MILK, DISODIUM PHOS-
      PHATE, CARRAGEENAN AND VITAMIN D3.
```

```
              NUTRITION INFORMATION
      PORTION SIZE: 4 OZ. (ABOUT 1 CUP)
      PORTIONS PER CONTAINER: 20
      CALORIES ......................... 400
      PROTEIN (g) ....................... 14
      CARBOHYDRATE (g) ................. 83
      FAT (g) ............................ 2
      SODIUM (mg) ....................... 0
      PERCENTAGE OF U.S. RECOMMENDED DAILY
      ALLOWANCES (U.S. RDA) PER PORTION:
      PROTEIN .......................... 20
      VITAMIN A .........................*
      VITAMIN C .........................*
      THIAMINE (B₁ ..................... 45
      RIBOFLAVIN (B₂ ................... 25
      NIACIN ........................... 30
      CALCIUM .......................... 20
      IRON ............................. 25
      PHOSPHORUS ....................... 10
      *CONTAINS LESS THAN 2% OF THE U.S. RDA OF THESE
      NUTRIENTS

      CONTAINS: UNBLEACHED WHEAT FLOUR, CALCIUM SUL-
      FATE, MALTED BARLEY FLOUR (IMPROVES YEAST BAKING,
      (NIACIN, IRON, THIAMINE MONONITRATE (VITAMIN B₁),
      RIBOFLAVIN (VITAMIN B₂), POTASSIUM BROMATE.
```

Figure 2-7 A label from evaporated milk and one from flour. The vitamin D in the evaporated milk is added, so the milk is a fortified product. Thiamin, riboflavin, niacin, and iron are substances lost in milling the flour, and are then added again making the flour an enriched product.

charged with the inspection of seafood beds. The EPA also has jurisdiction in certain areas.

The Delaney Amendment to the Pure Food, Drug, and Cosmetic Act requires removal from the market of any food containing a known or suspected carcinogen (cancer-causing agent). Stilbestrol, a suspected carcinogen, was banned under this amendment, as was cyclamate, a nonnutritive sweetener. The FDA does not need to go to court to remove products from the market under this amendment.

Food Fortification

Since 1958 the federal government has required, or in other cases allowed, some nutrients to be added to foods to increase their dietary value. Refined cereals *must* be enriched with thiamine, riboflavin, iron, and niacin equal to the amounts present in the original whole grain. Milk may have vitamins A and D added, and also calcium and some other nutrients. When a product is fortified, the label must state what has been added (Fig. 2-7).

Some people oppose fortification, because they regard it as the introduction of additives—supplementary food components, though no one has demonstrated that the body uses added nutrients any differently than it uses natural ones.

Whether whole-grain cereals are better than refined, fortified ones can be debated. Phytic acid is a component of whole-grain cereals that is lost in refining, but in the digestive tract phytic acid combines with some vitamins and minerals to form an insoluble phytate that cannot be absorbed. Thus, some nutrients in whole grains are lost that are still available in the refined fortified product, since phytic acid has been removed. However, some argue that there is not enough phytic acid in whole grains to do harm. The question has not been answered definitively.

WHAT IS NUTRITIOUS?

Thus far we have been talking about nutrition, nutritious food, food and health, and using other terms to indicate the relationship between eating well and promoting health. But what is nutritious food? We have various ways of making a judgment. The simplest method is to obtain the food's *nutrient density*, which is merely a method of apportioning the calories in the food among its various nutrients. Another, more complex, method gives the ratio of a food's nutrient content to its caloric (energy) value. It is called Index of Nutrient Density (IND). For our purpose of estimating the nutrient value of a food, the method of nutrient density is most suitable.

Nutrient Density

Suppose we wanted to know how nutritious each of four different foods was. By using the nutrient density method we would divide the calories into the various nutrient values for protein, fat, vitamins, and minerals. Table 2-2 shows selected nutrient values of skim milk, potato chips, baked salmon, and pure lard, and Table 2-3 evaluates the same foods for nutrient density. An examination of the nutrient densities indicates that, per calorie, skim milk gives a good yield of minerals and vitamins. Per calorie it gives the best nutrition. Salmon is next. Potato chips come in third—fat raises the calorie content. Lard is the least nutritious, since 100% of its calorie count comes from fat.

TABLE 2-2
Selected Nutrient Values of Four Foods

Food	Calories	Protein	Fat	Carbohydrates	Calcium	Phosphorus	Iron
Skim milk	36	3.6	0.1	5.1	121	95	Trace
Potato chips	568	5.3	39.8	50	40	139	1.8
Baked salmon	182	27	7.4	—	—	414	1.2
Lard	902	—	100	—	—	—	—

Food	Potassium	Vitamin A	Thiamine	Riboflavin	Niacin	Vitamin C
Skim milk	145	Trace	0.04	0.18	0.11	1.0
Potato chips	1130	Trace	0.21	0.07	4.30	16.0
Baked salmon	446	160	0.16	0.06	9.80	—
Lard	—	—	—	—	—	—

THINGS TO COME

In Part I we have presented a broad overview of some of the problems facing the foodservice industry along with a brief historical review of the situation. We

TABLE 2-3
The Nutrient Density of Four Foods

Food	Calories	Protein	Fat	Carbohydrates	Calcium	Phosphorus	Iron
Skim milk	36	0.1000	0.0028	0.0028	3.3611	2.6389	—
Potato chips	568	0.0093	0.0701	0.0880	0.0704	0.2447	0.0036
Baked salmon	182	0.1484	0.0457	—	—	2.2747	0.0066
Lard	902	—	100.0000	—	—	—	—

Food	Potassium	Vitamin A	Thiamine	Riboflavin	Niacin	Vitamin C
Skim milk	4.0278	—	0.0011	0.0050	0.0031	0.0278
Potato chips	1.9804	—	0.0004	0.0001	0.0076	0.0282
Baked salmon	2.4381	0.8791	0.0009	0.0003	0.0538	—
Lard	—	—	—	—	—	—

showed sources of reliable and unreliable information and indicated how foodservice personnel can sort the good from the bad and where they can go for reliable information. Some basic criteria have been set forth in these discussions on what the responsibilities of the foodservice industry may be in providing healthful food. Some government efforts to improve eating patterns have been cited, such as Standards of Identity, ingredient labeling, nutritional labeling, the *Dietary Goals* for the United States, and others. This is all in the way of an introduction.

In Part II we turn our attention to basic nutrition information. Personnel in the foodservice industry should know these basics if they are to perform effectively and knowledgeably in providing healthful food choices for patrons. The discussion is simplified, and many complex concepts have been omitted, because the discussion is not directed to those engaged in following precisely prescribed diets in a health-related facility but toward those serving the general public, for whom broad guidelines suffice.

In Part III, the core of the book, marketing, planning, and implementation of healthful food programs is discussed and concrete ways of doing this successfully are presented. Experience has shown that in order for foods to be healthful, they must be of high quality, lest people refuse to eat them. It is also true that not all patrons want healthful foods, so programs must be broad enough to appeal to all tastes. Starting up a successful program is not easy and is always challenging. Part III gives some pointers that may help make such a challenge more enjoyable.

SUMMARY

Food is very important to health and well-being, yet its role in health is not well understood by many people who are, however, concerned and want to eat well. Lacking good information, they may easily be misled by those who seek to profit from ignorance. There is much misinformation on how to eat for optimal health. To improve the eating standards in this country, a more effective education program is needed. While billions are spent giving food to those that need it, few dollars are spent telling Americans how best to use food.

Much money is also wasted on fad diets, dietary preparations, and unnecessary nutrient supplements. This waste also occurs because of the lack of accurate information. Magazines, newspapers, and other communications media should take greater responsibility for the kind of information they publish and should take more care to see that nutrition and diet information coming from them is authoritative.

The trend toward natural foods and improving the average diet indicates that people are waking up to the need for careful selection of food in order to obtain a balanced diet. This concern must be tempered by caution as there are persons who would misinform for personal gain. Some things advocated by natural food enthusiasts have little or no scientific support.

Much good information on how to eat healthfully is distributed by government agencies and private councils, associations, businesses, and schools. Laws and regulations empower government agencies to enforce sanitation and the nutritional quality of foods. The FDA must administer the Pure Food, Drug and Cosmetic Act, Standards of Identity, and nutritional labeling regulations. It must also see that ingredient information given about foods meets approved standards. The Delaney amendment to the Pure Food, Drug and Cosmetic Act is another responsibility.

The USDA, Department of HHS, and PHS are the main distributors of information on healthful eating in the federal government. The American Dietetic Association, the Nutrition Council of the Academy of Sciences, the American Diabetic Association, The American Heart Association, and the American Medical Association, among others, publish reliable information. The AHA works with foodservices planning menus, providing recipes, and otherwise helping to see that healthful food is served. Much food information is published by trade associations and businesses. Community education programs, colleges, and universities commonly offer nutrition courses. Where hotel and restaurant courses are taught, the curriculum usually includes a course in nutrition.

The fortification or enrichment of food with nutrients has been approved since 1958. Refined cereals must be enriched to equal the nutrients in the whole grain. Other foods may or may not be fortified, at the option of the producer. Not everyone agrees that fortification is desirable, but this dissention in no way is sufficient to stop the program.

Chapter Review

1. Bring to class examples of what you feel are advertisements that can contribute to having a poor diet. (Hint: Look at some tabloid newspapers.)
2. Do you know of anyone who has been harmed in any way by taking special diet pills or diet drugs or by going on a special non-medical diet?
3. What use could a person in the foodservice industry make of knowledge of misinformation about diets and dieting?
4. Why do people fall for gimmicks on how to eat for good health? Personal reasons? Lack of education? Cultural background?

5. Set up a list of the pluses and minuses you see in natural or organic food programs.
6. How effective do you think government and private information services have been in disseminating information on how to eat for good health? If they have been doing a good job, why is so much erroneous information around?
7. Take a label with nutrition information on it and see how much information you can obtain and understand.
8. Take another label with an ingredient list on it and see what information you get. Does it show amounts?
9. How would you define a nutritious food? A non-nutritious one?
10. What are the pros and cons of fortifying (enriching) foods?

SOME FEDERAL PUBLICATIONS ON NUTRITION:

Conserving the Nutritive Values in Foods, USDA Home and Garden Bulletin No. 90. (How to select and handle foods to get maximum nutrition from them.)

Family Fare, a Guide to Good Nutrition, USDA Home and Garden Bulletin No. 1. (The basics of a balanced diet with recipes to implement it.)

Family Food Budgeting for Good Meals and Good Nutrition, USDA Home and Garden Bulletin No. 94. *(How to select nutritional meals on a limited budget.)*

Food and Your Weight, USDA, G 74. (Selecting balanced meals that are low in calories.)

Food for the Young Couple, USDA G 85. (Getting a good diet at low cost.)

Food Guide for Older Folks, USDA G 17. (Balanced meals at low cost.)

Nutritive Value of American Foods in Common Units, USDA Agricultural Handbook No. 456. (An authoritative list of food values.)

Nutritive Value of Foods, USDA Home and Garden Bulletin No. 72. (Another good list of food values.)

Composition of Foods, Raw, Processed, Prepared, USDA Agricultural Handbook No. 8. (One of the best sources of food values of common foods.)

Part 2

Nutrition

Chapter 3
Eating for Optimal Health

Chapter Goals

- To discuss why and how to eat to be healthy.
- To briefly describe the basic nutrient groups and what they do for us.
- To describe how food is digested and nutrients absorbed.
- To describe various ways of calculating the adequacy of a diet using a food value table, the Basic Four Food Plan method and the Food Exchange Method.
- To present drawbacks in present methods of calculating dietary intake.

WHY EAT?

Our bodies cannot function without food. It is the fuel of the human machine. Some cars sputter or lose efficiency on low-octane gas; high-octane fuel makes them run better. Likewise, food must contain certain nutrients that enable the body to perform optimally.

Food provides substances that build and maintain the body; it furnishes heat and energy; it supplies substances necessary for physiological processes; and it yields regulatory substances that keep the body in good running order. If the food a person eats does not provide these things, the body functions poorly or stops functioning. Eating an adequate amount of all food (but not an excess) promotes health. It also makes life more enjoyable. We view life more positively when we have food that keeps us healthy and satisfied. Consuming food that provides all the 40-some nutrients the body needs can help us achieve our personal best and may help us avoid certain diseases.

Eating well means different things to different people. To some, eating well is eating foods they like and eating poorly is eating foods they don't like. To others, eating well is eating to satiation. Some people think they are eating well when they eat expensive or exotic food. In some cultures eating well is overeating and body fat is evidence of wealth; slimness is equated with poverty. In the United States many young women think eating well is eating food that keeps one thin and lithe.

All of these people may think they are consuming "the right food," but it may not contain the right nutrients. They may be misinformed, mislead, or apathetic. Eating for good health is eating foods that perform the four functions listed above, but there is more to eating than just meeting nutritional needs. Often food satisfies deep psychological needs. Eating is something to be enjoyed with others, a social experience; food can afford a feeling of communion. We frequently use food to enhance social gatherings and other functions. The importance of food as something other than a nutritional vehicle is especially relevant to those in the foodservice industry, who sell not only food but service, ambience, and a pleasant experience.

KINDS OF NUTRIENTS

Food must supply six kinds of nutrients in the proper amounts if the body is to be adequately nourished—carbohydrates, proteins, fats (lipids), vitamins, minerals, and water. Alcohol may be considered a nutrient because it provides energy or heat. Some classify it with carbohydrates and others, with fats. Actually it is neither; although, when the body uses it, it breaks down more like a fat than a carbohydrate. Because it provides energy, in this text it is classified as a fuel food.

The above nutrients work together, so every group must be represented if a balanced diet is to be the result. Most foods contain more than one kind of nutrient. Beef steak contains protein, fat, vitamins, and minerals; it has little carbohydrate. Bread contains largely carbohydrate and some fat, minerals, and vitamins and a little protein. Butter is mostly fat, with a few vitamins and minerals. A few foods contain only one nutrient: table sugar is all carbohydrate; all salad oils are virtually pure fat but some have a bit of vitamin E. A person who knows which nutrients are in different foods and how much there is can select foods that provide all the necessary nutrients in the right amounts (Fig. 3-1).

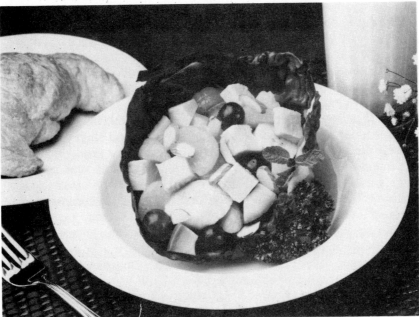

FIGURE 3-1 All six kinds of nutrients are in this turkey-fruit salad meal served with a croissant and milk. The croissant, fruit and milk contain carbohydrates; proteins are in the turkey, croissant and milk; fat is found in the milk and croissant and a slight bit in the turkey; vitamins and minerals are in all items and water liquid (liquid) is found in the milk, fruit, vegetables and even croissant. *(Courtesy Perdue Foods)*

Eating a variety of foods increases the chances of getting all the nutrient groups in their proper proportions. Eating only meat and potatoes does not do the trick. It is desirable to select a wide range of foods to be sure of getting all the nutrients in the right amounts. Old-fashioned as this may seem, it is most scientifically modern.

THE SIX NUTRIENT CATEGORIES

The Energy Nutrients

Three of the six nutrient categories provide calories, or energy: carbohydrates, proteins, and fats. These are the fuel foods.

Carbohydrates provide energy and fiber, whereas protein and fats have other jobs in addition. Fat and protein must be changed in the body before they can be used for energy. Fat or protein must be converted into energy-yielding units if there is not enough carbohydrate available for energy.

Carbohydrates   Carbohydrates are a large family of substances including starches, sugars, fiber, and pectin that are plentiful in grains and cereals, potatoes, legumes (beans and peas), sugar cane or beets, plant or fruit syrups, and fruits and vegetables. Many processed items such as pasta, flour, baked goods, and other products made from grains are also rich in carbohydrate.

There is one carbohydrate that we cannot digest but still need to consume; this is fiber, sometimes called roughage or bulk. Fiber is mainly a carbohydrate called cellulose, which is found largely in grains, fruits, and vegetables, where it forms much of their skeletal structure. Rabbits, cows, horses, and other ruminants can digest cellulose, but humans cannot. It adds bulk or volume to foods as they pass through the human digestive tract, and enhances absorption of nutrients by keeping the food from compacting. It also stimulates the bowel and helps in elimination of solid waste. We will discuss fiber at greater length in Chapter 4.

Protein   Besides providing energy, which is not its principal job, protein is needed to build new tissue and repair it. It is an important part of early bone and tooth structure. Blood, muscles, hormones, antibodies to fight disease, and other essential substances are made from protein. Meat, fish, poultry, eggs, dairy products, and soybeans are good protein sources. Some foods, such as legumes, nuts, and cereals can contribute significant amounts of protein. Not all proteins have the same value in the body, so a mixture of different ones is recommended. It is usually recommended that part of one's protein intake be animal protein and part, plant protein.

The body does not use proteins whole, but breaks them down into smaller units called *amino acids*. Certain ones must be in our food because the body cannot manufacture them. These are called "essential amino acids." Nonessential amino acids can be made by the body; we also obtain them from food.

Fats   Fats belong to a large family called lipids which includes substances such as waxes, resins, phospholipids, sterols and others. They are all insoluble in water. Lipids are concentrated energy-giving substances acting as a storage place for excess energy the body has obtained. Fat can be a protector of the body; a layer over muscle protects it; fat is also needed as padding around organs. It is an insulator and reduces body heat loss. Only one fat is known to be essential in our food and this is linoleic acid. Fat does many jobs such as to help transport fat-soluble products around the body. Dietary fats are found in vegetable oils, animal fats, butter, cream, cheese, seeds and nuts. A few other vegetable foods, such as the avocado and olive, are high in fat.

Non-fuel Nutrients (Maintenance, Regulatory, Enzymatic, etc.)

Vitamins, minerals, and water produce no energy. They are in the body to do a wide range of jobs as maintenance and regulatory agents.

Minerals Minerals make up teeth, bones, and other body structures. Some can transport nerve impulses. Minerals also help regulate body functions; they are important in maintaining a proper alkaline-acid balance and in muscle functioning. They work in combination with body substances to perform countless essential jobs. For instance, to stop bleeding, the mineral calcium must be present so the vitamin K can perform its work to coagulate blood. Certain minerals act outside or inside body cells helping to pull nutrients in and sending wastes out. Fruits and vegetables, dairy products, grains, cereals, meats, poultry, and fish; selections from each of these groups of food are good sources of minerals. Some foods provide specific minerals available from only limited sources, such as iodine which is in fish and seafoods.

Vitamins Vitamins are vital body regulators often acting in concert with minerals or other vitamins to carry out essential body functions. To get all the needed vitamins, one must eat a wide variety of foods—meats, dairy products, fruits, vegetables, whole or enriched grains or cereals, seeds, and nuts.

Water Water is a most essential component of our diet. It carries our nutrients to us, either in food or liquids. The human body needs 1-1/2 to 2 liters per day under normal conditions. Most of our vitamins, minerals and food components are water soluble. Water also is what brings food to plants and so, were it not for water, there would be no food because it is one of the basic components of life. Man can live without certain nutrients for days, weeks, months, or longer, but without water only a few days. Water is the medium in which most of our body functions are carried out, and it makes possible the work and transfer of substances and impulses throughout the body. Most of our body functions occur with the help of water. We need water to digest food, to transfer the nutrients digestion gives to the blood, and then to carry these nutrients throughout the body. Water is the medium in which body wastes are carried out via sweat, urine, and feces. The heat of energy is transferred to water, which distributes it around the body. Water in the form of sweat cools the body by evaporating on the skin. We will discuss the importance of water further in Chapter 9.

HOW FOOD IS REDUCED TO NUTRIENTS

If we must eat food to get the nutrients we need, how does the food give up its nutrients and how does the body take them and use them? This complex process has been studied for many years, and it is still incompletely understood. It starts out with hunger, a sensation that tells us it is time to eat. It is a persistent signal issued by the brain when the body's blood sugar level gets low. Hunger ends when the stomach is full. Psychological factors can also begin or stop hunger. An emotional upset or an aversion to a particular food may suppress hunger.

THE DIGESTIVE SYSTEM

To free nutrients from food for their essential roles in the body, after consuming food we must first digest it. Next we must absorb the nutrients, and finally, the nutrients are transported to the appropriate needy cells.

Food is digested and nutrients are absorbed in a part of the body called the *alimentary canal*, which is composed of the *mouth, esophagus, stomach, small intestine* (made up of the *duodenum, ileum,* and *jejunum)*, and the *large intestine* (made up of the *colon, rectum,* and *anus)*. The large intestine also stores waste after digestion until it is eliminated (Fig. 3-2).

The Mouth

The mouth is a sort of judge, ruling on the propriety of letting food introduced into it go farther. It can reject distasteful food or spoiled food. The tongue moves food around so the teeth can chew it, making it easier for digestive juices to break it down. While food is chewed, the mouth frees saliva, which contains *mucin* to make the food slippery, and *ptyalin* (salivary amylase), which starts the breakdown of complex carbohydrates. Saliva also moistens the food, allowing it to move more easily through the esophagus. Some few substances are dissolved by the water in saliva.

The Esophagus

The esophagus is little more than a canal between mouth and stomach through which food passes. It does little else in the digestive process.

The Stomach

The stomach contains a highly acidic gastric juice composed of hydrochloric acid, water, and a number of enzymes. The principal job of the stomach is to break down the protein in food into simpler units. The enzymes *pepsin, renin,* and gastric *lipase* do this job, aided by the acidic action of the gastric juice. Some hydrolization (adding water) of some of the simpler sugars occurs, and the ptyalin continues acting on the more complex carbohydrates, though the action is minor. The stomach can absorb water, alcohol, and some of the simpler dissolved sugars, but this also is a small-scale process.

Liquids leave the stomach faster than some more solid foods. Carbohydrate-rich foods leave faster than rich-protein or fatty foods, and combinations of fat and protein stay the longest. This is why a meal of hotcakes and syrup (carbohydrates) leaves one feeling hungry sooner than eating butter and pork sausage (fat) along with the hotcakes. Most food leaves the stomach within three hours.

The stomach moves food around in a churning action that helps break it up and mix it. The mixing also adds gastric juices that make the food more fluid. The mixed food is called

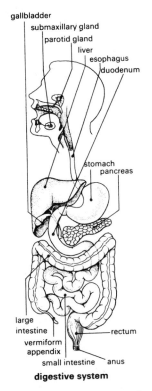

gallbladder
submaxillary gland
parotid gland
liver
esophagus
duodenum

stomach
pancreas

large
intestine
rectum
vermiform
appendix
small intestine   anus

digestive system

FIGURE 3-2 Schematic drawing of the digestive system.

chyme, and in this form it is forced out of the stomach into the duodenum, the first segment of the small intestine. It is in the small intestine that the real digestive process and most absorption occurs. This organ, about 20 feet long, has three parts: the duodenum, the ileum, and the jejunum. Because the chyme is acidic, the first digestion that occurs is hydrolysis of protein, which is enhanced in an acidic medium. But, as the chyme moves along the small intestine, the reaction becomes alkaline (nonacid), which favors the digestion and absorption of carbohydrates, fats, and some other substances.

The small intestine digestive juices contain three secretions from different sources: the pancreas, cells of the inner lining of the small intestine, and the liver. The pancreatic juices contain the enzymes *trypsin* and *chymotrypsin*, which break proteins down into *amino acids*; the enzyme *pancreatic amylase* changes starch and dextrins to maltose; and the enzyme *pancreatic lipase* helps break down fats. The intestinal cells supply *peptidase* enzymes that help break down proteins; *maltase* to change maltose to glucose; *sucrase* to change sucrose to glucose and fructose; and *lactase* to change lactose to glucose and galactose.

The liver supplies *bile*, which is stored in the gallbladder until needed. Bile acts to reduce the chyme, making it alkaline. Bile does not contain any enzymes but is essential in orchestrating the digestion and absorption of fats. By the time bile has mixed with chyme, it is essentially a mixture of emulsified fats (fat and water blended), simple sugars, amino acids, vitamins, and minerals. Absorption of these is the next step.

Digestion and Absorption in the Small Intestine

The nutrients in the chyle are now reduced to molecules. Some smaller molecules are absorbed by a process called *diffusion*; they just pass through the intestinal walls by themselves. Other larger molecules cannot do this. They must be pulled in by some kind of force. The intestinal wall has certain agents that pick up these larger nutrients and carry them through. Some kinds of molecules are surrounded with a slippery coat that enables them to slip through as a greased pig would through a small aperture. Absorption is an interesting and multifaceted process.

While the small intestine is only about 20 feet long, its inside surface area is large enough to cover half a basketball court. This surface area is possible because the walls of the small intestine are covered with tiny furlike fingers called *villi* (Fig. 3-3). They are about 1 centimeter (cm) long (0.04 inch) and wave back and forth. They come in contact with the nutrients and pick them up, transferring them inside to the crypts of the villi *(receptaculum chyli)*, where either blood or lymph picks them

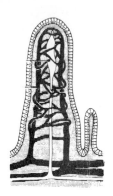

FIGURE 3-3 A simplified drawing of the intestinal villi. These villi are tiny furlike fingers extending from the small intestine wall (a) into the chyle, where they pick up nutrients. The capillary vein (solid black line) extends up into the villus where it picks up nutrients the villus absorbs. These nutrients are then carried to a vein in the wall of the small intestine where they make their way eventually to the portal vein, which carries them to the liver. The lymph vessel (white line) also extends up the villus and picks up other nutrients that are carried to the lymphatic system.

up and carries them around for use by the body. This large surface enables the small intestine to come in contact with a lot of the nutrients and select the ones needed. Different nutrients are pulled in from the small intestine by different mechanisms. According to signals from the body, the villi can be very selective. At times they may pick up iron and at other times they may not if the body has not signaled them to bring it in.

The blood carries its nutrients to the liver, which redistributes them to the various cells. The lymph carries its nutrients to the junction of the portal and subclavian veins and dumps them there where the blood picks them up and carries them around the body. Eventually some may return to the liver, which may determine that certain fuel nutrients are in excess and must be converted to calorie storage forms or be eliminated.

Absorption and Elimination in the Large Intestine

The colon is largely an area where food that is not digested or absorbed is stored in the form of feces until it is eliminated through the rectum and anus. Water and electrolytes are absorbed in the colon causing the chyle to become more solid feces. Too much water absorption can occur. The fiber content of feces is most important because it holds water, and this bulk facilitates elimination and avoids constipation. The colon is colonized by bacteria that produce vitamins, some of which are absorbed but not significant amounts.

After absorption into the body, nutrients are either stored or used in a process called *metabolism*. The body also breaks down substances to get rid of some nutrients. When we speak of nutrients being utilized for construction processes, we call this *anabolism* and when substances are broken down to eliminate nutrients it is called *catabolism*. Metabolism is both anabolism and catabolism. Metabolism will be discussed later with various nutrients.

HUMAN NUTRIENT NEEDS

To many people calories are things in food that make them fat. We may avoid eating a piece of cake because it gives us 400 calories. But what is a calorie? In scientific terms, under certain conditions, it is the amount of heat (energy) needed to raise the temperature of 1 gram of water 1°C. Some scientists, such as biochemists and nutritionists, find this unit too small to be practical, so they speak in terms of "large" calories, one of which raises the temperature of 1 gram of water 1000°C; or of 1000 grams (a kilogram; kg) 1°C. In this text when we use the term "calorie" we mean the large calorie. Sometimes the small calorie is called "gram calorie" and the large calorie, the "kilocalorie." The fuel foods furnish calories. Carbohydrate yields four calories per gram of pure carbohydrate; pure protein yields four calories per gram, and fats, nine (some authorities say eleven). Alcohol yields seven per gram.

Different people need different amounts of calories and other nutrients. A baby may need a limited amount of calories but considerable protein, minerals, and vitamins because it is growing quite fast. In comparison, a young active male might need about 3000 calories per day (about 14 cups of cooked rice), which should include about 56 grams of protein (about two ounces, the amount in 7 1/4 ounces of roast beef), 60 milligrams (mg) of vitamin C, and 3 micrograms (µg) of vitamin B_{12} and other nutrients.

Calculating an Adequate Diet

In order to determine what nutrients people need every day and in what quantities, studies have been made. After this *average* need was found, a safety factor was calculated in. Thus, 60 mg is the adults' standard for vitamin C, including the safety factor. The standards used today are thought to cover 97% of the population. Different standards had to be set for persons at different stages of life. There is a different standard for calorie and other nutrient requirements of infants, children, youths, adult males and females, pregnant and lactating females, and elderly persons. Although we know the needs for some nutrients, we may not know how much, so no standard amount for a daily intake has been set for these nutrients. We are also not sure that some substances found in the body are needed or what they do, but since they are commonly found we assume a need. Scientists probably have not discovered all the nutrients. As we gain new information, we add to the standards or revise them.

The most frequently used recommended amounts to consume per day are the Recommended Dietary Allowances (RDA) established by the Food and Nutrition Board of the National Academy of Sciences to "provide standards serving as a goal for good nutrition." They are revised from time to time as new information is learned. The latest revision was in 1980. The RDAs give nutrient values needed per day for people of various ages and different stages of life. Not all vitamins and minerals known are represented, but persons who eat to meet the RDAs without taking supplements are likely to be obtaining adequate quantities of the nutrients for which a definitive RDA has yet to be established.

Another much used set of dietary intake recommendations is the U.S. Recommended Daily Allowance, a set of values used by the FDA and other government agencies as a baseline for human nutrition requirements. It is used by the government to evaluate the nutritional value of foods. The US RDAs are the values used in the nutrition labeling of food products that were discussed in Chapter 2. Tables 3-1 and 3-2 show the RDAs and US RDAs. The US RDAs are based on the RDAs.

Many people in foodservice cannot understand what the RDAs and US RDAs mean, because they seem too technical for them. A simpler method is needed to allow the average person to know what to eat every day to be well nourished. The

TABLE 3-1
Food and Nutrition Board, National Academy of Sciences— National Research Council Recommended Daily Dietary Allowances,[a] Revised 1980

	Age (years)	Weight (lb)	Height (in)	Protein (g)	Vitamin A (μg RE)[b]	Vitamin D (μg)[c]	Vitamin E (mg α-TE)[d]	Vitamin C (mg)	Thiamin (mg)	Riboflavin (mg)	Niacin (mg NE)[e]	Vitamin B6 (mg)	Folacin (μg)[f]	Vitamin B12 (μg)	Calcium (mg)	Phosphorus (mg)	Magnesium (mg)	Iron (mg)	Zinc (mg)	Iodine (μg)
Infants	0.0-0.5	13	24	kg×2.2	420	10	3	35	0.3	0.4	6	0.3	30	0.5	360	240	50	10	3	40
	0.5-1.0	20	28	kg×2.0	400	10	4	35	0.5	0.6	8	0.6	45	1.5	540	360	70	15	5	50
Children	1-3	29	35	23	400	10	5	45	0.7	0.8	9	0.9	100	2.0	800	800	150	15	10	70
	4-6	44	44	30	500	10	6	45	0.9	1.0	11	1.3	200	2.5	800	800	200	10	10	90
	7-10	62	52	34	700	10	7	45	1.2	1.4	16	1.6	300	3.0	800	800	250	10	10	120
Males	11-14	99	62	45	1000	10	8	50	1.4	1.6	18	1.8	400	3.0	1200	1200	350	18	15	150
	15-18	145	69	56	1000	10	10	60	1.4	1.7	18	2.0	400	3.0	1200	1200	400	18	15	150
	19-22	154	70	56	1000	7.5	10	60	1.5	1.7	19	2.2	400	3.0	800	800	350	10	15	150
	23-50	154	70	56	1000	5	10	60	1.4	1.6	18	2.2	400	3.0	800	800	350	10	15	150
	51+	154	70	56	1000	5	10	60	1.2	1.4	16	2.2	400	3.0	800	800	350	10	15	150
Females	11-14	101	62	46	800	10	8	50	1.1	1.3	15	1.8	400	3.0	1200	1200	300	18	15	150
	15-18	120	64	46	800	10	8	60	1.1	1.3	14	2.0	400	3.0	1200	1200	300	18	15	150
	19-22	120	64	44	800	7.5	8	60	1.1	1.3	14	2.0	400	3.0	800	800	300	18	15	150
	23-50	120	64	44	800	5	8	60	1.0	1.2	13	2.0	400	3.0	800	800	300	18	15	150
	51+	120	64	44	800	5	8	60	1.0	1.2	13	2.0	400	3.0	800	800	300	10	15	150
Pregnant				+30	+200	+5	+2	+20	+0.4	+0.3	+2	+0.6	+400	+1.0	+400	+400	+150	h	+5	+25
Lactating				+20	+400	+5	+3	+40	+0.5	+0.5	+5	+0.5	+100	+1.0	+400	+400	+150	h	+10	+50

a The allowances are intended to provide for individual variations among most normal persons as they live in the United States under usual environmental stresses. Diets should be based on a variety of common foods in order to provide other nutrients for which human requirements have been less well defined.

b Retinol equivalents. 1 retinol equivalent = 1μg retinol or 6 μg β-carotene.

c As cholecalciferol. 10 μg cholecalciferol = 400 iu of vitamin D.

d α-tocopherol equivalents. 1 mg d-α tocopherol = 1 α-TE.

e 1 NE (niacin equivalent) is equal to 1 mg of niacin or 60 mg of dietary tryptophan.

f The folacin allowances refer to dietary sources as determined by Lactobacillus casei assay after treatment with enzymes (conjugases) to make polyglutamyl forms of the vitamin available to the test organism.

g The recommended dietary allowance for vitamin B12 in infants is based on average concentration of the vitamin in human milk. The allowances after weaning are based on energy intake (as recommended by the American Academy of Pediatrics) and consideration of other factors, such as intestinal absorption.

h The increased requirement during pregnancy cannot be met by the iron content of habitual American diets nor by the existing iron stores of many women; therefore the use of 30-60 mg.of supplemental iron is recommended. Iron needs during lactation are not substantially different from those of nonpregnant women, but continued supplementation of the mother for 2-3 months after parturition is advisable in order to replenish stores depleted by pregnancy.

(Reprinted from *Recommended Dietary Allowances*, ed. 9, 1980, with permission of the National Academy Press, Washington DC.)

saying is, "One eats food, not nutrients." The average person needs to learn what foods to select daily, and how much to eat. We have two simple methods. One is the Basic Four Plan and the other is the Exchange Method (often used by persons who must balance their diet very carefully, such as those who have diabetes). Another more complex method is to make calculations using tables of food values. Let us examine how such tables and the Basic Four Plan and the Exchange Method work.

Table of Food Values Method Tables of food values tell how much of the various nutrients 100 grams, a serving, a pound, or another amount of food contains. For instance, a 1-cup portion of cooked spaghetti is found to contain 155 calories, 5 grams of protein, and 1 gram of fat. Other nutrients in the spaghetti are also measured. Adding up all the nutrients in all foods consumed in a day would yield the entire daily intake of each; Table 3-3 is a sample tabulation. If the first were for an adult female, the diet would be adequate except for niacin and iron. (Check this with the RDAs in Table 3-1 and see what the nutrient yield is with this diet.)

Calculating a diet manually using the table of food values is a time-consuming task, but a computer can do in minutes what used to take hours. (See Figure 12-5.)

A table of food values taken from *Home and Garden Bulletin*, No. 72, 1981, USDA can be found in Appendix A of this book from which the quantity of specific nutrients in a particular food can be ascertained. Other reliable tables of food values

TABLE 3-2
U.S. Recommended Daily Allowances (U.S. RDA)*

	Adults and Children Over 4 yrs.	Children Under 4 yrs.	Infants Under 13 months	Pregnant or Lactating Women
Protein†	65 grams	28 grams	25 grams	65 grams
Vitamin A	5,000 IU	2,500 IU	2,500 IU	8,000 IU
Vitamin C	60 mg	40 mg	40 mg	60 mg
Thiamin	1.5 mg	0.7 mg	0.7 mg	1.7 mg
Riboflavin	1.7 mg	0.8 mg	0.8 mg	2.0 mg
Niacin	20 mg	9.0 mg	9.0 mg	20 mg
Calcium	1.0 grams	0.8 grams	0.8 grams	1.3 grams
Iron	18 mg	10 mg	10 mg	18 mg
Vitamin D	400 IU	400 IU	400 IU	400 IU
Vitamin E	30 IU	10 IU	10 IU	30 IU
Vitamin B$_6$	2.0 mg	0.7 mg	0.7 mg	2.5 mg
Folacin	0.4 mg	0.2 mg	0.2 mg	0.8 mg
Vitamin B$_{12}$	6 μg	3 μg	3 μg	8 μg
Phosphorus	1.0 grams	0.8 grams	0.8 grams	1.3 grams
Iodine	150 μg	70 μg	70 μg	150 μg
Magnesium	400 mg	200 mg	200 mg	450 mg
Zinc	15 mg	8 mg	8 mg	15 mg
Copper	2 mg	1 mg	1 mg	2 mg
Biotin	0.3 mg	0.15 mg	0.15 mg	0.3 mg
Pantothenic acid	10 mg	5 mg	5 mg	10 mg

* For use in nutrition labeling of foods, including foods that also are vitamin and mineral supplements.
† If protein efficiency ratio of protein is equal to or better than that of caseine U.S. RDA is 45 grams for adults and pregnant or lactating women, 20 grams for children under 4 years of age and 18 grams for infants.

are Bowes, Church, and Remington, *Table of Food Values of Portions Commonly Used*, J.B. Lippincott, 1986; USDA *Agricultural Handbooks No. 8 and No. 456*, and *Home and Garden Bulletin, No. 2*, USDA, 1976.

The Basic Four Food Group One of the simplest ways to calculate the adequacy of a diet is to use what is called the Basic Four Plan (also known as the Four Food Group Plan and the Daily Food Guide). Originally there were 10 groups—some say 17—then the scheme was modified to include seven, and then four groups. There is talk of further refinement that would produce a five-group plan.

The four basic food groups are: (1) milk or its derivatives, (2) meats or protein equivalents, (3) fruits and vegetables, and (4) grains, breads, and other cereal and grain products. The fifth group would be composed of sweets, fats, and other high-calorie foods of low nutrient density (Fig. 3-4).

TABLE 3-3
Nutrient Values of a Sample Day's Food Intake

	Energy cal	Protein grams	Fat grams	Carbohydrates grams	Calcium mg	Iron mg	Vitamins A IU*	B1 mg	B2 mg	Niacin mg	C mg
Breakfast											
Orange, sliced	65	1	—	16	54	0.5	260	0.13	0.05	0.5	66
Puffed wheat	55	2	.	12	4	0.6	—	0.08	0.03	1.2	—
Milk, ½ cup	80	4	4	6	144	0.1	175	0.03	0.20	0.1	1
Poached egg	80	6	6	—	27	1.1	590	0.05	0.15	—	—
Toast, 2 slices	140	4	2	26	42	1.2	—	0.12	0.10	1.2	—
Butter, 2 tsp	70	—	8	—	2	—	340	—	—	—	—
Coffee Cream 2 tbsp	60	2	6	2	30	—	260	—	0.04	—	—
Total	490	19	26	62	303	3.5	1,625	0.41	0.57	4.0	67
Lunch											
Tomato soup	175	7	7	23	168	0.8	1,200	0.10	0.25	1.3	15
Saltines, 4	50	1	1	8	2	0.1	—	—	—	0.1	—
Choc. milk, 1 cup	190	8	6	27	270	0.5	210	0.10	0.4	0.3	3
Pineapple, canned, 1 slice	90	—	—	24	13	0.4	50	0.05	0.03	0.2	8
Total	505	16	14	82	453	1.8	1460	0.25	0.32	1.9	26
Dinner											
Chicken pie, 1 cup	535	23	31	42	68	3.0	3020	0.60	0.26	4.1	5
Cauliflower, 1 cup	25	3	—	5	25	0.8	70	0.11	0.10	0.7	66
Cucumber slices	5	5	—	2	8	0.2	—	0.02	0.02	0.1	6
Biscuits, 2	210	4	10	26	68	0.8	—	0.12	0.12	0.2	—
Butter, 2 tsp	70	—	8	—	2	—	340	—	—	—	—
Jelly, 1 tbsp	50	—	—	13	4	0.3	—	—	0.01	—	1
Pumpkin pie	275	5	15	32	66	0.7	3210	0.04	0.13	0.7	—
Wine, dry 7 ounces	170	—	—	8	18	0.8	—	—	0.02	0.2	—
Total	1340	40	64	128	259	6.6	6640	0.89	0.66	6.0	78
Total day's nutrient intake	2335	75	104	272	1015	11.9	9725	1.55	1.55	10.9	171

* International units

TABLE 3-4
Basic Four Food Plan Portions for Various Persons

Food Group	Serving	Minimum Servings per Day				
		Children	Teenagers	Adults	Pregnant Women	Lactating Women
Milk	1 cup milk, yogurt or buttermilk, etc. Some equivalents: 1½ ounces cheese 2 cups cottage cheese 1¼ cup ice cream 1 cup milk-base pudding or 1 cup milk base soup	3	4	2	4	4
Meat	2 ounces cooked, lean meat, poultry, or fish, or 2 eggs 2 ounces cheese 1 cup cooked legumes 4 tbsp peanut butter ½ cup cottage cheese 1 cup chili, stew or casserole meat dish ¼ 14" meat pizza with cheese 1 taco	2	2	2	3	2
Vegetable-Fruit*	½ cup cooked vegetable or fruit 1 cup raw vegetable or fruit ½ cup juice 1 medium apple, banana, orange, peach, pear, etc. ½ grapefruit ¼ canteloupe	4	4	4	4	4
Grain†	1 slice bread, roll or biscuit 1 cup macaroni, etc. 1 cup ready-to-eat cereal ½ cup ready-to-eat cereal ½ cup cooked cereal, rice, or grits	4	4	4	4	4

Supplemental
Select other foods such as butter, margarine, salad dressings, pie, cake, cookies, sugar, jam or jelly, carbonated beverages, wine, beer, etc., to give adequate calories and to provide for menu palatability.

* Select a fruit or vegetable each day that gives a good yield of Vitamin C; select a leafy green or yellow vegetable or a yellow or orange fruit every other day to provide adequate vitamin A.

† It is recommended that grains be enriched or whole grain.

Note: For the adult group, selecting the first four groups as suggested with no supplemental foods will give about 1200 calories a day.

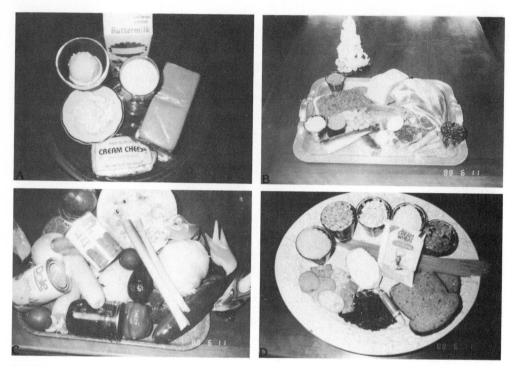

FIGURE 3-4 Examples of foods in the four basics groups: A, dairy; B, meats; C, fruits and vegetables; and D, grains.

The simplicity and easy application of the Basic Four recommends it. Complicated calculations required for using tables of food values are avoided. One has only to eat a specific number of portions (Table 3-4) from each of the four groups every day, depending on age and special conditions such as pregnancy or lactation, to be well nourished.

The Milk Group Milk and other dairy products such as cheese and yogurt are in this group. Low-fat, low sugar products should be used by those who want to reduce calories. Chocolate milk and unreconstituted condensed or evaporated milk are high in calories. Dry milk is least expensive, canned milk is next, and low-fat fluid products, next. Young children should have four portions a day from the milk group but not more, or they may not have the appetite to consume the variety of foods they need. It is very important that adults, especially older ones, consume at least two milk portions daily. Some elderly persons may need to eat more portions or to take supplemental calcium to guard against osteoporosis (brittle bones). For those who cannot tolerate the lactose in milk, some lactose-free milk products are available. Some may be able to eat yogurt or sweet acidophilus milk, but soybean curd (tofu) is an adequate substitute for milk in protein, calcium, and phosphorus.

The Meat Group Animal protein foods may be substituted for by legumes such as dry beans, and peas. Some seeds and nuts also can be an adequate substitute. Soybeans almost equal meat in protein value. All flesh should be measured lean without bones. Beef, veal, pork, lamb, poultry, fin and shellfish are acceptable, but fatty products such as bacon, salt pork, and certain processed delicatessen meats provide much less protein per ounce. Eggs are an adequate meat substitute. A cup of cottage cheese or 3 ounces of cheddar or Swiss cheese from the dairy group contributes as much protein as 3 ounces of meat. Often half a portion of meat is served with half a portion of a substitute, as in chili con carne with beans.

The Fruit and Vegetable Group Fruits and vegetables contribute many of the vitamins and minerals needed in the diet and they are important sources of dietary fiber. Vegetable selections should include a large assortment of root vegetables (carrots, radishes, turnips, beets), leafy green ones (spinach, broccoli, chard, and other members of the cabbage family), and others such as tomatoes, peppers, celery, lettuce, and squash. Though potatoes, sweet potatoes, and yams are considered to be vegetables, for energy comparisons it is better to regard them as grain or as extra-calorie foods, since they contain more calories than other vegetables. Fruit should also be varied. In the U.S. vitamins A and C are sometimes lacking in the diet. Melons, papayas, strawberries, and pineapple are adequate substitutes for citrus fruit in providing vitamin C. If tomatoes, cabbage or Irish potatoes are among the vegetables consumed, the vitamin C requirement can be fulfilled without eating fruits. Some yellow fruits, including cantaloupe and apricots, are good sources of vitamin A. Yellow, orange, or leafy green vegetables are good sources of vitamin A.

Fresh, frozen, dried, and canned fruits all satisfy the fruit recommendations. It is often best to use fresh fruit and vegetables at the peak of their season, when they have the highest nutrient quality and lowest price.

It is not difficult to meet the four-portion daily requirement for fruits and vegetables or consistently to include good sources of vitamins A and C. A fruit or fruit juice for breakfast, a hamburger with lettuce, onions, tomato, and pickles for lunch, a mixed green salad for dinner, along with another vegetable satisfies the daily requirement. Applesauce, a lower calorie fresh fruit cup, or a slice of cantaloupe counts as a fruit portion.

The Grain Products Group Grain products, especially whole-grain or enriched ones, can contribute vitamins and minerals as well as bulk and carbohydrate for energy. Wheat, rice, barley, rye, corn, oats, and other grains can be used to meet this requirement. Thiamine, riboflavin, niacin, iron and other nutrients are furnished by grain products which also furnish good dietary fiber if they contain whole grains.

The Other Group Often when additional calories come from a fifth group (sometimes called the "other group," of foods—fats, desserts, jams, jellies, alcoholic beverages, and other high-calorie foods), the plan is called the Daily Food Guide. The Basic Four Plan amounts to around 1200 to 1400 calories a day, and many people need more than that. The extra foods provide these calories, and often added nutrients. Of course, extra calories are better obtained by eating additional portions of the Four Food Groups.

The Exchange Method The Exchange Method is designed as a guide not only to obtain a balanced diet but to control intake to meet special dietary needs. It began as a calorie-control, flexible method for dietary control of diabetes, but it has since been adapted and expanded for use in weight-control, low-sodium, low-cholesterol, low-fat, and other diets. It is also used frequently for every day food intake planning.

The Exchange Method has the advantage of seeing that persons consume a variety of foods, which the Basic Four Plan does not do as well.

The method uses seven food groups: vegetable, fruit, grain or starch, meat, fat, skim milk and freely allowed foods. The vegetable group differentiates between low, moderate, and high-carbohydrate items. The bread and cereal group includes high-starch vegetables such as dry legumes, winter squash, potatoes, and corn. Some nuts, legumes, seeds, and other nonanimal high-protein foods are included in the meat group. Sometimes the meat group is subdivided into low-, medium-, and high-fat items. The fat group includes fats and oils, butter, and margarine, salad dressings, cream, nuts, olives, avocadoes, bacon and other high-fat items. The milk group exchange is based on skim milk. If whole-milk products are consumed, two fat exchanges are added for each milk exchange. A number of low-calorie vegetables, such as spinach, lettuce, mushrooms, summer squash, many spices, vinegar, coffee, tea, bouillon, and low-calorie pickles, are in the freely allowed group. One exchange from a group is equal to one clearly defined portion of food; for example, one fruit exchange equals one half of a medium banana.

In 1986 the Food Exchange Lists were revised. Fats were subdivided into saturated and unsaturated types, and other slight changes were made, such as showing what foods are high in sodium or fiber. The complete revised list of foods for the Exchange Method is presented in Appendix B.

For a specific meal, a given number of items from various exchange groups is specified. Thus, breakfast might have the selections in Table 3-5:

TABLE 3-5
Sample Breakfast Selected by the Exchange Method

Selection Allowed	Foods Selected	Portion Size
1 fruit exchange	Sliced oranges	½ cup
2 bread exchanges	Whole wheat toast	2 slices
1 meat exchange	Boiled ham	1 ounce
1 milk exchange	Nonfat milk	1 cup
2 fat exchanges	Margarine	2 pats (2 teaspoons)
Free list as desired	Coffee, black	

Every item or exchange from a given group provides approximately the same amount of carbohydrate, protein, fat, and calories as others in the group. Table 3-6 shows the yield of carbohydrate, protein, fat, and calories from the various exchanges:

The fuel nutrients provide calories at the following levels: protein or carbohydrates, 4 per gram: alcohol, 7 per gram; and fat, 9 per gram. The total calories and fuel nutrient quantities in the sample breakfast are shown in Table 3-7.

The Exchange Method is not as simple to use as the Basic Four Plan, but it guides selection of a variety of foods in the major food groups. It may be necessary to take care to see that vitamin intakes are adequate. Also, many of the foods we eat are not listed in the Exchanges, though some lists now include Chinese and other ethnic food exchanges, which is a help. Foods such as chicken pie or meat and spaghetti are still a problem; it would be almost impossible to formulate exchanges

TABLE 3-6
Nutrient Values of Exchanges

Exchange	Serving Size	Carbohydrate	Protein	Fat	Calories
Vegetable	½ cup	5 grams	2 grams	—	25
Fruit	varies, see list	15 grams	—	—	60
Bread/starch	1 slice	15 grams	3 grams	trace	80
Meat, lean	1 ounce	—	7 grams	3 grams	55
Milk, skim	1 cup	12 grams	8 grams	trace	90
Fat	1 teaspoon	—	—	5 grams	45

owing to the variety of ways such dishes can be prepared. Overall, the attributes of the Exchange Method outweigh the drawbacks, and the result is a useful method of planning a good diet. Understanding the Exchange Method can provide an excellent foundation for selecting balanced, healthful meals and snacks and for planning menus.

TABLE 3-7
Nutrients and Calories in Exchanges for a Sample Breakfast

Food Item	Carbohydrate	Protein	Fat	Calories
Orange (2½" across)	15 grams	—	—	60
Toast (2 slices)	30 grams	6 grams	trace	160
Meat, lean (1 oz.)	—	7 grams	3 grams	55
Milk, skim (1 cup)	12 grams	8 grams	trace	90
Butter (2 teaspoons)	—	—	10 grams	90
Total	57 grams	21 grams	13 grams	455

IS AN IDEAL DIET POSSIBLE?

We have been discussing different plans for selecting a balanced diet that provides excellent nutrition, but is it really possible to select *all* the nutrients one should have *all* the time? Some authorities say that, our resources notwithstanding, there are limitations. They say that planning precisely to achieve a completely adequate diet is an impossible dream.

One of the problems in planning an optimal diet is that a single set of standards must be adopted although the objective is to satisfy the needs of a group of unique individuals. The RDA sets standards according to sex, age, and body size. Do all males between ages 19 and 22 have exactly the same nutrient needs? The same energy output? Of course not. Some people need more nutrients than others; we don't know why. People's needs also differ from day to day. It is not possible, therefore, to set up a single diet that will be the best possible for everyone. A sliding scale to meet individual variations is not feasible. RDAs are designed to apply to persons whose needs are as much as two standard deviations above the mean, which should include 97% of the population. But what about the other 3%? How are their needs to be met? The RDAs must be written as they are if we are to have standards at all. The intent was to provide standards that cover most persons' needs (Fig. 3-5).

The method of calculating nutritional yields from tables of food values is not for the ordinary person. They do not understand how to use them, and the method is too complex. Any plan that laymen are to use should specify foods rather than nutrients. People can understand food though they may not understand nutrients, and even those who understand how to use tables of food values, the Basic Four, or the Exchange Method, may not be getting a proper diet. For example, there are wide variations among foods: 4 ounces of freshly squeezed orange juice should contain about 60 mg of vitamin C, but it well might contain half that, or half again as much. Seasonal differences in the quality of fresh foods, marketing practices, varietal differences in fresh foods, effects of processing, and other factors contribute to this variability. Nutrient loss during storage, handling, preparation, and holding of foods in foodservices can be significant. A study in one college dormitory foodservice determined that only 5% of the original amount of vitamin C in potatoes remained when the mashed potatoes finally were served.

Diets should not only meet physical needs but should also satisfy psychological and social ones. Food is to be enjoyed, and when the enjoyment factor is lost, the dietary cause may be also. Many elementary school feeding programs learned this the hard way. The food they served was very nutritious, but the children would not eat it. Even food that is well prepared may be unacceptable owing to certain religious, ethnic, cultural, or lifestyle values. It is poor practice to select and prepare food only for its nutritional value and to ignore the very important factors that make food acceptable and appealing. A foodservice must first of all be concerned with pleasing patrons. Some notable failures in recent years occurred when foodservices programs emphasized nutrition but failed to follow through to see that patrons approved of the offerings. Nutrition is good only when diners willingly eat the food.

It is a mistake to think it possible to produce a menu replete with optimally healthful foods. Nutritional needs are so different from person to person that all a foodservice can do is try to design a program that meets the standards generally advocated by respected authorities and then to support patrons within that baseline. A foodservice that tries to be too nutritionally rigorous, if it is not a healthcare-related operation, usually is found wanting.

SUMMARY

Food should provide the building blocks that maintain or promote good health, productivity, and longevity. It should also be tasty and meet psychological and social needs. So, to eat well, one should eat an adequate diet that is, at the same time, satisfying and enjoyable.

Six categories of nutrients are needed: carbohydrates, proteins, fats, vitamins, minerals, and water. Carbohydrate, protein, and fat produce energy. Protein is needed to build tissues, bone, and teeth and the cellular components of blood, antibodies, and lymph. Fat protects, insulates and stores energy. Vitamins and minerals are body regulators; minerals also help build tissue and perform other functions. Water provides the place and the means for bodily nutrient action.

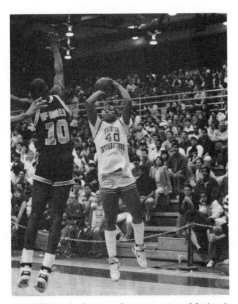

FIGURE 3-5 Star performance in athletics is built upon a well-balanced diet. Without it, the ability to perform at top level is lessened. Star basketball player Sylvester Wigham, Florida International University. *(Courtesy Florida International University Athletic Department)*

Digestion starts in the mouth where saliva moistens food, mucin makes it more slippery, and pytalin starts to break down some carbohydrates. Chewing macerates food, helping to promote digestion. The stomach acts largely to digest proteins. Most digestion and absorption occur in the small intestine. Acidic chyme from the stomach is gradually converted in the small intestine to alkaline chyle. With these changes, different digestive and absorptive actions occur.

Nutrients in the form of amino acids, simple sugars, emulsified fats, vitamins, and minerals are absorbed into the body through villi in the small intestine. Different mechanisms are needed to absorb different nutrients. Villi work to take in certain nutrients and exclude others according to signals from a central physiological regulator in the body.

The colon acts as a storage depot, and in it water and some electrolytes are absorbed. Solid waste is eliminated through the rectum and anus.

To have optimal nutrition, one must consume certain quantities of over 40 nutrients, which are found in different foods in varying quantities. To obtain a truly adequate, healthful diet one must know which foods are good sources of specific nutrients and how much of them to eat. Nutrient intake can be estimated by keeping track of food consumed and determining its nutrient yield from a table of food values. Computer programs are now available to do the calculations, so the task has been simplified considerably. It is the most accurate method. Using the Basic Four Plan is simpler; though it is not always possible to know exactly how much of various nutrients is being obtained. Following the Basic Four Plan is a fairly reliable way to get an adequate diet. The Exchange Method also can be used to provide a balanced diet and is especially effective for persons who must control intake of certain foods for some special physiological reason.

Chapter Review

1. Why do people eat? List reasons why some people eat when they are not hungry. Describe the basic needs food meets for humans.
2. Define "eating well."
3. List the six major nutrient categories. What function does each perform?

4. Identify which of the major nutrient categories do each of the following: 1) furnish energy for heat and power, 2) build and maintain the body, 3) provide regulators that "run" the body.
5. What are the dietary functions of water?
6. What is the Recommended Dietary Allowance list? Using this list, find your approximate needs for protein, vitamin C, iron, thiamine, riboflavin, and calcium.
7. What are the RDAs and the US RDAs?
8. What is the difference between a small calorie and large calorie?
9. What is the Basic Four Plan?
10. Using the table of food values in this or another reliable text, compile a nutrient evaluation of a day's diet for yourself. (You will need to keep a 24-hour diary of everything you consume and its measure.)
11. What is the Exchange Method? What are some of its advantages and disadvantages?
12. If each exchange group is matched with a corresponding Basic Four Plan group what exchange group is left out?
13. What is the alimentary canal?
14. What phases of digestion occur, respectively, in the mouth, esophagus, stomach, small intestine, and colon?

Chapter 4
Carbohydrates

Chapter Goals

- To describe how carbohydrates are made in nature and the kinds of carbohydrates in our food—their nature and some of their properties.
- To show what kinds of carbohydrates we should eat and how much.
- To describe how the body uses carbohydrates and what functions they perform in the body.
- To describe the good and bad effects carbohydrates can have in the body.
- To show how to select carbohydrates from exchange lists.
- To discuss alcohol as a fuel food.

THE PRINCIPAL ENERGY SOURCE

"Carbohydrate" is not the name of a specific food. It is a form of nutrient. Some foods such as bread, pasta, and potatoes are known as carbohydrates or starches, because they contain a lot of carbohydrate. Of the four nutrient groups contributing food energy (carbohydrate, protein, fat, and alcohol), carbohydrates occur in the greatest number of foods. Carbohydrates are unique among the four groups, because it is generally believed that most people who want to eat healthfully should **increase** their carbohydrate intake. Patrons are often interested in the carbohydrate content of foods because they want to follow a weight control program or they have diabetes or they want to increase the fiber in their diet or they have other needs that require it. Carbohydrate foods are popular, often inexpensive, and they are an essential part of a healthful eating plan. In addition, they are versatile and come in many forms and an enormous spectrum of flavors, textures, and colors.

Many people believe that foods high in carbohydrate are more fattening than other foods. This is not true. In the pure state, a gram of carbohydrate provides four calories, a gram of protein four, a gram of fat nine, and a gram of alcohol seven. If we do not get calories from carbohydrate, we must get them from protein or fat, which often are not as good for us and are a more expensive way of getting energy. Carbohydrates in our body burn cleanly; protein and fat leave residues, which are sometimes troublesome to the body's food-burning system.

THE CARBOHYDRATE FAMILY

Carbohydrates belong to a large family of organic saccharides (sugars). They are made by plants taking water from the soil and carbon dioxide from the air and combining them together to make basic CH_2O units. They then link six of these basic units to make a simple saccharide, such as glucose or fructose; or they join 12 of the basic units to make a disaccharide such as maltose or sucrose (table sugar). Starches and fiber consist of many saccharides formed into countless combinations (polysaccharides). Carbohydrate names often end in -ose (e.g., glucose, fructose, sucrose, cellulose).

Most carbohydrates exist in plant foods as a mixture of simple and complex carbohydrates. Simple carbohydrates (sugars) are made up of one or two monosaccharide chains; examples are sucrose (table sugar), maltose and fructose. Complex carbohydrates contain many monosaccharides, for example starches and carbohydrates that contain fiber (See Figs. 4-1 and 4-2, Table 4-1). Foodservice personnel are not bio-chemists, but a basic understanding of simple and complex carbohydrates enhances awareness of different types of carbohydrates in foods, the ways they overlap and blend in different foods, the ways they change during refinement or processing, and the various ways different types are broken down by the body to produce energy. Knowing about these differences makes it possible to eat carbohydrates in a more healthful way.

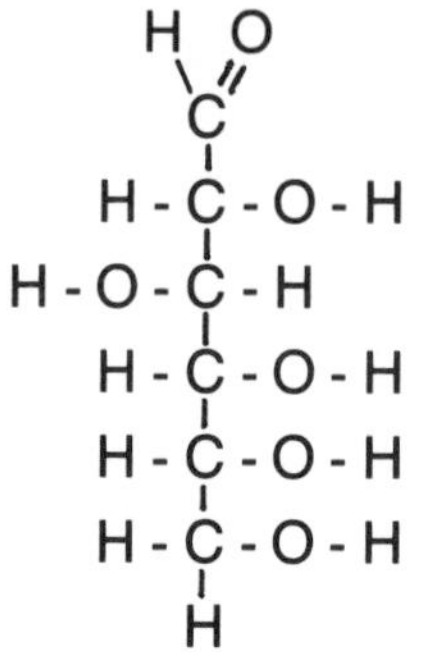

FIGURE 4-1 This is a graphic presentation of how oxygen and hydrogen atoms are grouped around carbon atoms to make glucose. Fructose, galactose, and mannose (rarely found in foods) are only slightly different from glucose, so they can easily be converted from one to another.

How Simple Sugars (Monosaccharides) Form Disaccharides or Polysaccharides

The Simple Sugars

G   = Glucose
F   = Fructose
Ga = Galactose

can be joined to make disaccharides as follows:

G + F   = Sucrose
G + G   = Maltose
G + Ga = Lactose

They join to make polysaccharides as follows:

G + G + G + G + G + G + G etc. = Starch
(many glucoses joined together)

G + G + G + G + G + G + G etc. = Cellulose (fiber)
(again many glucoses joined together)

G + G + G + G + G + G + G etc. = Glycogen
(animal body starch)
(again many glucoses joined together)

FIGURE 4-2 Monosaccharides (the basic molecule is shown on the left) join together as shown to form disaccharides. Thus sugar (sucrose) is made of one glucose and one fructose; and lactose from one glucose and one galactose. Starches, cellulose, and glycogen—complex carbohydrates—are composed of many, many glucose molecules.

TABLE 4-1
Classification of Carbohydrates

Simple Carbohydrates	Complex Carbohydrates	
Monosaccharides*	Disaccharides*	Polysaccharides*
Glucose	Sucrose (glucose and fructose)	Starches
Fructose	Maltose (glucose and glucose)	Fibers
Galactose	Lactose (galactose and glucose)	Cellulose Hemi-cellulose Pectin Gums Lignin

*Mono = one, di = two, poly = many

The Making of Carbohydrates

Carbohydrates are the major source of energy for human beings. They are manufactured in the green substance of plants known as *chlorophyll* in a process called *photosynthesis*. The energy in sunlight is captured by chlorophyll to join carbon dioxide and water, creating saccharides, which are formed into simple (sugars) or complex carbohydrates (starches). Animals and man consume these sugars and starches and break them down again into carbon dioxide and water, extracting in the process the sun's energy captured there. Figure 4-3 shows this cycle, which is basic to all life.

Simple Carbohydrates, or Sugars

Simple carbohydrates, or sugars are either monosaccharides or disaccharides. Glucose, fructose, and galactose are monosaccharides (mono = one): each is composed of only one distinctive type of saccharide. Glucose may also be called dextrose, and fructose, levulose. Sucrose, maltose, and lactose are disaccharides: they are each made up of two monosaccharides.

Monosaccharides   Whatever the form of digestible carbohydrate the body takes in, it is eventually converted to glucose, the only form of carbohydrate the body can directly convert to energy. So the breakdown of all carbohydrates in the body eventually produces glucose. Body enzymes, minerals and vitamins make this change.

Fructose, a monosaccharide, is responsible for much of the sweetness of fruits; and is sometimes called grape sugar because grapes contain so much of it. Fructose is sweeter than sucrose, and it has been touted as a lower-calorie sweetener, but the difference is not great enough to be effective for weight reduction or control. Sucrose's sweetness is indexed at 100% and fructose's at 120%. Some say fructose is a natural fruit sugar, but taking *pure* fructose has no advantage over consuming any other sugar. All are natural. The body still has to turn fructose into glucose. Fructose is no better than other sugars for persons with diabetes, which is essentially an intolerance to glucose. All sugars contain four calories per gram. Galactose is most plentiful in

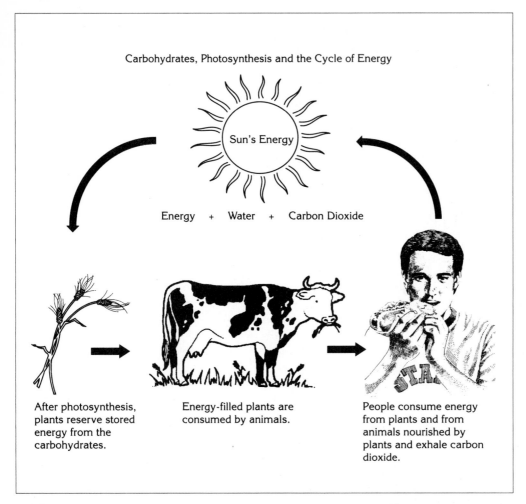

Carbohydrates, Photosynthesis and the Cycle of Energy

Sun's Energy

Energy + Water + Carbon Dioxide

After photosynthesis, plants reserve stored energy from the carbohydrates.

Energy-filled plants are consumed by animals.

People consume energy from plants and from animals nourished by plants and exhale carbon dioxide.

FIGURE 4-3 The production and use of carbohydrates: the sun's energy is used by plants to make carbon dioxide and water into saccharides. Man and animals consume these saccharides in foods and extract the energy after breaking down the saccharides into carbon dioxide and water again, which are now again available for making saccharides.

milk and milk products. It is a component of lactose. Galactose does not occur alone in nature, but is always coupled with at least one other monosaccharide. Mannose, another monosaccharide, is seldom found in our food.

Disaccharides Disaccharides consist of two monosaccharides bonded together to create a new sugar such as sucrose, maltose, or lactose. Sucrose is formed by the joining of glucose and fructose; maltose, by two glucose molecules; and lactose, by galactose and glucose. Maltose is often called "malt sugar," because it is obtained from the starch in barley when barley sprouts. Lactose is also called "milk sugar," because it is the natural sweetener of milk. When lactose turns to lactic acid, we say the milk is sour.

Complex Carbohydrates, or Polysaccharides

Complex carbohydrates are also divided into two groups, starches and fiber-related substances. Complex carbohydrates are called polysaccharides because they contain many (poly) molecules.

Starch Plants make starch by taking many glucose units and joining them together in a complex network. Starch in a plant is usually used to nourish developing new plants (in fruits or seeds) and to fuel life's ongoing demands (roots). If the plant tried to store glucose as glucose, it would wash away as soon as dew or rain hit it. Most starch foods store their starch, or energy reserve, in seed kernels or pods (grain, fruit), in roots (carrots), or tubers (potatoes).

Glycogen Animals and human beings manufacture a starch called *glycogen*. It is used as an energy reserve. In an adult man, the reserve may be around one third to one half of a day's energy expenditure, 800 to 1000 calories or about 200 to 250 grams of carbohydrate. Most of the glycogen is concentrated in the liver and in a certain type of skeletal muscle (muscles that move the body).

Fiber Plants also package many glucose units into long, branched chains known as cellulose, a type of *fiber*. These chains may be hundreds or even thousands of units in length. Cellulose, hemicellulose, lignins, gums, dextrins, and some pectins comprise the group we call fiber. Plants use these carbohydrates to make up the fibrous outer covering of grains (bran) and the "skeletons" that give plants rigidity, shape, and strength. Upright stems and stalks, and even the most delicate leaves depend on a "backbone" of fiber. Humans can derive energy from starch, but not from fiber. Cows, horses, rabbits, and some other animals can get energy from cellulose. Though fiber is not classified as an essential nutrient, it alone contributes beneficial roughage to the diet.

Fiber physically separates food particles in the digestive tract and so aids digestion and absorption. It also helps in waste elimination by drawing water into the digested matter and giving feces bulk. Fiber is also thought to effect more regular absorption of glucose, which is beneficial to diabetics. It is also thought to reduce the risks of diverticulosis, appendicitis, and bacterial infections in the digestive tract. There are mounting reasons for believing that specific sources of fiber can reduce the risk of certain types of cancer such as colon cancer (wheat fiber), and of heart diseases (oat fiber). Good sources of fiber are bran, whole grains, fruits, nuts, vegetables, and legumes.

Fiber values can be expressed in two ways. Formerly a value for crude fiber was derived by subjecting food to acid and alkaline treatments. The more common way today is to express fiber values as *dietary fiber*, which is usually about three times the value of the crude fiber in a given food. Nutritionists recommend a daily intake of 15 to 18 grams of dietary fiber or six grams of crude fiber. A recent study shows most Americans usually get less. It can be difficult to know how much fiber—or other kinds of carbohydrate—are in a food. Only the **total** amount of carbohydrate is required to be given in nutrition labeling. Some cereal manufacturers and others are beginning to furnish information on the quantities of different kinds of carbohydrate, including fiber, in response to growing interest among consumers. Figure 4-4 shows an example of voluntary disclosure of carbohydrate information on a cereal package. Tables of food values are also beginning to include this information for many common foods. Figure 4-5 shows the ingredient label of a bread rich in fiber.

RECOMMENDATIONS FOR CARBOHYDRATE INTAKE

The *Dietary Guidelines for Americans* recommend that we eat foods with adequate starch and fiber and avoid too much sugar. According to the *U.S. Dietary Goals*, 58% of total calories should come from carbohydrate, up to one tenth of total calories might be from sugars and nearly half from complex carbohydrates. Thus a person who consumes 2000 calories per day should get roughly 1200 calories from carbohydrate—about 200 from sugars, and 1000 from complex carbohydrates (See Fig. 4-6).

The situation today is not good. Only 48% of our calories, on average, come from carbohydrate and over 50% of that is from sugar and under 50% from complex carbohydrates. We not only eat too few carbohydrate calories proportionally (48% instead of 58%), but we eat two and one half times as much of the wrong kind (simple) as we should, and less than half as much as we should of complex carbohydrates. Simple carbohydrates are usually higher in calories and lower in nutrients per measure, whereas complex carbohydrates usually provide more nutrients per calorie (higher nutrient density) and, so, are better for us.

A WORD ABOUT FIBER

The importance of fiber in our diets is a popular topic. U.S. Dietary Guidelines encourage Americans to increase their consumption of foods containing fiber. Cheerios, low in sugar, has always been a good source of fiber. Each 1-ounce serving contains 2g (7.5% by weight) dietary fiber, including 4g (1.4% by weight) non-nutritive crude fiber.

CARBOHYDRATE INFORMATION

	Cheerios	
	1 ounce	with ½ cup milk
STARCH AND RELATED CARBOHYDRATES, GRAMS	17	17
SUCROSE AND OTHER SUGARS, GRAMS	1	7
DIETARY FIBER, GRAMS	2	2
TOTAL CARBOHYDRATES, GRAMS	20	26
VALUES BY FORMULATION AND ANALYSIS.		

FIGURE 4-4 The label from a box of Cheerios gives detailed information on what kinds of carbohydrate are in the product. (CHEERIOS is a registered trademark of General Mills, Inc. for breakfast cereal. Reprinted with permission of General Mills, Inc.)

USING CARBOHYDRATES

Carbohydrate foods end up in the body as glucose. A physician who measures our *blood sugar* is measuring the amount of glucose in the blood. If glucose is naturally present in a food, it can be absorbed readily and used. If we eat fruit, the fructose may be converted in digestion to absorbable glucose or the fructose may be absorbed and converted in the liver to glucose or glycogen. If we eat table sugar (sucrose), the digestive system splits it into glucose and fructose, which then follow the pathways described above. Similarly, lactose in milk is split into galactose and glucose. The glucose is absorbed and used that way and either the digestive system or the liver changes galactose to glucose for body use. (Some persons lack the enzyme needed

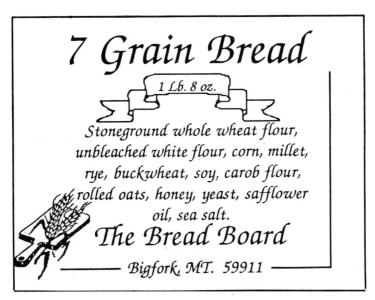

7 Grain Bread

1 Lb. 8 oz.

Stoneground whole wheat flour, unbleached white flour, corn, millet, rye, buckwheat, soy, carob flour, rolled oats, honey, yeast, safflower oil, sea salt.

The Bread Board

—— Bigfork, MT. 59911 ——

FIGURE 4-5 Products such as this whole grain bread have become popular because they yield a good supply of minerals, vitamins, fiber, carbohydrate, and protein. (Courtesy Bread Board)

to change galactose to glucose and may have a reaction if they eat dairy products. This condition is called *lactose intolerance.)* If we eat bread (starch, dextrins, and some other digestible complex carbohydrates), the digestive juices change the carbohydrate to maltose and then into glucose. It is then absorbed and used that way.

The body stores a small amount of glucose in the body tissues, most in the blood. The liver can convert limited excess glucose into glycogen, which is stored in the liver and body tissues for quick energy, or it can make the excess glucose into fat.

If carbohydrate is lacking, protein is used for energy, rendering it unavailable for other vital needs. To use protein for energy, the body must use enzymes and vitamins to first *deaminize* it, a process in which the nitrogen fraction of protein is removed. It then follows its own pathway to become energy. When a person suffers from starvation, the use of protein from the tissues of heart, lungs, and other muscles can be very harmful. Ideally the body should get enough carbohydrate so that it can be used for energy, and the valuable protein spared for uses to which it is better suited. Carbohydrate may be called "protein-sparing" because of this. If too much protein is broken down, some people have difficulty getting rid of the nitrogen fractions. These excess fractions go to the kidneys, which attempt to eliminate them in the urine; if the fractions remain in the body, they can cause a serious acid condition called uremic poisoning.

Because fat is highly concentrated carbon and hydrogen, with little oxygen, the body must have oxygen to convert it to energy. This it gets from carbohydrate, so people who wish to lose body fat safely still must have carbohydrate. Otherwise, ketone bodies can accumulate causing a serious condition called "ketosis." Diabetics

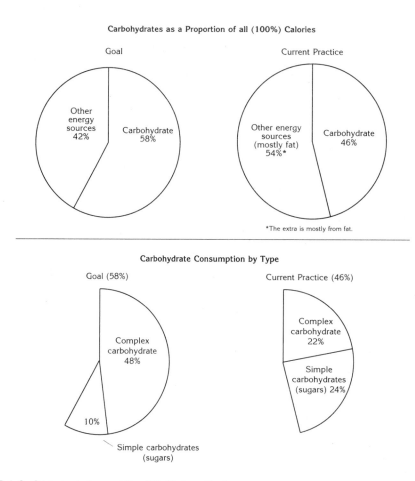

Carbohydrates as a Proportion of all (100%) Calories

Goal

Other energy sources 42%

Carbohydrate 58%

Current Practice

Other energy sources (mostly fat) 54%*

Carbohydrate 46%

*The extra is mostly from fat.

Carbohydrate Consumption by Type

Goal (58%)

Complex carbohydrate 48%

10%

Simple carbohydrates (sugars)

Current Practice (46%)

Complex carbohydrate 22%

Simple carbohydrates (sugars) 24%

FIGURE 4-6 Carbohydrates and the *U.S. Dietary Goals.*

are at risk for ketosis if they don't get enough carbohydrate: the body begins to burn its fat, and ketone bodies are the byproduct. Normally, a person should get at least 500 calories a day from carbohydrate (about 120 grams of pure carbohydrate, the equivalent of seven slices of bread). Fat is converted to energy in a complex process in which enzymes and vitamins break down molecules a few units at a time and change their form. The result of the series of changes is energy.

When glucose is transformed to energy, it goes through a number of changes in which the vitamins thiamine, pyridoxine, niacin, and pantothenic acid, the hormone insulin, and a phosphorous (mineral) substance work together, splitting off oxygen and hydrogen atoms, producing energy (the stored sunlight we mentioned previously) and residues of water and carbon dioxide. The water is used by the body or eliminated, and the carbon dioxide is carried by the blood to the lungs where it is exhaled. The complex process that breaks down glucose to produce energy is known, variously, as the *Krebs cycle*, the *citric acid cycle*, or the *tricarboxylic acid cycle*. So much thiamine is needed to develop energy that a person's need for it is sometimes calculated by counting the number of calories burned. An athlete who burns a lot of calories needs thiamine to go along with it.

CARBOHYDRATE ISSUES

Simple carbohydrates are of special interest today because of their involvement in tooth decay, in displacing needed nutrients, and in the non-nutritive and alternate sweeteners we employ.

Dental Health

Tooth decay, or caries (cair'-eez), and gum disease are the most prevalent disorders in the civilized world. A high incidence of tooth decay long has been associated with a diet high in sugar. The typical soft diet that is high in sugar and is consumed in frequent snacks favors the development of tooth decay and gum disease. While simple carbohydrates are considered to be the main culprits, all carbohydrates, even complex ones, can contribute to dental caries.

Tooth decay begins with plaque (plack), a sticky whitish material that builds up on teeth and harbors bacteria that thrive on the carbohydrates in it. These bacteria produce acids that eat into the tooth enamel, eventually breaking it down. Brushing and flossing teeth within 10 minutes after consuming carbohydrates is an excellent tactic that physically removes plaque and reduces the amount of sugar available for bacteria to consume. The type of carbohydrate and the length of time it is in contact with the teeth actually are more important than the overall amount of carbohydrate in the diet. For example, fiber is less harmful than starch, which is much less destructive than refined sugar. How long carbohydrate is in contact with the teeth—the shorter the better—involves a combination of factors. Sticky and chewy foods that tend to cling to the teeth are prime decay promoters. Foods high in sugar—dried fruit, honey-baked granola—also tend to cling to the teeth, and should be removed quickly.

In 1985 the *Journal of the American Dental Association* reported a study which showed that the frequency with which people consumed sugary soft drinks is more significant than is how much they drink. Sipping soda every now and then all day can be more damaging than consuming the same amount during a meal. Likewise infants should not be given a bottle of milk or fruit juice and allowed to suck on it for hours. The same principle applies to all sugary foods: the longer the teeth are exposed to carbohydrate, the more acid the bacteria produce, and the more time they have to attack tooth enamel.

Overconsumption of Sugar

According to a United States Department of Agriculture (USDA) study, the average intake of caloric sweeteners is over 125 pounds per year per person. Consumption of sucrose (table sugar) actually dropped from 103 to 71 pounds between 1972 and 1983, but consumption of other forms of sweeteners more than filled the gap. During the same period, the use of corn sweeteners, such as corn syrup, more than doubled. Estimates for the late 1980s predict that the new high-fructose corn syrup (HFCS) often used in carbonated beverages will be consumed at a rate of 40 pounds per person per year. And that is just *one* sugar source!

Can eating so many sweets fill us up and "crowd out" other foods? Can it add calories and weight? Yes. Consider that 125 pounds of sugar per year works out to about 600 calories per day! For a person with a moderate daily calorie need of 2000 calories, this is 30% of it as empty calories. The Dietary Goals recommend limiting intake of refined carbohydrates to 10% of total calories; again, a mere 200 calories from all refined sugar sources should be the ceiling for a 2,000 calorie diet.

Some people don't always **trade** calories from other foods for empty-calories. They often **add** them. Another tendency with sugar-rich foods simply is to eat large amounts; they are tasty, go down easily, and some claim they can be wickedly habit forming. Calories taken, from *any* source, in excess of the amount the body needs to maintain itself, are stored as fat. For every person there is a natural allowance of calories that allows him or her to maintain weight. Tempting snack foods and desserts that are high in sugar and fat and low in other nutrients are the ones that are abused and overused in spending the calorie allowance. Table 4-2 shows the amounts of sugar in some common foods.

Body weight is one link between sugar and life-threatening illnesses. Overweight is associated with a higher incidence of such problems as diabetes, heart and blood vessel diseases, and cancer, among others, and imprudent consumption of refined carbohydrates often plays a large part in becoming overweight. Another danger is that sweets are eaten preferentially instead of nutritious foods.

It is not uncommon for a child to consume 25 to 50% of his or her calories in low-nutrient density foods. A youngster who should consume 1600 calories to support growth would then consume 400 to 800 calories as soft drinks, pre-

TABLE 4-2
Examples of the Amount of Sugar
in Some Ready-to-Eat Cereals*

0—1%	1—5%	6—10%	11—34%	35—44%	45%+
Shredded Wheat	Chex cereals	Rice Krispies	A wide variety fit in this middle ground	Sugar Frosted Flakes	Sugar Smacks
Puffed Rice	Cheerios	Total		Cocoa Krispies	Apple Jacks
Puffed Wheat	Kix	Grape Nuts		Cap'n Crunch	Sugar Crisp
	Corn flakes	Wheaties		Lucky Charms	Fruit Loops
		(Plus all the "health" cereals)		Alpha Bits	Sugar Pops
				Trix	
				Sweetened granolas	

* Total sugar by percent of dry weight

sweetened cereals (Table 4-2), candy, and ice cream. This scenario is typical: a child munches on sweets late in the afternoon, then is too full to eat nutritious foods at dinner. Later in the evening, parents concerned that the child should eat something, offer ice cream. The sweets have crowded out nutritious foods. Even dietitians find it close to impossible to plan a diet youngsters like that provides all the needed nutrients in the small appetite and calorie allowance that remains after all those refined carbohydrates have been consumed.

A mature office worker may have a Danish for breakfast, taking empty calories in place of a balanced breakfast. Attention to calories is important for weight control, but how about the nutrient trade? The Danish gives a lot of calories but few other needed nutrients. Will foods eaten later in the day make up for the lack of nutrients? It isn't likely.

Finally, simple sugars, whether natural or concentrated, are associated with raising the levels of cholesterol in the blood of vulnerable persons, and elevated blood cholesterol levels are a risk factor for heart and blood diseases.

Non-nutritive and Alternative Sweeteners

If sugar is considered less than healthful, why not use artificial sweeteners? This seems reasonable, and many patrons are in favor, but there are some shortcomings.

Three non-nutritive sweeteners have been used on a large scale in foods. Saccharin has had the longest use; cyclamates came next, and then aspartame. Because saccharin is thought to cause bladder cancer in rats, the Food and Drug Administration (FDA) has banned it under the Delaney Amendment. Congress later overruled the FDA and allowed continued use of saccharin, because at the time no other inexpensive non-nutritive sweetener was on the market, and it was decided to let consumers choose whether or not to use it. Next cyclamates were banned as potential carcinogens. Interestingly, in Canada, saccharin has been banned as a potential carcinogen but cyclamates have not. It has never been proven that either substance produces cancer in human beings. Saccharin is used by millions of people. It is in many processed foods. Until the artificial sweetener aspartame (NutraSweet is a brand name) began to be used widely, saccharin was the principle sweetener in diet soft drinks.

Some sugar alcohols such as xylitol, maltitol, sorbitol, and mannitol are used as sweeteners. These are found naturally in fruits but can be synthesized from dextrose. Xylitol is as sweet as sucrose, but the others are not. They are metabolized in the body differently from the way carbohydrate sweeteners are, although their calorie contribution may be very similar to that of sugar. If some of these alcohols remain in the digestive tract too long they can produce diarrhea.

Aspartame consists of two protein amino acids, phenylalanine and aspartic acid, bound together. Under the trade name NutraSweet it is used widely to sweeten diet drinks and processed foods (Fig. 4-7, B). It is 200 times sweeter than sugar. It is sold in packets as Equal brand (Fig. 4-7). Since it is mixed with lactose, a one-gram packet contributes about four calories, and is about as sweet as two teaspoons of table sugar, which would have about 30 calories. In the body aspartame breaks down into its two amino acids, and the carbon fraction forms methyl alcohol, which in large amounts can damage the optic nerve and even cause blindness. Aspartame has been blamed for health problems such as dizziness, nervous disorders, vision problems, menstrual problems, seizures, and other functional problems in some persons, and persons with an intolerance to phenylalanine cannot use it. Aspartame breaks down easily in hot foods such as tea or coffee, especially if acids are present.

The FDA has set the safe standard of aspartame intake as 34 milligrams (mg) per day per kilogram (kg; 2.2 pounds) of body weight. This allows a 132-pound person to use 60 one-gram packs of Equal or drink 11 12-ounce drinks sweetened by it. One study concluded that most persons could use six times more without harm.

Given the fact that some alternative sweeteners are suspected of being associated with cancer and other health problems, the risk may not be worthwhile if the objective is to reduce calories. Sugar alcohols save few calories, if any. They are nutritive—they do supply energy—so for weight reduction they are no better than regular sugars. Persons may use more of these products to get a desired degree of sweetness and end up taking in slightly more calories. There is serious doubt about

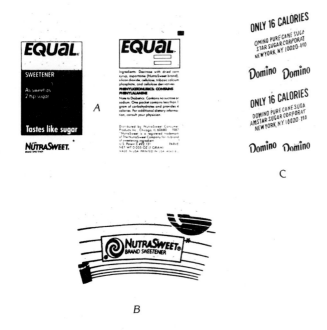

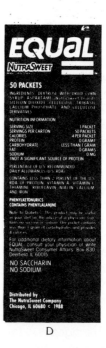

FIGURE 4-7 A, the face of a packet of Equal®, the low-calorie tabletop sweetener, which contains NutraSweet® brand sweetener. B, How NutraSweet brand sweetener is advertised on a bottle of cola. C, The face of a packet of a packet of sugar which contains about one teaspoon of pure sucrose giving from 15 to 20 calories. D, Some nutritive information given on Equal sweetener on a box containing 50 packets. (A, B, & D courtesy of The NutraSweet Company, Deerfield, IL 60015. NutraSweet and the NutraSweet symbol are registered trademarks of The NutraSweet Company for its brand of sweetening ingredient. Equal is a registered trademark of the NutraSweet Company.)

whether using non-nutritive sweeteners reduces total calories in the end. Studies show that when they are used there is usually a compensatory addition of other high-calorie foods. For example, using an alternative sweetener may prompt a person to rationalize having a piece of chocolate fudge cake that he or she would otherwise avoid.

MANAGING CARBOHYDRATE INTAKE

For persons who must reduce or otherwise manage carbohydrate intake, such as those on low-calorie diets and diabetics, the Exchange Method is readily used to monitor carbohydrate in the diet. This explanation should contribute to an understanding of carbohydrate differences among foods and of what is entailed in following such a control plan. Table 4-3 shows how to calculate the calories from information given on a package label. The label was on a bread wrapper. This method may also be used for calorie calculation for foods on the exchange lists. See also chapter 3.

Four of the seven exchange lists offer items with plentiful carbohydrate: vegetables, fruits, bread (including legumes and starchy vegetables), and skim milk. The three other lists (meat, fat, and things that may be taken in unlimited quantities) include some foods that provide various types of carbohydrates, but appropriate ones must be selected from among the listed items. Not everything in these lists is a good source of carbohydrates, but some can be almost *all* carbohydrate. For example, on the meat list, only the legumes—not the meat—provide carbohydrate. Dried legumes (dried peas, beans, and peanuts) appear on both the bread and meat lists. They are rich sources of complex carbohydrate. Most foods in the fat list, other than pure fat or oil, contribute carbohydrate. Finally, many of the low-calorie vegetables, such as lettuce, noted on the unlimited list, are excellent sources of fiber and, so, contribute highly desirable complex carbohydrates. But unlimited items like coffee, herbs, and spices do not provide carbohydrate in significant quantities. Candies, syrups, and sugar contribute only sugar and no complex carbohydrates. Table 4-4 indicates the carbohydrate yield and characteristics of typical sources.

TABLE 4-3
How to Calculate Calories in Food

Whole wheat bread*			Calories per gram		Calories from each nutrient ÷ Total Calories		Percent Calories from each nutrient
Label		×		=		=	
Per Serving:							
Serving size	1 ounce (1 slice)						
Protein	2 grams	×	4	=	8÷73	=	11%
Carbohydrate	14 grams	×	4	=	56÷73	=	77%
Fat	1 gram	×	9	=	9÷73	=	12%
					73 Total		

* This information was obtained from the bread label. The formula can also be applied using information from food exchange lists.

One problem is that the refined, concentrated carbohydrates, which are present in our daily fare in thousands of disguises, are not accounted for in the exchange lists because most prepared foods are not included. The exchanges list fresh foods (an apple) and foods that have been minimally processed, such as canned, cut green beans. They omit most processed foods, and foods that we eat as ingredients in dishes rather than whole. For instance, processors extract, concentrate, and purify the pulp of sugar beets to make table sugar, but sugar and its refined cousins are not in the exchange lists because they are now in an empty-calorie form, yet they are surely in the dishes we serve.

TABLE 4-4
Carbohydrates: Using the Dietary Exchange Lists vs. Refined Foods

Carbohydrate-Rich Exchange Lists	Exchange Example or Serving Size	Grams of Carbohydrate	Type(s)	Notes
Bread, grains, starchy vegetables and legumes	1 slice bread or 1 small potato or ½ cup cooked legumes	15	High in complex carbohydrates; some high in fibers	Grain products that are refined (white rice, flour) will contain much less fiber
Vegetable (low-calorie)	½ cup	5	High in complex carbohydrates; good source of fiber	High in bulk or fiber for calories
Fruit	½ banana	15	Some starch, fiber; simple natural sugar also	Processed products with added sugar and/or eaten without edible peels are less fiber-rich.
Milk, skim	1 cup	12	Simple, natural sugar (lactose)	Not considered concentrated unless processed into flavored beverages, yogurt, ice cream, etc.
Unlimited	"Lettuce...in reasonable quantities"	2 to 4	Mostly undigestible fiber	Usually low in calories giving them good nutrient density
Refined, Concentrated foods				
Sugar	1 tbsp.	11	Concentrated simple sugar	Contributes no other nutrients
Pie, pecan	1/7 of 9 inch pie	61	Mostly concentrated simple sugar	Of nearly 500 calories, 50% are from concentrated sugar; empty, refined calories

ALCOHOL

Though alcohol provides energy—and little else—it is not an essential nutrient. Alcohol provides seven calories per gram or five and one-half calories per milliliter (ml). This totals over 60 calories for every ounce of 80-proof spirit or 4-ounce glass of table wine, and over 70 calories for a 12-ounce can of 4% beer. Because alcohol provides energy it has been classified with carbohydrates, but it breaks down in the body more as a fat. Here we shall consider it as carbohydrate-like, in the traditional manner.

The amount of alcohol in a beverage is stated as *proof* or as percent. The proof is simply twice the percentage of alcohol a beverage contains. Thus, an 80-proof whiskey is 40% alcohol. The alcohol content of beers and wines is usually given in percent; that of spirits is stated in proof. If the percent is by weight, there is more alcohol per unit than the same value in volume. Normally, one can say a two-ounce portion of an 80-proof spirit contains about 125 calories. The amount of calories in an alcoholic beverage can be considerable. Eight ounces of regular beer has approximately 114 calories; 12 ounces of light beer has from 72 to 135 calories. A Manhattan cocktail (three and one half ounces) gives 164 calories, an old fashioned (4 ounces), 190. A three and one half ounce portion of dry dinner wine has 85 calories.*

The problem is that alcohol is empty calories. Some alcoholics consume it almost exclusively and, as a consequence, are undernourished. A four-ounce glass of red wine gives 0.4 mg of iron. Beer has some niacin and thiamine, but not much. Some mixed drinks with fruit juice contribute a bit of vitamin C and other nutrients.

Alcohol is one of the major causes of malnutrition in this country. Over 20,000 people enter hospitals every year because of alcohol (over 7.5 million hospital days). Diseases associated with excessive alcohol consumption are a major health problem. The life expectancy of an alcoholic is reduced by eight years. Working alcoholics have twice the health problems, absenteeism, accidents, and interpersonal problems with other employees as those who are not alcoholics, and they are less productive. In the U.S. today there is a trend toward drinking more moderately, and many people have switched from spirits to beverages that have a lower alcohol content. This may help reduce the heavy price we pay for being a drinking nation—in health and in dollars.

Alcohol is a narcotic. If the liver cannot immediately metabolize all the alcohol a person consumes, it goes into the bloodstream and then, to the brain. Alcohol reaches the outer areas of the brain first, causing impairments of judgment and reasoning; next it penetrates deeper, affecting vision and speech. If more alcohol is consumed, the muscles are affected: the person may not be able to walk a straight line. Finally, when alcohol penetrates deep into the brain, the drinker passes out. If this does not happen and still more alcohol is consumed, death could occur if the alcohol affected the part of the brain that controls heartbeat and breathing. Liver enzymes break alcohol down first into an aldehyde, the "cause" of hangovers. The aldehyde is broken down to an acetate, and then to a carbohydrate-like product. If the demand on the liver to metabolize alcohol is too great, fatty deposits develop,

*The calories given here for beer and wine are not at variance with those given above. The above figures are for *just* alcohol calories.

then fibrosis, and finally cirrhosis (hardening), occurs, which can be fatal. An excess of alcohol interferes with the liver's ability to metabolize properly many nutrients. Because the liver is overburdened and a diseased liver functions imperfectly, there can be an overall reduction of vitamin absorption in the body. The liver may become so busy metabolizing alcohol or so functionally impaired that it cannot properly metabolize vitamin D and, for instance, make bile for digestion. Glucose metabolism is also retarded, so ketones and lactic acid may build up in the body, producing gout, and other disorders. The body's use of vitamin A is also impaired, which can cause night blindness and, in males, sterility. Alcohol can interfere with vitamin A and D utilization in bone maintenance. It causes zinc deficiency, one effect of which is loss of sex drive (since zinc is needed to make male sex hormones). Anemia and blood clotting problems (due to vitamin K deficiency) also are possible. Because alcohol is a diuretic, an excess of minerals may be lost in the urine. Nerve and brain cells are damaged by alcohol: some chronic alcoholics become "rum-dumb" (mentally impaired from drinking too much alcohol). Alcohol is also fairly high in calories, and prolonged use can cause obesity.

The incidence of alcohol use by foodservice personnel has been found to be high; it causes problems in the quality of the work, absenteeism, productivity, and their general health. Supervisors and managers of such personnel need to understand that alcoholism is a disease that requires treatment. Many alcoholics know they have a problem and want help. With appropriate assistance and encouragement they can recover and resume a normal life. It takes tolerance, patience (often professional help), and an understanding of people and of alcoholism.

Alcohol has many drawbacks and very few benefits, though it can be an enjoyable social accompaniment. A small amount can whet the appetite and a drink can be relaxing. There is even some evidence that drinking a moderate amount every day may reduce the risk of heart attacks. Consumed in moderation it causes few problems because the body can handle moderate amounts. Taken in excess it is extremely harmful.

SUMMARY

Carbohydrates are the major source of body energy. There are simple sugars and complex (starch and fiber) carbohydrates. All carbohydrates are made up of what is called a hexose, a saccharide unit of six carbons in a chain to which hydrogen and oxygen are attached. It is the basic unit of monosaccharides, such as glucose, galactose and fructose, and of disaccharides, such as sucrose, maltose, and lactose. Starches and fiber—complex carbohydrates—are polysaccharides. Some complex carbohydrates may have more than 2000 single saccharide units in one molecule.

Fifty-eight percent of the total calories in a normal diet should come from carbohydrate; 10% from simple carbohydrates and 48% from complex carbohydrates (about 20% and 80%, respectively, of total carbohydrate intake). Gram for gram, carbohydrates are no more fattening (caloric) than protein, and they are less fattening than fat or alcohol. Carbohydrate has four calories per gram, protein four, fat nine, and alcohol seven.

All carbohydrate in food must be broken down to simple sugars to be absorbed in the digestive tract, and all carbohydrate must be converted to glucose to be used by the body for energy. The conversion of glucose to energy is a complex reaction that requires oxygen for its completion and produces water and carbon dioxide in addition to energy. Fat and protein are also reduced to energy. If the body lacks glucose and tries to burn only fat, substances called ketones are formed. The condition in which there is an excess of ketones—ketosis—can cause coma and death. The body makes a starch called glycogen out of glucose units. A limited supply of glycogen is stored in the liver and skeletal muscles.

Cellulose, pectins, and some other complex carbohydrates (fiber) that cannot be digested by humans are nevertheless important, because they furnish bulk in the digestive tract which aids digestion, absorption, and elimination. Fiber is also thought to produce more regular absorption of glucose, which is beneficial to diabetics. It is also thought to reduce the risk of diverticulosis, appendicitis, and bacterial infection in the digestive tract. Fiber from specific sources even appears to reduce the risks of certain types of cancer and heart disease. High-fiber foods have the additional benefit of filling the stomach without supplying concentrated calories, and most are nutritious. Good sources of fiber are bran, whole grains, fruits, nuts, vegetables, and legumes.

Foods that contain sugar—candy, desserts, sweetened fruits, jams and jellies, and syrups—are sources of simple carbohydrate. Starchy foods—whole grains, flour products, legumes, and corn—are sources of complex carbohydrates, which are considered more healthful than simple ones. Both types can initiate tooth decay, so moderation of intake and regular brushing and flossing of teeth are advised. Sugar is not a bad nutrient since it provides energy, but it is not uncommon to eat so much sugar that we lack the appetite for other foods we need. Foods that contain only sugar and no other nutrients are called empty-calorie, or junk, foods. Eating too much of this kind of food and *then* trying to eat enough to supply needed nutrients can lead to overweight. If one does not eat enough other food to supply needed nutrients, one becomes undernourished.

One of the principal sources of sweets in Americans' diets is carbonated beverages. Candy is another. Artificial sweeteners may not be entirely good things. Cyclamate is banned in the U.S.—but not in Canada—because it is suspected to cause cancer. Saccharin also was banned, but Congress lifted the ban. Aspartame is 200 times sweeter than sugar, but it too *may* be harmful. It breaks down in the body into phenylalanine, aspartic acid, and methyl alcohol, the latter being highly toxic. When lightly heated, aspartame breaks down into possibly harmful substances. People who use alternative sweeteners seem to treat themselves to other foods that make up for the calories "saved." The sugar alcohols are not low calorie: they contain about as many calories per measure as table sugar.

Alcohol gives seven calories per gram. Consuming too much alcohol to the exclusion of other nutrients can cause malnutrition and many other health problems. Alcohol is metabolized in the liver; overloading it with alcohol can harm the liver and impair its functioning. The health and social costs of alcohol consumption in the U.S. are enormous.

The Exchange Method is usually recommended for controlling carbohydrates in the diet. Exchange lists also guide the user to foods rich in complex carbohydrates.

Chapter Review

1. What is the basic unit of carbohydrates? What elements comprise this unit?
2. What are simple sugars and what are complex carbohydrates?
3. What is fiber and what good is it in the diet if we cannot digest it?
4. What proportion of total calories in a normal diet should be carbohydrate?
5. What proportion of total calories should come from simple carbohydrates and what proportion from complex carbohydrates? What proportion do we get of each type today?
6. Name the three simple sugars most common in our foods. What sugar is table sugar? What is maltose and how is it made? What is lactose and where is it found?
7. About how much dietary fiber does a normal person need per day? Does the average American get more or less than this? About what is the ratio of difference between the measure of crude fiber and that of dietary fiber?
8. How many calories does a gram of pure carbohydrate have? Of protein? Of fat? Of alcohol?
9. How is alcohol burned in the body?
10. How might you indicate on the menu that carbohydrates are essential and healthful foods without doing a publishing bit on it?
11. How might a restaurant manager help patrons select high complex carbohydrate foods from a normal menu that offers a variety of foods?
12. Name two reasons why foodservice personnel trying to meet nutritional needs of patrons should know something about the Exchange Method.
13. Does alcohol have any beneficial effects? What are some negatives of over-consumption?
14. Why are carbohydrates considered culprits in causing dental caries and gum disease?
15. Why is an excess of simple sugars undesirable in a normal diet?
16. What happens when a person eats too much of the simple carbohydrates and not enough of the complex ones?
17. Why might foodservice guests like alternative sweeteners to be available? What are two arguments against their use, in general?
18. Which four Exchange Method lists are most representative of foods that can contribute carbohydrate to the diet? Name four foods from each list.

Chapter 5
Proteins

Chapter Goals

- To realize the importance of protein in maintaining life and supporting essential body functions.
- To understand the makeup of protein and amino acids.
- To be able to select the proper amount and kind of dietary protein at a desirable cost.
- To know what the terms "limiting," "complete," "incomplete," "essential," "nonessential," and "nutrient density" mean when applied to proteins.

What Is Protein?

Carbohydrate keeps the body fueled and functioning; protein builds. Next to water, protein is the most plentiful body constituent, making up about half the body's nonwater weight. About 40% of this protein is in body fluids and tissues other than muscle, 30% in muscle, 20% in bones and cartilage, and 10% in skin.

Protein is a basic substance in living cells. From proteins come amino acids, the building blocks of cells and tissues. All life must have protein to carry out essential life functions; nothing living does not contain it. Early investigators understood protein's importance; "protos" is Greek for "primary", or "first."

Protein is an essential nutrient, and, as we will see, it is incredibly versatile. To appreciate protein's unique abilities and the body's need for protein, it is necessary to understand the architecture of protein molecules. Carbon, oxygen, and hydrogen are the basic components of protein, just as they are of carbohydrates, fats, and alcohol, the other energy nutrients, but the characteristic element of protein is nitrogen. The word "amine," meaning ammonia, is the term used to refer to organic molecules formed by nitrogen atoms. *Amino acids are building blocks.*

We know of 20 some common amino acids, which, as the letters of the alphabet are combined in infinite variations to make words, are combined in countless combinations to make different proteins. Protein chains typically are long and complex, containing anywhere from several dozen amino acids to hundreds. The way amino acids are put together determines the protein character. Thus, proteins that make up flesh are quite different from those in blood or fingernails.

Certain of the 20 some common amino acids are called essential amino acids (Table 5-1) because the body cannot make them or make them fast enough to meet protein needs. To support life, these essential amino acids must be in the foods consumed. There are 10 amino acids considered essential, but one called arginine may not be essential for human beings and one called histidine may not be essential for adults. (Source Dunn, *Nutrition: An Applied Science*). The other amino acids can be built by a healthy well-nourished body if all the necessary components are available, so they are called nonessential.

TABLE 5-1
Essential Amino Acids

arginine	methionine
histidine*	phenylalanine
isoleucine	threonine
leucine	tryptophan
lysine	valine

* Adult requirement not clearly established.

Protein Value

All proteins are not created equal. Some are of more benefit to the body than others. They do a better job of promoting tissue growth, maintenance, and repair. Those that are most efficient contain all the essential amino acids in good supply. They are called *complete* proteins. Proteins that lack some essential amino acids are called *incomplete* (Fig. 5-1).

Fruits and vegetables have incomplete proteins, and very small amounts, so they are poor sources of protein (Fig. 5-2). Legumes—peas, beans, garbanzos, and soybeans—have a high protein content, but the protein is incomplete, though much less so than that in fruits and vegetables (Fig. 5-3). Seeds and nuts contain incomplete protein, like legumes. Grains and cereals contain considerable protein that is also incomplete, but in a different way from that in legumes, seeds, and nuts. Animal protein, such as that in eggs, milk, meat, fish, seafood, and poultry, is complete and present in high concentrations. It is worth noting that the protein value of soybeans almost equals that of beef, so soy protein can be considered nearly complete, if not complete.

Legumes, seeds and nuts lack the essential amino acids of tryptophan and methionine, but have other essential amino acids in good supply. Because this lack makes it impossible for their protein to adequately support reproduction, growth, maintenance and the repair of tissues, their amino acids are called *limiting*. It is not complete. Grains have all essential amino acids in good supply except lysine and isoleucine. They too have limiting amino acids because of this. However, if we combine grains (cereals) with legumes we get a complete protein. The addition of only a small quantity of complete protein such as that in eggs, milk products or flesh foods makes either of these limiting amino acid foods (legumes or cereals) also complete. The need for complete protein has thus been met by many

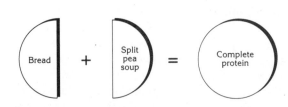

FIGURE 5-1 Particular food forms of incomplete protein can form a complete protein.

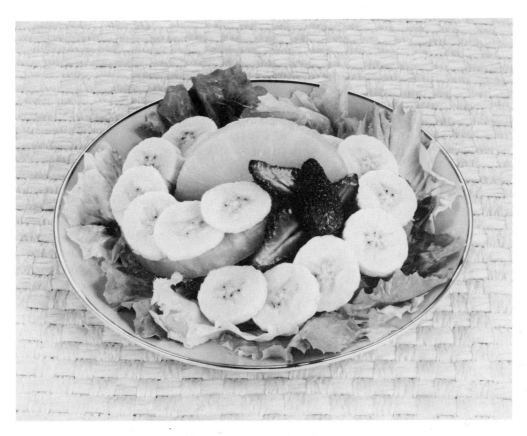

FIGURE 5-2 A fruit salad provides little protein and what protein the fruit has is not complete.

population groups over our history by either of these combination methods. Figure 5-1 shows how incomplete proteins can be combined with legumes and grains to make a complete one. For centuries the Chinese have prospered on a diet of soy and other legumes plus rice or wheat. Basics of the diet of millions of East Indians who eat no meat are dahl, a legume, and grains. Many people in Mexico and South America subsist on black or brown beans and corn products. The Irish and Poles eat huge quantities of potatoes and add enough animal protein to make complete protein. Americans eat many dishes that contain legumes, seeds, or nuts. In Boston, baked beans and brown bread are popular. In the South a dish of rice and beans and a bit of spice called Hoppin' John is popular. Even a peanut butter sandwich furnishes complete protein. (See also, chapter 15.)

Because so many people live largely on grains, scientists have been trying to develop grain that provides more complete protein. Corn and wheat have already been improved considerably in that respect. People who traditionally consume principally grains are being encouraged to grow legumes, seed foods, and nuts to complement the limiting amino acids in the grain. A very inexpensive cereal product made largely from cottonseed flour called *incaparina* has become popular in Central and South America. It is fortified with animal protein, which makes it quite complete. Protein food sources are being improved worldwide.

Calculating Protein Value

How is the growth, maintenance, and tissue repair value of a protein determined? We have three ways of calculating this: biological value (BV), net protein utilization (NPU), and protein efficiency ratio (PER) (Table 5-2).

TABLE 5-2
Three Ways of Calculating Protein Values

Method	Definition
Biological value (BV)	The amount of protein digested and absorbed of what we eat
Net protein utilization (NPU)	The amount of protein the body uses of what we eat
Protein efficiency ratio (PER)	The product's protein value compared with that of milk casein protein*

*Under nutritional labeling we noted the FDA set a recommended intake of 45 grams of protein a day for an adult, if the food was equal or better in its protein content compared to milk casein, and 65 grams per day if it was not.

These highly technical methods of calculating protein value are rarely used in ordinary dietary calculations. A value called *nutrient density*, which was discussed in a previous chapter, is simpler and adequate for the needs of foodservices.

To obtain the *nutrient density ratio* of a food's protein, we divide the number of grams of protein in a serving of the food by the number of calories. Thus, if a portion of pizza gives 145 calories and six grams of protein, the nutrient density is 0.0414 (6/145). It must be remembered that nutrient density in this case refers to the amount of protein, but tells nothing about its quality. Table 5-3 lists the nutrient density of

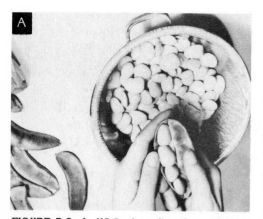
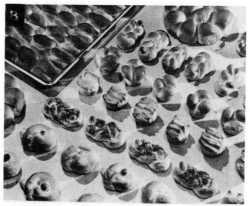

FIGURE 5-3 A. While these lima beans furnish a good supply of protein, the protein is lacking in methionine and tryptophan, two essential amino acids. B. If the limas are combined with a cereal product such as bread that contains a fair amount of methionine and tryptophan, then one gets all the essential amino acids in good supply. Cereals provide what the legumes lack, and the legumes provide what the cereals lack. (USDA photos).

TABLE 5-3
The Protein Nutrient Density of Selected Foods

Food	Protein (grams)	Calories	Nutrient Density
Gelatin, dry*	85.0	335	0.2537
Cod, raw	17.6	78	0.2256
Chicken, raw	23.4	117	0.2000
Shrimp, raw	18.1	91	0.1989
Spinach, cooked*	3.2	26	0.1231
Cooked lean beef rib	28.2	240	0.1175
Soybean curd	7.8	72	0.1083
Milk, skim	3.6	36	0.1000
Egg, whole, raw	12.9	163	0.0791
Cabbage, raw*	1.3	24	0.0542
Spaghetti, cooked*	5.0	148	0.0338
Bread, white*	8.7	269	0.0323

* Protein is not complete.

protein in some foods. Unless you know that gelatin and spinach protein, with respective values of 0.2537 and 0.1231 are incomplete, you might think they were superior to the protein in whole eggs, cooked lean rib beef, and skim milk, the respective densities of which are 0.0791, 0.1175, and 0.1000. Gelatin and spinach have more protein per calorie, but their protein alone will not support life. It is not complete.

Science and technology are doing many fascinating things to increase and improve protein in foods. Soybean protein can be processed to resemble nuts, bacon, ice-cream, chicken, ham, beef, veal, and pork. Soybean curd (tofu) is successfully marketed as an up-scale frozen dessert or meal. It is prepared in a number of delicious ways by companies such as Legume, Inc. Surimi, made from pollock, a plentiful, inexpensive fish, can be made into forms that imitate fish steaks, shrimp, lobster, crab legs, and other products. There are cholesterol-free egg imitators. Yeast is a protein food that can be cultivated very easily from waste carbohydrate products like sawdust and other cellulose. We are studying ways to make this very inexpensive protein into palatable foods. (Yeast strains are even being used to produce insulin, among other valuable nutrition substances.) Enzyme manipulation and protein cloning give promise of such new products as peach yogurt that is cultured, flavor and all, from a special strain of bacteria developed through enzyme engineering (no peaches or flavoring needed); and imitation blue cheese salad dressing with the flavor and mouthfeel of the real thing without the fat and calories. Similar genetic engineering techniques are prominent in the news. By switching genes among different kinds of wheat, the very nature of the grains is being changed, and new types of flour are being milled. The opportunities for new and excellent protein from low-cost sources are endless. In the future we may utilize the protein in alfalfa, grass, tree leaves, kelp, and algae. Insects could be a potential source, or, we may be able to synthesize protein directly from nitrogen, oxygen, carbon and hydrogen. If legume plants do it, why can't we?

How Much Protein?

If nutrient density does not tell us the value of the protein and BV, NPU, and PER are too complex to use, how do we know what to eat in order to get balanced protein? It's easy. For animal protein, about two to four ounces of cooked, lean meat or its equivalent daily is sufficient if we eat a variety of other foods. The *Dietary Goals for the United States* say we should get 12% of calories from protein, and the U.S. Department of Agriculture (USDA) says *animal* protein should constitute one fourth of this 12%. Persons who do not eat animal protein must take care to eat complementary proteins that provide complete protein.

If a young man of 19 who needs 3600 calories a day followed the recommendation of getting 12% of his calories from protein, a fourth of which is animal protein, he should get 432 calories from protein (3600 x 12%) and this would mean the total protein intake should be about 108 g (432/4 calories per gram of protein = 108), one fourth of which is 27 g of animal protein (108 x 1/4). Just an eight-ounce broiled choice grade (57% lean, 43% fat) porterhouse steak would give nearly 40 grams of animal protein, and the rest (108 g - 40 g - 68 g) could come from plant sources. Actually the RDA says this young man needs only 56 grams of protein a day; thus, only 14 grams need be animal protein (56 x 1/4).

In practice, we get much of our protein from plants. Excluding cheese, we get a larger share of our protein from grains and vegetables than from milk products. The USDA also reports that the intake of protein from plant foods is twice that provided by all the chicken eaten in the U.S. This proportion is likely to increase as more foodservices respond to patrons' interest in healthful eating and offer appealing alternatives to meat dishes.

One of the best ways to ensure that protein intake is adequate is to follow the Four Food Groups Plan or the Exchange Method and to select a variety of foods from each list. In the Basic Four Plan, the two servings of meat plus the protein in the milk and bread and cereal groups gives a more than adequate supply of quality protein. In the Exchange Method, one exchange from the meat list provides approximately seven grams of protein; a milk exchange, eight grams; and a vegetable or bread exchange, two grams. Selecting a balanced diet from the list ensures getting an adequate amount of good-quality protein.

Protein needs vary with sex, diet, health, size, and stage of life. During the first year, infants need nearly a gram of protein a day for each pound of weight. By age 10 the child needs a bit over one half gram per pound. The requirement drops slowly and levels off at around 23 years of age. Physically, senior citizens need less protein, but they also digest, absorb, and use it less efficiently. Because they often consume fewer total calories than others, the protein density of their food is especially important. Elderly persons often tend to choose starchy items that are easy to buy, prepare, and eat but which may also lack adequate protein.

During pregnancy and lactation, a women's protein needs rise. This is seen in the Recommended Dietary Allowances (RDA). Trauma, such as major surgery, a bad burn, fever, or an infection, also increases the body's need for protein. Protein loss, coupled with increased demand in these and other situations, may result from inefficient use of protein, from inability to consume enough protein, from muscle wasting due to forced inactivity, from blood loss, and from extraordinary demands to repair and build tissue. Incidentally, hard work or strenuous exercise does not increase protein need. The body needs only the usual amount.

The Cost of Protein

Protein foods can be some of the most expensive ones, or they can be relatively low in cost. It all depends upon the source. To calculate what protein costs in food, the cost per unit weight and the percentage of protein in the product must be known. If ground beef costs $1.89 a pound and is 17.9% protein, divide the cost per pound by the percentage of protein to determine the cost per pound of protein: $1.89/0.179 = $10.56. To derive the cost per ounce of protein, divide the protein price per pound ($10.56) by 16 (the number of ounces in a pound): $10.56/16 = $.66.

Table 5-4 shows the cost of the protein in six different foods calculated by this method. Note that a dozen eggs weighs 24 ounces, a quart of milk weighs two pounds, and the canned corn has a net weight of 17 ounces.

Functions of Protein

Protein performs many functions in the body. Every body cell contains proteins, and they work not only to build muscle, blood, and other tissues, but to perform other functions. Protein is a sort of jack-of-all-trades, but all of the jobs it does are vital to life. Some of the most important ways the body uses protein are to produce enzymes, hormones, antibodies, and conjugated proteins, and to provide a proper balance of fluids and electrolytes, proper acid-base balance, tissue growth, repair, and maintenance, and energy.

Misconceptions About Protein

Many people think that a high-protein diet has particular benefits. Protein is not all good, nor does it do some of the things some people think it will for them. Like so many things, in excess, protein can cause problems.

Meat, for example, provides complete protein but is not a complete food. Eating too much to the exclusion of a variety of foods may produce vitamin or mineral deficiencies and will not provide enough carbohydrates and fiber. Overloading the kidneys with protein can damage them permanently, and a liver that must process too much protein may be unavailable to perform other functions necessary for optimal health. Damaged kidneys cannot maintain a proper acid-base balance.

Some people erroneously believe that eating a lot of meat avoids calories; that carbohydrate is the fattening food. Others say that a high-protein diet is so monotonous that a person who eats to satiety will consume fewer calories than if he or she were to eat a balanced diet; this is not true.

TABLE 5-4
The Cost of Protein in Some Foods*

Food	Cost per Unit Weight	% Protein	Cost per Ounce
Flour, wheat	.27/pound	10.5	·.16
Eggs, large	$.72/doz (24 ounces)	12.9	$.23
Cornmeal	.60/pound	7.9	.47
Milk, whole	.65/qt (2 pounds)	3.5	.57
Beef, ground	1.89/pound	17.9	.66
Corn, cream style	.45/can (17 ounce)	2.1	1.26

* Note that these protein costs are only as found in the food; not the true cost as the body uses it. This changes the cost because not all the protein in the product is used. Some proteins are absorbed and used better than others.

High-protein liquid diet foods that contain not more than 600 calories a day are available, but for most normal people, they do not contain enough carbohydrate and other essential nutrients. Consuming them exclusively has caused fatal organ dysfunction. Some of these diet foods contain harmful substances or large quantities of unneeded nutrients.

Athletes are often sold on high-protein preparations by false claims that they enhance muscle strength and stamina. A high-protein diet can result in a loss of strength and stamina. Appropriate exercise with a *high carbohydrate* diet build strength and stamina. The exercise should burn excess calories and train the muscles to store more glycogen and glucose. It is exercise and increased glycogen storage, not a high-protein meal, that give athletes extra power and endurance. While muscle is made from protein, no amount of protein-forcing builds muscle unless a need is created by using the muscles in work, play, or exercise.

A common misconception about protein foods is that they are pure protein. Far from it. Figure 5-4 illustrates the protein-to-fat relationship for a 6-oz portion of ground sirloin. Of its 660 calories, 500 (76%) are from fat and 160 (24%) are from protein. Along with its high-quality protein comes a hefty complement of fat. This can interfere with fat intake moderation and weight control if a dieter chooses meats and full-fat dairy products as protein sources.

Proteins can cause intolerance reactions. Sensitivity to the protein of milk, eggs, shellfish or wheat is not unusual. Some people even react to very small quantities of protein in a fruit or vegetable. The responses vary from hives to nasal congestion to swelling in the throat that can obstruct breathing. Such reactions can occur if the body lacks the ability to separate all the amino

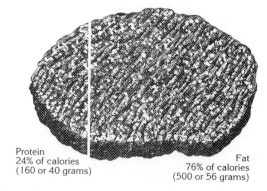

Protein
24% of calories
(160 or 40 grams)

Fat
76% of calories
(500 or 56 grams)

Figure 5-4 Ground Sirloin Steak, lean and fat, 6 ounces— Total calories: 660

acid links from certain proteins and those fragments cross through the intestinal wall and get into the blood, where antibodies attack them as if they were bacteria. One physical sign is evidence of the battle going on—inflammation.

Protein Metabolism

Once in the body, amino acids may be taken up by any cell, or they may travel to the liver, where they become a part of the protein pool. It takes about four hours for ingested protein to be available for use in the body. The body selects the proteins it needs to do the necessary jobs—building muscle, bones, or teeth, making enzymes or hormones. A common myth is that the body uses extra protein for strength. This is not true. Since the body is unable to store extra protein as such, it deaminizes (breaks off the nitrogen fraction) any extra and uses it to supply energy, or converts it to glycogen or fat, which is stored.

The body is constantly replacing protein in body structures with new protein. After the nitrogen fraction is taken off (the amino acid is *deaminized*) the nitrogen part becomes *ammonia*, which is toxic to the body and is converted into *urea* in the liver. This urea is then sent to the kidneys, where urine is manufactured. Sometimes the ammonia fraction is attached to another carbon chain to make one of the nonessential amino acids. After deamination the carbon chain is broken down to produce energy; the carbon and oxygen are exhaled as carbon dioxide and the hydrogen and other oxygen form water, which the body uses or excretes.

Certain substances in the body encourage protein synthesis (anabolism) while others encourage its breakdown (catabolism). A person is said to be in *positive nitrogen balance* when absorbed amino acids are retained and used in the body. When more catabolism is going on than anabolism, a person is said to be in *negative nitrogen balance*. People recovering from surgery, burns, or other illnesses often go into negative nitrogen balance and require extra complete protein. Rapid growth, pregnancy, and other extra-ordinary conditions also increase demands for protein. Again, the diet must have extra, complete protein so that the period of negative nitrogen balance is eliminated or reduced to a minimum.

SUMMARY

Proteins are basic building blocks for body tissues and for substances such as vitamins, antibodies, enzymes and hormones. Protein is responsible for growth, repair, and maintenance of tissue. It is also important in regulating acid-base balance and fluid balance. It can bond with other substances to form molecules such as lipoproteins. The body can use it for energy, convert it to glucose or glycogen, or make it into fat and store the fat for future energy needs. The latter is an inefficient way of using protein, however.

The ordinary adult needs from 45 (women) to 56 (men) grams of protein per day. Infants need the most protein per pound of body weight, and from then on to adulthood the need drops, reaching a plateau about age 23. Pregnant and lactating women need more protein than usual. The amount of protein needed by the body depends upon the protein's quality and how well the particular protein is digested, absorbed, and utilized. Protein needs vary according to age, sex, health status, and overall diet. Heavy work or exercise does not increase protein demand. Usually it is adequate to take about 12% of the day's calories as protein and to see that about one fourth of this comes from animal sources.

The basic units of protein molecules are amino acids which are made up of hydrogen, oxygen, carbon, and nitrogen. There are over 20 known amino acids, all of which the body needs. Some it can make, but those it cannot must come from food (*essential* amino acids). There are eight or nine essential amino acids needed by noninfants and nine or 10 needed by infants. We call protein that contains all essential amino acids in good supply *complete* and protein that does not contain all of them, *incomplete*. If a protein lacks one or more essential amino acids, the missing amino acids are called *limiting* ones, because they limit the ability of the protein to meet the body's needs. We can combine foods with complementary limiting amino acids to provide complete protein if they are eaten at a single meal. They must be consumed within the same time period to become complete in the body. The various proteins combined to make a complete protein must together supply all essential amino acids in adequate amounts to promote growth, repair, and maintenance of the body.

When cost is a factor in choosing, it is good to understand the quantity of protein in various foods and its quality or value in meeting body needs, so as to obtain maximal protein for the amount spent. We are doing much through science and technology to improve the world's protein supply.

Chapter Review

1. Why do you think the Greek word "*protos*," meaning primary, was used to name protein?
2. What percentage of the human body's nonwater weight is protein?
3. How do a carbohydrate and a protein molecule differ in basic elements?
4. What is deaminization? When a protein is deaminized, can it be used to create energy?
5. What is an amino acid? What are essential and nonessential amino acids?
6. What is a complete protein? An incomplete protein?
7. How can two limiting amino acid foods be combined to provide a complete protein food? Give an example.
8. List the jobs of protein in the body?
9. What do the *Dietary Goals* suggest as the amount of protein we should eat in relation to our total calories?
10. How much of the protein we consume should come from animal sources?
11. What factors determine your protein RDA category (e.g., gender)?
12. How many grams of protein per day should you have? (Find this in the RDA tables.)

13. What conditions increase the need for protein?
14. If you were in charge of a large institution feeding many elderly people and wanted to get into the diet as much protein that can be *utilized* in the body at a low cost, what would you have to know about each food?
15. Can eating a lot of meat produce strength and stamina? If not, what kind of program does this?
16. Can eating a lot of meat be harmful? Why might it not assist in weight loss? What's wrong with a 600-calories per day liquid-protein diet?
17. How can proteins cause intolerance reactions?
18. What do you think lies in the future of synthetic proteins?

Chapter 6
Fats and Oils: The Lipid Family

Chapter Goals

- To indicate why fat is a focus of attention today in nutrition.
- To know the makeup of lipids, especially fats and oils, and how different lipids do different things in the body.
- To understand how lipids break down in the body and how the body uses them.
- To understand the meaning of "saturated," "unsaturated," "monounsaturated," "polyunsaturated," "hydrogenation," "cholesterol," "glycerol," "fatty acid," "lipoprotein," and "phospholipid" as they apply to lipids.
- To know how much lipid we should consume and what kinds.
- To be able to select foods so as to control the amount and kinds of lipid in the diet.
- To understand current thought on the relationship of lipids to cardiovascular diseases and on lipids in nutrition.

FAT: GOOD OR BAD?

Fat has a reputation as quite a villain in dietary circles. It is little wonder since eating too much fat is associated with such conditions as high blood pressure, stroke, heart attack, kidney failure, diabetes, certain types of cancer, and obesity, which carries yet other health problems. Americans spend more money and time on weight reduction than on any other nutritional problem. Next to calories, fat is perhaps the most frequently used word in discussions of food and eating.

Still, we could not live without fat. It performs many necessary body functions. It also helps to make our food more flavorful, tender, and enjoyable. Fat gives food a satisfying quality. It is energy in reserve that can be converted to fuel when we don't eat enough or when we need extra energy. Properly managed, fat is a beneficial part of a balanced diet; improperly managed it creates problems. Some people have to watch their fat intake more closely than others. Other people struggle to control their weight, because they do not understand how to manage food fat. To them, fat is the villain.

Dietary patterns in the United States include foods containing more fat than in other countries, largely in processed foods—chocolate cheesecake, potato chips. The foodservice industry discovered that people like food fairly high in fat and has offered

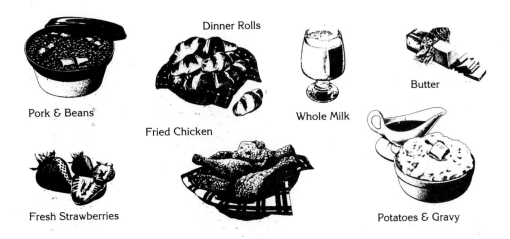

FIGURE 6-1 Can you find the food fats in this picture? (Hint: One item is virtually fat free.)

menu items that are rather high in fat to satisfy the demand. We in foodservices butter, fry, cover with rich sauces, and in other ways add fat to foods to please the customer. It has been stated that America's favorite flavor is "crisp." Millions crave the crunch of products fried in fat, from fried chicken to zucchini tempura. French fried potatoes are the number one selling side dish. Deepfried shrimp is the number one shellfish dish. Test your awareness of fat on the menu by finding the hidden and obvious food fats in Figure 6-1. One restaurant chain recently began trying to meet conflicting demands of patrons who wanted fried food that was lower in fat and calories. The firm now offers poultry from which they remove the skin and fat layer below it, then batter and deepfry it. The batter soaks up more fat than if the chicken had been broiled with the skin and fat on. Often fat in food is hidden and people don't know it is there.

Fat often is the crowning adornment. What's a baked potato without butter or sour cream? A mound of fatty tartar sauce served with fish usually supplies more calories than the fish. Who wants a tossed salad without some nice creamy dressing? When vegetables are served, they frequently swim in butter or huddle under a hollandaise or cheese sauce. Bread without butter? No cream in coffee? How about a fudge sundae?

From a foodservice viewpoint, fats take on a special value, because fat adds so much to a food's richness. It's the aroma carried by the fats we smell when hamburgers are on the barbecue, bacon on the grill, or butter sizzling in the pan. Fats provide, carry, and help keep flavors distributed; consider the rich flavor of peanut oil, or the way a salad dressing clings to a salad. Fats have everything to do with the texture of baked goods; their flakiness (pie crust), tenderness (cake), and crumb (biscuits) depend largely upon the amount, type, and manipulation of various fats used as ingredients. Meat without any fat would be dry, tough, and less tasty. The meat tissue we use most often is muscle, which is marbled with a fine network of fat

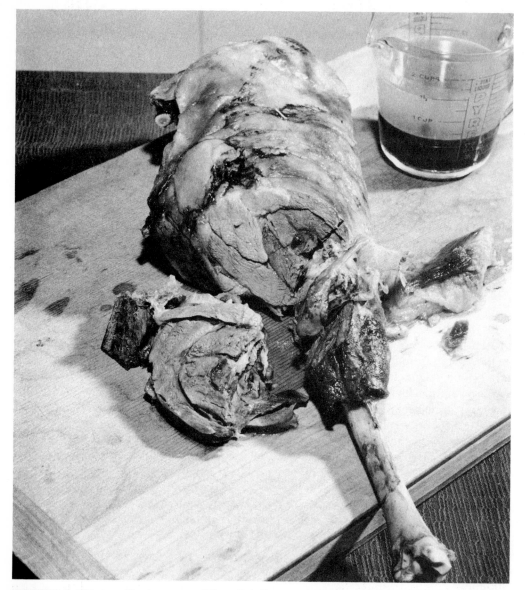

FIGURE 6-2 This leg of lamb roast would have little flavor and richness without the fat found in its juices and the meat. Its juiciness also depends on moisture carried in the fat.

flecks. The better meat grades place a premium on such fat. Some fat is needed to give meat better palatability or to make it perform better in roasting or broiling; such fat marbling helps to keep meat moist and succulent, if it is handled and cooked properly (Fig. 6-2).

Why shouldn't we serve fats that are so popular? Study after study demonstrates dietary fat is associated with our most devastating diseases. Cardiovascular (heart [cardio] and blood vessel [vascular]) diseases (CVDs) are thought to be linked to a high fat intake, and they can lead to many complications, including strokes and heart attacks, which are responsible for one-half of all deaths in the U.S. Evidence is also accumulating that some cancers may be associated with diets high in fat. (Such diets typically are also high in fat-rich animal protein and low in important fiber.) With some understanding about fats and oils and their types, roles, food sources, and intake guidelines, it is not hard to make menu changes to reduce fat.

THE LIPID FAMILY

Fats and oils belong to a large family called lipids, a family that also includes lipoproteins, waxes, resins, sterols, and some other substances. Cholesterol is a relative. All lipids are insoluble in water. Most are made up of chains of a dozen or more carbon atoms, each carbon having hydrogen and oxygen atoms attached just as do carbohydrates and proteins. Differences in the length of the carbon chains and the number and kind of other substances attached to the carbons make the lipid what it is. Thus, the temperature at which margarine liquefies or the firmness of a shortening used in making a pie crust is determined by the characteristics of these carbon chains.

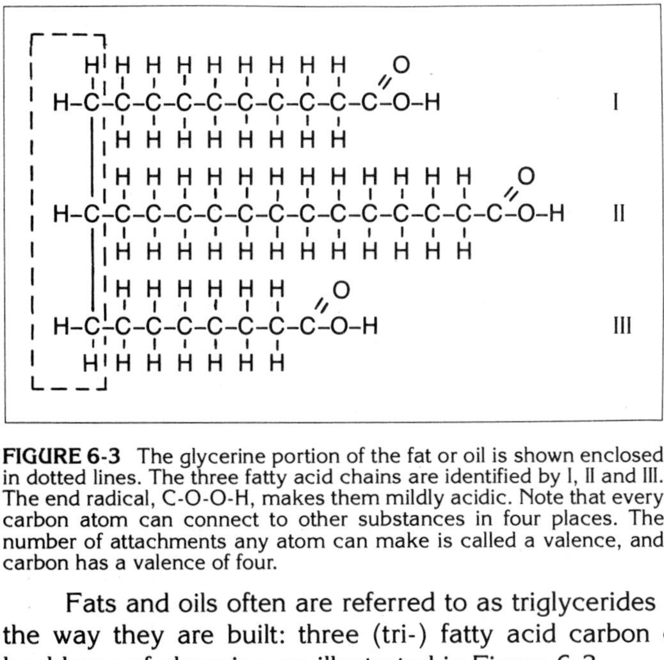

FIGURE 6-3 The glycerine portion of the fat or oil is shown enclosed in dotted lines. The three fatty acid chains are identified by I, II and III. The end radical, C-O-O-H, makes them mildly acidic. Note that every carbon atom can connect to other substances in four places. The number of attachments any atom can make is called a valence, and carbon has a valence of four.

Fats and oils often are referred to as triglycerides because the word describes the way they are built: three (tri-) fatty acid carbon chains are attached to one backbone of glycerine, as illustrated in Figure 6-3.

Dietary Lipids: Food Fats and Oils

Dietary lipids are the fats and oils in foods we eat. They provide nine calories per gram, over twice that provided by a gram of protein or carbohydrate. A teaspoon of pure oil or fat weighs about five grams and provides approximately 45 calories. Dietary lipids are those that are built into foods and those we use in cooking or otherwise consume. Some are easily identified (margarine, fat on a steak); some are hidden (in salad dressing, pastries, or French fried potatoes).

Saturated and Unsaturated

Mass communication media and advertisers make many references to "saturated," "unsaturated," "monounsaturated," "polyunsaturated," and "hydrogenated" fat. These different words describe how the carbon atoms are joined in the fats and oils.

If each carbon atom bonds to two hydrogens, it is said to be saturated, because all four links, or valences, where the carbon can attach itself to other substances are filled. But if two carbons are joined by a double bond and each carbon is attached to only one hydrogen atom, it is said to be unsaturated. Each carbon could hold more hydrogen. If the carbon chain has only one unsaturated point, it is said to be monounsaturated, but if there are two unsaturated points or more on the carbon chain, it is polyunsaturated (Figs. 6-4, 6-5, and 6-6).

$$
\begin{array}{c}
\text{H\ \ H\ \ H\ \ H\ \ H\quad O} \\
\text{H–C–C–C=C–C–C–O–H} \\
\text{H\ \ H\qquad\ \ H}
\end{array}
\qquad\qquad
\begin{array}{c}
\text{H\ H\ H\ H\ H\ H\ H\ H\ H\ H\ H\ H\quad O} \\
\text{H–C–C–C–C=C–C–C–C–C=C–C–C–O–H} \\
\text{H\ H\ H\qquad\ \ H\ H\ H\qquad\ H}
\end{array}
$$

(monounsaturated)   (polyunsaturated)

FIGURE 6-4 Schematic diagrams of a monounsaturated and a polyunsaturated fatty acid.

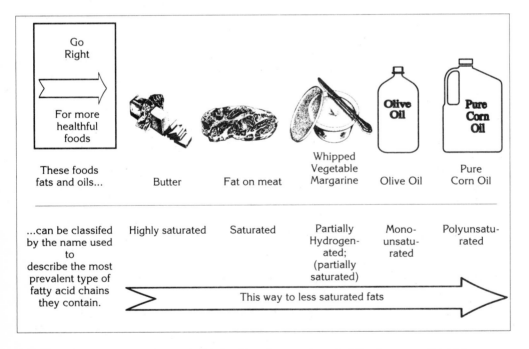

FIGURE 6-5 The above indicates the kinds of fats that are characteristic of common food fat sources.

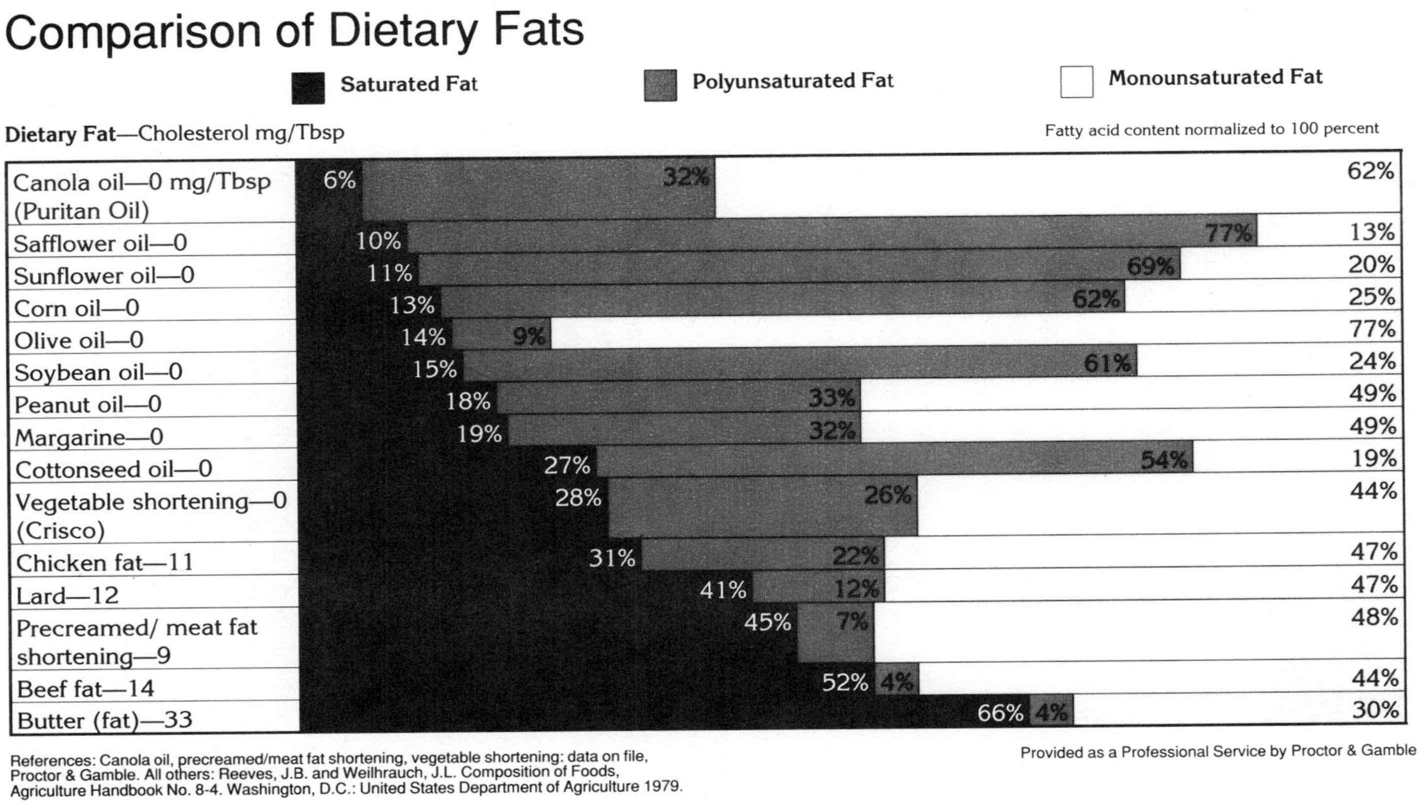

Comparison of Dietary Fats

Legend: ■ Saturated Fat   ▨ Polyunsaturated Fat   □ Monounsaturated Fat

Fatty acid content normalized to 100 percent

Dietary Fat—Cholesterol mg/Tbsp

Dietary Fat—Cholesterol mg/Tbsp	Saturated Fat	Polyunsaturated Fat	Monounsaturated Fat
Canola oil—0 mg/Tbsp (Puritan Oil)	6%	32%	62%
Safflower oil—0	10%	77%	13%
Sunflower oil—0	11%	69%	20%
Corn oil—0	13%	62%	25%
Olive oil—0	14%	9%	77%
Soybean oil—0	15%	61%	24%
Peanut oil—0	18%	33%	49%
Margarine—0	19%	32%	49%
Cottonseed oil—0	27%	54%	19%
Vegetable shortening—0 (Crisco)	28%	26%	44%
Chicken fat—11	31%	22%	47%
Lard—12	41%	12%	47%
Precreamed/meat fat shortening—9	45%	7%	48%
Beef fat—14	52%	4%	44%
Butter (fat)—33	66%	4%	30%

References: Canola oil, precreamed/meat fat shortening, vegetable shortening: data on file, Proctor & Gamble. All others: Reeves, J.B. and Weihrauch, J.L. Composition of Foods, Agriculture Handbook No. 8-4. Washington, D.C.: United States Department of Agriculture 1979.

Provided as a Professional Service by Proctor & Gamble

FIGURE 6-6 Vegetable oils are lower in saturated fat and higher in monounsaturated and polyunsaturated fat. It is possible to remove saturated fat and do other things to make the use of oils and fats better nutritionally (Adapted from a graph of Proctor and Gamble and published with permission).

Hydrogenation An unsaturated fat can be made into a saturated one by placing the fat, usually an oil, in a chamber and then heating it under pressure. Then ground nickel is added, and hydrogen gas is bubbled up though the melted fat or liquid oil. The nickel takes hold of a hydrogen atom and fixes it to the carbon, breaking the double bond, changing it from (=) to (-). This happens many times, making the product more saturated. The nickel is not a part of the reaction but only helps it: it is a catalyst. When saturation has gone far enough, the process is stopped, the nickel is drained off, and the product is cooled. At room temperature the fat is more firm, or solid, than it was before. Thus can liquid oils be made into solid fats, which is often done with soybean oil, to make margarine, and with cottonseed oil, to make a solid shortening. We call such treatment of lipids hydrogenation. We often see on the ingredient list for a food the words "hydrogenated oil," which means an oil that was once unsaturated has been treated to be at least partially saturated. The processor can stop the hydrogenation process at any point, depending on what form is desired: pourable, spreadable, semi-solid, or firm.

For foodservices purposes the hydrogenation of fats and oils can be quite desirable. A relatively inexpensive vegetable oil, such as cottonseed oil, can be made into a substitute for a more expensive solid fat for baking or cooking. We can take some fats and convert them to a more plastic form that is more suitable for some food preparation processes.

Importantly, hydrogenated fats also are less perishable. Double or unsaturated bonds are easily occupied by oxygen and the fat becomes rancid. Unsaturated oils must be used fairly soon or must contain antioxidants such as vitamin C or E or butylated hydroxy-anisole (BHA).

From a health standpoint, we know saturated fats tend to raise blood cholesterol whereas unsaturated ones seem not to. Thus, some health benefits are lost when an oil is hydrogenated. While processors may claim health benefits for a product made from vegetable oil, hydrogenation nullifies the "unsaturation," something they may neglect to say. The fact is that the hydrogenated fat is now more saturated than it was.

As noted, the more solid a fat or oil, the more saturated it usually is. Beef suet and mutton tallow, both rather saturated fats, harden at a fairly high temperature, while some unsaturated oils have to be chilled considerably before they solidify. In olive oil and some vegetable oils used in salad dressings and other products this is undesirable. Processors often winterize oils to counteract the tendency to solidify when refrigerated: the oil is centrifuged, which throws out the heavy saturated molecules to be drained off. Only the lighter molecules are left, which do not solidify as easily. This process appears to be safe and is, perhaps, beneficial, since the oil now has less saturated fat.

For health reasons, it is better to avoid saturated fats when possible. In this regard it is advisable to consider the source of the fat or oil. Nonhydrogenated vegetable and fish oils tend to be less saturated than animal fat (Table 6-1). Olive oil is pretty much mono-unsaturated. Coconut, palm, and palm kernel oil and cocoa butter are somewhat saturated; unfortunately, since they are relatively inexpensive, they are used widely in such processed foods as nondairy cream substitutes and in

TABLE 6-1
Oils & Fats
It's the Difference That Counts

Type of Oil or Fat	Polyunsaturated Fat (%)	Saturated Fat (%)
Safflower oil	74	9
Sunflower oil	64	10
Corn oil	58	13
Average vegetable oil (soybean plus cottonseed)	40	13
Peanut oil	30	19
Chicken fat (schmaltz)	26	29
Olive oil	9	14
Average vegetable shortening	20	32
Lard	12	40
Beef fat	4	48
Butter	4	61
Palm oil	2	81
Coconut oil	2	86

All fats and oils are equally high in calories, so see how little you can use. When you do use fats and oils, choose those high in polyunsaturated fats—the ones at the top of the chart.
Source: U.S. Department of Health and Human Services Public Health Service, Jan. 1985.

confections. Many fish oils contain a high proportion of polyunsaturated fats. Another clue is consistency at room temperature: in general, the softer a lipid is at room temperature, the more polyunsaturated it is. An oil usually has a greater proportion of polyunsaturated carbon chains than a solid fat such as that on a lamb chop (see Fig. 6-6).

Adipose Tissue, or Body Fat

Some bodily padding of moderate degree; adipose tissue on muscles and bones is beneficial, but in excess, it is considered detrimental to health. Body fat is stored for possible later energy needs. A pound of adipose tissue represents roughly 3500 calories. (Since it contains some water and protein, it does not yield the 4000 calories that a pound of pure animal fat or oil would.) When an excess of food is consumed, the body usually takes the calories that the body does not need at the time and turns them into body fat for storage. If the excess is in the form of dietary fat or oil, 97% of it is converted to body fat; if it is carbohydrate or protein, only about 77% is directed to body fat. The reason for this is that the body must use energy to convert nonfats into body fat; when fat is consumed to be stored as fat, this energy need not be expended.

Blood, or Serum, Lipids and Related Substances

Blood lipids and related substances can be subdivided as (1) simple lipids, (2) lipids joined with other substances, and (3) cholesterol.

The simple lipids, or glycerides, and related substances circulate in the blood. A physician monitoring or treating the heart and blood vessel (cardiovascular) system may routinely measure serum triglycerides. There is much talk today about triglycerides in the blood and about recommendations on the types and amounts of dietary fat that could affect cardiovascular health.

Fatty acids also combine with other substances that are of increasing interest to medical researchers interested in more healthful eating. Lipids bond with phosphorus to make the hard-working emulsifiers called phospholipids. Protein combines with fat to make lipoproteins. Cholesterol is not a lipid, but a sterol, a member of the alcohol family. It is discussed here because its presence in the blood is associated with CVD. It is presently the subject of intense study and controversy in relation to these diseases. Recommendations on healthful levels of cholesterol have been changed recently and not all authorities agree.

Throughout this chapter, we will discuss how lipids are involved in some of our health problems. Building from this we discuss at this chapter's end the potential relationships between lipids, cholesterol, and CVD. After all, isn't this really among the principal motivations of consumers who demand low-fat, low-cholesterol food choices?

THE ROLES OF LIPIDS

The Roles of Fat

While linoleic acid is the only essential fatty acid (one the body cannot manufacture), many different fatty acids participate in a range of tasks lipids perform. Linoleic acid itself is associated closely with physical growth and with skin maintenance. Without it, children's growth is retarded and they develop dermatitis (skin inflammation). Other fatty lipids are credited as being the sources of hormones responsible for regulating a broad range of physical functions, such as blood pressure and stomach and other smooth muscle functions. Fat surrounding organs supports and protects them. Adipose tissue can help protect the body from blows and also acts as an insulator, helping the body to retain heat. Fat is a reserve of energy we can draw on if we need it. For this reason, some authorities feel that persons who are extremely thin might be at a disadvantage if they become ill. If glucose and glycogen reserves run low and there is a demand for more energy, fat can be metabolized to provide it. Another unique contribution of lipids and related substances is their importance as part of the membrane, or envelope, surrounding every body cell. Fats are also the natural vehicle for the fat-soluble vitamins (A, D, E, and K), both in foods and once the nutrients are in the body. Because fats remain in the stomach longer than alcohol, carbohydrate, or protein, they offer a lingering feeling of satiety. Satiety value, as this is known, is an expression of how long one remains satisfied following a meal. Even persons on weight-loss diets do well to include some fat for this reason. For persons who have a hard time maintaining or gaining weight, eating high-caloric fats and oils may be helpful.

Phospholipids

The phospholipids are excellent emulsifying agents; that is, they help fat and liquids to blend, as, normally oil and water do not mix. To effect emulsification, the phosphorus portion of a phospholipid molecule attracts water, and the lipid portion of a phospholipid molecule attracts other lipids. They assist in digestion, absorption, and transportation of lipids in the body. The retention of body moisture, especially in the skin, is one of their many tasks. They form parts of the cell walls and nerve coatings and are part of the clotting factor of blood.

Lecithin, a phospholipid present in every normal cell, exerts its excellent emulsifying power to assist in transporting and utilizing fatty acids. Lecithin is added to margarines to give them a smooth, uniformly blended quality and to help produce foam when they are heated. Lecithin contributes to emulsification of salad dressings, whipped toppings, and a host of other processed foods. Many claims are made of the power of lecithin to restore memory loss, to melt body fat, and to lower blood lipid levels, among other benefits, but there is no scientific evidence that lecithin works such miracles. We get plenty of lecithin if we eat a varied diet, and the body can produce lecithin and other phospholipids if more is required, so they are nonessential. Taking kelp mixtures, or other forms of lecithin supplements seems to be a pointless waste of money.

Lipoproteins

Lipoproteins help transport many lipids in the blood. Three of the four types of lipoproteins are of special interest in cardiovascular disease, because they appear to be related to the deposition of cholesterol and other substances along the arterial walls, a possible prelude to heart attack or stroke. These are discussed later.

Cholesterol

Our bodies need cholesterol. It is an important part of brain and nerve cells, it is a part of bile needed to emulsify fats and oils in the digestive tract, and it is involved in the synthesis of sex hormones, and others. When the ultra-violet rays of sunlight strike cholesterol in the skin the essential vitamin D is formed. Thus, some cholesterol must be in our food or our bodies must manufacture it to meet all these needs.

LIPID METABOLISM

About 95% of the lipids we eat are triglycerides. In the digestive system, lipases (fat-breaking enzymes) do one of four things:
1. Leave the triglyceride as is,
2. Take off one fatty acid leaving a diglyceride (two fatty acids attached to the glyceride portion) and one free fatty acid,

3. Take off two fatty acids leaving a monoglyceride (one fatty acid attached to the glyceride portion) and two free fatty acids,
4. Take off three fatty acids leaving a free glycerol and three free fatty acids.

The products are then absorbed from the small intestine in this form. The free fatty acids, monoglycerides, diglycerides, and triglycerides next are carried into the bloodstream. Since they cannot mix with blood, lipoproteins pick them up and carry them throughout the body so that the cells can use them for energy. A lot of these fatty acids and glycerides get back to the liver, where they are either broken down to make energy or are re-formed into fat and stored as reserve energy. Physicians measure triglycerides and cholesterol in the blood to determine a person's risk status for heart disease and other problems. The glycerol portion gets to the liver and starts on its way toward making energy or fat. (Glycerol is a form of alcohol.)

Most body cells have little ability to store fat, but certain ones are built for it. In some people these cells continue to absorb fat until they are vastly expanded. The fat cells in obese people are larger than those of a thin person by a hundredfold or more. This ability to store great quantities of fat in fat cells is thought to be an inherited characteristic.

As we have noted earlier, fats and oils supply nine calories per gram; alcohol seven, and carbohydrates and proteins four. Why is this so? Now that we know the makeup of a fatty acid chain and a glucose chain, we can note in Figure 6-7 that fat has a lot of hydrogen atoms attached to it but not a lot of oxygen atoms. Glucose has many more oxygen atoms with its carbons and hydrogens. This is the answer to the difference in calorie yield. When fat is broken down for energy many more oxygen atoms must be added to the carbon and hydrogen to reduce them to the end products, water (H_2O) and carbon dioxide (CO_2). These oxidation reactions give off energy—the more oxidation reactions there are, the more energy is produced. (It is the same oxidation that occurs when wood is burned in a fire.) Thus, when fat is broken down, we get more than twice the energy than we do from carbohydrate or protein.

To create energy from a lipid, the liver begins by using enzymes to disassemble the acid portion. Enzymes break off two carbon atoms at a time until the carbon chain is split apart completely into two-carbon units. The two-carbon units are broken down much like carbohydrate is. If a lot of fat is broken down but no glucose is available to supply oxygen, two two-carbon units can join together to form what is called a "ketone body." An overload of ketone bodies, "ketosis," if not controlled can cause coma and even death. Alcohol breaks down in a

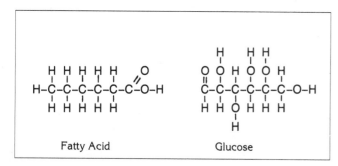

Fatty Acid   Glucose

FIGURE 6-7 Contrast the structure of a fatty acid and glucose carbon chains for energy yield. Note that the fatty acid contains 12 hydrogen atoms only two of which are bound to oxygen. This leaves 10 hydrogen and six carbon atoms to be oxidized. Glucose has 12 hydrogen and six oxygen atoms, leaving only six hydrogen and six carbons to be oxidized.

fashion similar to the way fat does. While there are differences between the two processes, this is basically true. Alcohol, like fat, has many hydrogen atoms to oxidize but not quite as many per carbon as fat does. Therefore alcohol provides only seven calories per gram; still this is almost twice the yield of carbohydrates and proteins.

Like lipids, alcohol is broken into energy in the liver. A healthy person whose nutritional state is good and who drinks a moderate amount of alcohol has no trouble metabolizing alcohol. But if liver function is compromised by alcohol overload, malnutrition, or illness can occur. If a heavy drinker eats poorly or doesn't eat at all, the body's supply of amino acids drops and a deficiency of the enzymes that break down alcohol develops. The liver of a heavy drinker may fail to metabolize proteins well, which can add to the protein deficit. It is wise always to consume some protein food while drinking alcohol.

Some people enjoy alcohol, but it can have unhappy consequences. The best thing is not to drink at all or to follow the advice of the Dietary Goals for the United States and drink in moderation.

HOW MUCH FAT AND CHOLESTEROL?

Fats and oils have no RDAs, but related recommendations suggest a number of guidelines. Based on a balanced diet of adequate calories, linoleic acid is the only essential lipid, and the amount needed can come from a mere tablespoon a day of vegetable oil. All polyunsaturated vegetable and fish oils contain good amounts of linoleic acid. Saturated fats also contain some linoleic acid, because all fats are a blend of at least some saturated and unsaturated fatty acid chains.

In most developed countries too much fat is consumed. Here in the U.S. we need to drop our average of 42% of our calories in fat to around 30%. We need to also observe the guidelines set forth for selecting the most healthful sources and types for the fat we do eat.

Dietary Goals for Lipid Intake

Some of the recommendations in the Dietary Guidelines for Americans were directed toward the concerns of a population in which one in five males and one in 17 women has heart disease. The objective of the recommendation to reduce calories is to avoid overweight, which increases the risk of cardiovascular disease. About fat the Guidelines state; "Avoid too much fat, saturated fat, and cholesterol."

How much is too much is put into perspective by the Dietary Goals. The recommendation in the Goals is that not more than 30% of total daily calories come from fat (Fig. 6-8). Some feel it should be 20 to 25%. The diet popularized by the late Dr. Nathan Pritikin contains 10% fat. The average American now obtains around 45% of total calories as dietary fat: a person who consumes 2000 calories per day takes in 90 grams or 800 calories, of fat. This is like eating a stick (1/2 cup) of butter every day. Americans lead the world in per capita consumption of fat. If one follows the Dietary Goals, on a 2000-calorie daily diet, the fat calories must drop to 600, a decrease of 300 calories, or 33 grams (over an ounce of fat), per day.

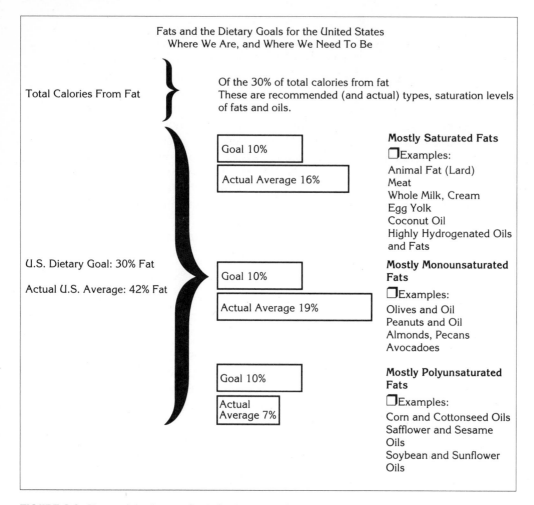

FIGURE 6-8 Fats and the Dietary Goals for the United States.

The Goals further suggest that the fat we consume should be taken in equal proportions of polyunsaturated, monounsaturated, and saturated fat sources. The actual pattern currently is to consume much more saturated fat than mono- and polyunsaturated fats combined. Thus, we need to lower total fat intake and increase the proportion of mono- and polyunsaturated fats while reducing the balance of saturated fat. This could mean shifting a sizeable proportion of our fat food choices (see Fig. 6-8).

Dietary Exchange Method

The Dietary Exchange Method is good for monitoring the amount of fat in the diet. The number of fat exchanges (one exchange is 1 teaspoon, or 5 grams, of fat, 45 calories) are listed for the food lists: fat, milk, bread and starchy vegetables, and meat and meat alternatives lists. Table 6-2 indicates where fat usually is found in the

TABLE 6-2
Dietary Fats in Exchange Lists

Contains Fat or Oil?			
Always	Sometimes	Rarely	The two faces of a fat exchange
Fats	Milk products (unless skimmed)	Vegetables	1. As an item on the Fat List, e.g., butter.
Meat/meat alternatives list	Bread products, some grains and legumes	Fruits	2. As part of the makeup of and item on a list, e.g., the marbling of fat in ground beef.

various lists. Note that there is always fat in meat and fats, sometimes in milk products and in bread, and rarely in vegetables and fruits.

The Basic Four Food Groups

The Basic Four Food Plan calls for two portions of milk (18 grams of fat if whole milk) and two two-to-three ounce portions of lean meat (16 grams of fat). This gives 34 grams of fat, 306 calories from fat alone. The fat content of other foods and dressings, such as butter, is not monitored; a person can easily consume more than the recommended amounts. Some caution, therefore, is recommended. Unlike the Food Exchange Method, the Basic Four does not indicate upper or lower limits of dietary fats, a fact that might be considered a weakness of that plan.

American Heart Association (AHA) Recommendations

The AHA recommends limiting intake of meat and cheese to no more than five to seven ounces a day and taking less than 30% of total calories as fats. Table 6-3 shows the fat exchanges in a typical day's foods. It is not uncommon for people to take in even more fatty foods in a day. As a result, many Americans' diets run to about 45% fat—over 1200 calories, or 40%, of a 3000-calorie diet.

The AHA emphasizes limiting cholesterol in the diet, publicizing that an average maximum of 300 milligrams (mg) per day should be the goal. An egg (250 mg cholesterol) and a glass of whole milk (34 mg) almost meet the cholesterol allowance, so that no other animal food should be consumed on the same day. The average male adult needs 900 to 1000 mg of cholesterol per day. The average daily intake from dietary sources is about 600 mg; the body manufactures the remainder. It is easy to get the cholesterol we need; it is present in all animal foods.

WHAT TO DO ABOUT IT

In planning menus and preparing food, how is it possible to satisfy consumers' desires and meet the responsibility of the facility for serving foods that are both tasty and healthful? Undoubtedly some menu items must be changed, or at least some ingredients (egg substitute for fresh eggs, for instance), and preparation methods

TABLE 6-3
Fat Exchanges of Some Items in One Day's Food*

Food Item	Fat Exchanges (No.)	Fat (grams)	Calories from Fat
Rib steak, no bone, 8	8	40	360
Bacon, 3 strips	3	15	135
Egg, poached	1	5	6
Butter, 3 tsp	3	15	135
Cream, heavy, 1 tbsp.	1	5	45
Mayonnaise, 2 tsp.	2	10	90
French fries, 3 ounces	3	15	125
Hamburger, 3 ounces	4	20	160
Cheddar cheese, 1 ounce	1	8	72
Almonds, shelled, 10	1	5	45
Total	17	138	1222

Using the exchange method, if one had an intake of fatty foods such as presented in Table 6-3, note the fat contribution. It is not uncommon to see such a group of foods with even more fat-yielding foods consumed in one day. This is what makes our diets go to around 45% of total calories in fat. It is also over 1,200 calories or 40% of a 3,000 calorie diet.
*These values have been calculated from values quoted in USDA, AHA and other source materials.

must be modified. Garnishes and sauces may have to be "rethought" (serve the salad dressing or gravy on the side so the patron controls how much goes on the food). It is important that foodservice providers think about how fats will be included as healthful foods—the logistics of the changes *and* how patrons will be informed of what is being done and what is available. The goal of the foodservice must be identified: is it menus with 30% fat or less? Low-cholesterol menu alternatives? The program must be directed toward identifying the market demands vis-à-vis fats and menu selections and in achieving the objectives of both the patrons and the operation. (In later chapters the marketing and planning efforts are discussed.)

Controlling Cholesterol

Presenting low cholesterol foods is not difficult if the sources and amounts of cholesterol in foods are known. Plant foods contain no cholesterol unless we add some animal source food such as butter or egg to a spinach timbale. All animal foods contain cholesterol, but the amounts differ (8 ounces of whole milk contains 34 mg of cholesterol, skim milk, only 5). Meat, fish, and poultry have about the same amount of cholesterol (Tables 6-4 and 6-5).

What is the difference in cholesterol in serving a 3-ounce portion of poached cod, cooked lean veal, or cooked lean beef? Not much, but there is a big difference between these and organ meats. Shellfish have the reputation of being high in cholesterol: some are, but others are not. The source of cholesterol is also important. An ounce of whole-milk cheddar cheese contains about 25 mg of cholesterol but an equal portion of skim-milk cheddar has about 15 mg. Table 6-5 gives the cholesterol values for some other foods.

Controlling Fat

Controlling fat in menu offerings, preparation, and service is accomplished in a manner similar to that recommended for cholesterol control. It can come also from choosing different menu selections, modifying recipes, substituting ingredients and altering presentation, as by serving the high-fat components on the side. A protein-based product has recently been announced which has qualities similar to fat but has fewer calories and may be more healthful than saturated fat. In the future this may be substituted for fat in some prepared foods. The Exchange Method can also be used to control fat, as many of the lists besides that of fats give the quantity of fat or direct the user to omit one or two fat exchanges if this food is served. The Exchange Method, however, fails to list many foods that one might wish to serve; for those foods, tables that list fat content must be consulted.

In later chapters we will discuss in menu planning, recipe development, preparation, and service how healthful foods can be offered on the menu. As a general strategy, either menu items are chosen that can be just as palatable as higher fat versions, or popular low-fat alternatives are offered. It is no use trying to compete with high-fat items. Making up a list of foods high in fats (especially saturated fats) and cholesterol can be helpful, as is a list of menu alternatives. Replacing a formerly high-fat lasagna with food that has lower total fat, saturated fat, and cholesterol yields can be a big step in fat and calorie reduction with minimal compromise in appeal. Table 6-6 shows how to reduce fat intake by changing food selections.

TABLE 6-4
Amount of Cholesterol in Three Ounces of Some Animal Foods

Food	Cholesterol	Food	Cholesterol
Beef, cooked, lean, fat trimmed	77	Liver, chicken	480
Veal, cooked, lean	86	Abalone	200
Rabbit, domestic	52	Lobster	96
Salmon, cooked	40	Oysters	67
Sardines, 3¾ ounces	109	Pork, cooked, lean	77
Kidney	690	Turkey, light meat	65
Heart	274	Turkey, dark meat	86
Crab	138	Haddock	51
Scallops	75	Herring	83
Lamb, lean cooked	83	Brains	810
Chicken, light meat	54	Sweetbreads	396
Cod	72	Shrimp	160
Flounder	43	Clams	92
Liver, beef	372		

TABLE 6-5
Amount of Cholesterol and Calories per Serving of Some Foods

	Serving Size	Cholesterol (mg)	Food Energy (calories)
Milk			
Whole	1 cup	34	165
2% (Nonfat milk solids added)	1 cup	22	145
1%	1 cup	14	103
Skim	1 cup	5	90
Cheese			
American	1 ounce	25	105
Cheddar	1 ounce	28	115
Cream	2 tbsp.	16	60
Mozzarella	1 tbsp.	5	26
Swiss	1 ounce	28	105
Ice Cream	1 cup	53	255
Yogurt (plain)	1 cup	17	125
Meat			
Lean beef, lamb, pork and ham	3 ounces	77	189
Lean veal	3 ounces	84	177
Poultry	3 ounces	74	150
Fish	3 ounces	63	126
Shellfish			
Crab	½ cup	62	85
Clams	6 large	36	65
Lobster	½ cup	62	68
Oysters (6)	3 ounces	45	53
Shrimp (11 large)	½ cup	96	100
Liver (beef)	3 ounces	372	136
Eggs, chicken	1 large	250	80
Bacon, cooked crisp	2 slices	14	90

The following may be a helpful summary on how to reduce fat or cholesterol in the foods served:

1. Substitute low-fat items for the higher-fat ones. Use yogurt instead of sour cream in a recipe. Rather than trying to cook up a low-fat egg-sausage-cheese on a buttered bun breakfast sandwich, offer an unrelated choice, such as cold cereal, fruit, and low-fat milk all packaged to eat in or to go.
2. Choose lean cuts of meat and trim as much fat as possible. Serve skinless chicken or turkey and fish in place of higher fat beef, lamb, or pork. Allow drippings to separate from meats and juices. Add the juices to the stock pot. If you use juices for gravy or sauces, chill, then skim off the fat.
3. Legumes, grain products, and other plant foods are very low in fat and can be made into popular dishes. Avocadoes and olives are exceptions and are relatively high-fat.

TABLE 6-6
Making Less of Fat on the Menu:
Simple Steps: Before-and-After Comparison

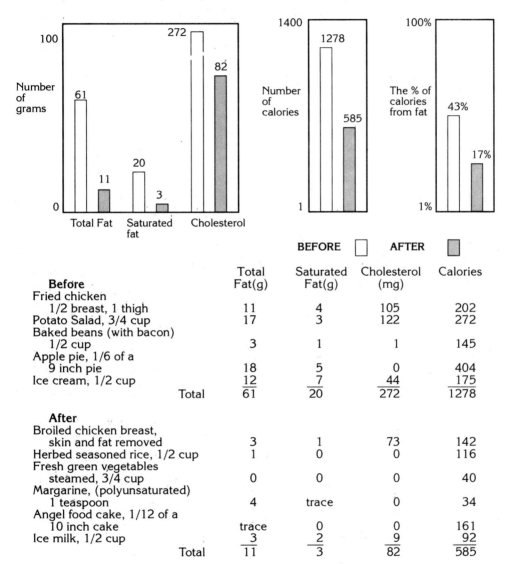

BEFORE □   AFTER ▨

	Total Fat(g)	Saturated Fat(g)	Cholesterol (mg)	Calories
Before				
Fried chicken				
1/2 breast, 1 thigh	11	4	105	202
Potato Salad, 3/4 cup	17	3	122	272
Baked beans (with bacon)				
1/2 cup	3	1	1	145
Apple pie, 1/6 of a				
9 inch pie	18	5	0	404
Ice cream, 1/2 cup	12	7	44	175
Total	61	20	272	1278
After				
Broiled chicken breast,				
skin and fat removed	3	1	73	142
Herbed seasoned rice, 1/2 cup	1	0	0	116
Fresh green vegetables				
steamed, 3/4 cup	0	0	0	40
Margarine, (polyunsaturated)				
1 teaspoon	4	trace	0	34
Angel food cake, 1/12 of a				
10 inch cake	trace	0	0	161
Ice milk, 1/2 cup	3	2	9	92
Total	11	3	82	585

4. Provide at least one alternative to high-cholesterol choices per meal; offer a low-fat soup and sandwich combination or low-fat salad and sandwich combination for lunch; provide selections such as skinless broiled chicken breast dressed with lemon juice and tarragon for dinner.

5. Offer low-fat and skim dairy products. Offer low-fat meatless or low-meat main dishes regularly.

6. Unnecessarily large additions of oil, shortening, lard, cheese, butter, cream, mayonnaise, bacon, salt pork, etc. turn a fat-free main ingredient such as pasta into a high-fat dish. Adapt recipes that use reasonable amounts of such ingredients on a portion basis. Some recipes for Mexican refried beans add over a tablespoon of fat (often saturated) per four-ounce serving, making even a legume dish a high-fat choice.

7. Replace saturated fats with polyunsaturated oils or polyunsaturated fatty acid (PUFA) products. A simple application of this would be to substitute for the quart of mayonnaise two to three cups of a reduced-fat and -cholesterol mayonnaise made from safflower or another polyunsaturated oil.

8. Frying adds fat. Avoid pan-frying, sauteing, deep-frying, and oven frying. Consider whether a food can be broiled, roasted, steamed, poached, or prepared in a low-fat manner. Use the greaseless type fryer equipment or use a vegetable oil-alcohol-lecithin spray to reduce fat needs. Stir-frying reduces the amount of fat needed to fry food.

9. Basting with large quantities of fats (butter, sauces, or meat drippings) is another way to add fat and should be avoided. For similar results, try increasing the moistness in meats by using more appropriate cooking techniques. Marinating foods before they are cooked or using a basting mixture that delivers less fat can impart wonderful flavor.

10. Offer reasonable portion sizes. The quickest way to get half the fat of a quarter-pound hamburger (4 ounces) is to have a 2-ounce one instead. The smaller burgers we are accustomed to seeing in fast food outlets actually weigh about 1.6 ounces before cooking. Listen to guest reactions to portion sizes. Watch the platewaste (food returned from the dining room to be thrown away). Consider offering two or more portion sizes: a mini-portion of a cup of soup and

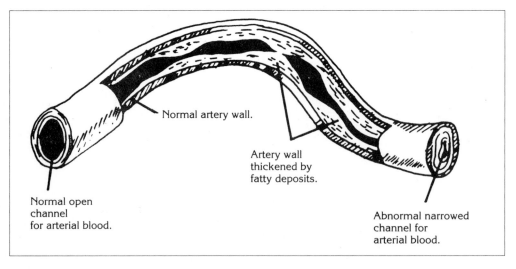

FIGURE 6-9 Schematic diagram of a normal artery wall thickened by plaque.

half sandwich with a melon slice; and a regular portion of a bowl of soup, a whole sandwich, and a more substantial salad.

11. Over-doing rich toppings is no favor. It can add fat and calories, not to mention overwhelming the recipe's intended light quality. It is common to see an extra portion of salad dressing or gravy sloshed over an item, but it is not always a courtesy to patrons. Most people will ask for extra if they want it.

12. Be prepared to offer foods that help patrons control fat and calories or at least to honor special requests. Honor requests to hold the butter; serve salad dressing on the side; provide an extra plate to share portions; or "people bags," to take uneaten food home. Even requests for measuring utensils in such self-serve areas as a salad or pasta bar might be honored. Properly structured, such efforts can be cost-effective and well received.

13. Substitutions of particular products that are lower in fat, saturated fat, or cholesterol also may be requested: skim milk instead of whole, milk instead of half-and-half or highly saturated nondairy "creamer," cholesterol-free egg substitutes, reduced-fat, polyunsaturated margarine and salad dressing. Most likely, what a foodservice operator makes available will evolve and change as customer expectations change and stocking such products becomes profitable.

CARDIOVASCULAR DISEASE (CVD)

Over half of all Americans who die succumb to *cardiovascular disease*. A half million deaths annually result from heart attacks. Cardiovascular disease is the Number 1 killer in the United States. Over 43 million people suffer from some form of it—high blood pressure, heart attacks, senility, kidney disease, and others—still, it used to be worse. The United States Public Health Service reported that between 1970 and 1978 deaths from cardiovascular disease dropped 18%, and we know this favorable trend has continued.

Cardiovascular disease begins with the deposition on artery walls of clumps of waxy material called *plaque* that narrow the channel and sometimes plug it completely. With time, these deposits harden, robbing the arteries of their flexibility (see Fig. 6-9). Both conditions make the heart work harder to pump blood throughout the body, evidenced by what we call high blood pressure (the pressure of blood against the stiff vessel walls). If a vessel is blocked by plaque or if a blood clot blocks an area where plaque has formed (thrombosis), blood and oxygen cannot get to vital tissue, which dies (infarction). In the brain the result is a cerebral infarction or stroke. In the heart, it is a coronary infarction, a heart attack. Partial blockage of a vessel reduces blood supply to tissues and organs, causing heart pain (angina pectoris) or kidney failure, or, when blood flow to the brain is compromised, onset of senility. Sometimes the high pressure causes a weak area of a vessel to balloon out. If the balloon bursts there is massive internal bleeding that can be rapidly fatal.

The AHA has increased public awareness of the dangers of cardiovascular disease, and many people are trying today to avoid it, but are not always sure how to do so. One problem is that different studies have produced conflicting data. Some say diet can help prevent cardiovascular disease, others say it can't. Let us take a look at some of the facts.

The Part Cholesterol Plays

A large part of plaque is cholesterol. For a long time the assumption was that eating foods high in cholesterol would result in high levels of cholesterol in the blood (serum cholesterol), which would increase the risk of plaque build up. Some researchers now dispute this. Let's look at some of the different viewpoints.

The AHA asserts that reducing dietary cholesterol can reduce serum (blood) cholesterol and recommends that the average adult consume not more than 300 mg of cholesterol per day. The actual average intake is somewhere between 500 and 600 mg. Thus, the AHA says, most persons should reduce their cholesterol intake by nearly half. The AHA also says serum cholesterol should not be over 160 mg per 100 milliliters (ml) of blood. Others feel that 210 mg should be the upper limit; others, 195. Only a third of American males have a cholesterol serum level of 210 mg or less.

Among those who do not agree with the AHA's stand is the Food and Nutrition Board of the National Academy of Sciences. They feel that the hazards of cholesterol vary from person to person and that making blanket recommendations for everyone, as the AHA has done, is not the best way to handle the problem. Why advise everyone to watch cholesterol when only those with CVD (15% of the population) and those at risk need to? They also question whether dietary cholesterol can do much to raise or lower serum cholesterol. There is, however, much common ground between these divergent views, and some prominent medical authorities and nutritionists can be found in both camps.

Other groups, such as the American Council on Science and Health and the Harvard Medical School, have taken the middle ground: they doubt that diet alone can do the job of reducing cholesterol but agree it does no harm to reduce it and until we know more we should not take any chances. Limiting dietary cholesterol can't hurt, and who knows *who* will develop cardiovascular disease?

Does Limiting Dietary Cholesterol Work?

It has been difficult to prove that diet can be effective in reducing serum cholesterol. Certainly over the years our attempts to reduce cholesterol by diet have not been too successful because the problem is still with us.

Several massive studies have been made; one studied 12,000 males over five years. It showed an average serum cholesterol reduction of 3% by diet control, which is not much: a person whose count was 300 mg would reduce that by 9 points, and 291 is still in the high-risk range. Most authorities feel that the best we can do with diet is to reduce the cholesterol level by 5 to 10%, which again may not be significant for those at high risk. Some animal studies have shown that a high-cholesterol diet does raise blood cholesterol, but there is some question of whether the animals were fed oxidized cholesterol, which would make the results invalid. Other studies have been questioned because the animals were fed cholesterol in amounts so great they were not typical of the normal human diet.*

*See Hamilton, Whitney, and Sizers: *Nutrition: Concepts and Controversies*, Ed 3, pp 114-121, and Ed 4, pp 131-142, 1988, St. Paul, West Publishing Co. for a fuller explanation of this questionability of these test results.

People Are Different. The fact that there is a wide difference in people and in the way they react to cholesterol also argues against a broad recommendation like the one made by the AHA. We saw this in the stand of the Food and Nutrition Board of the National Academy of Sciences. Age can be a factor: serum cholesterol level rises with age. Sex is also a factor. Males have higher cholesterol levels than premenopausal females. After menopause women's levels "catch up." Race can also be a factor, as can heredity. Cardiovascular disease can run in families. Plaques sometimes start to build up in infants, who, by the time they reach adulthood, are at high risk. In 1987 one medical authority made the statement that 95% of the heart attacks in the U.S. occur in only 5% of the families!

Another factor is that we don't get our cholesterol only from food. Our bodies can manufacture it. (Rabbits eat no cholesterol at all, but they have it in their blood.) The average male needs about 900 to 1000 mg of cholesterol a day to make bile, hormones, and other products the body uses. If dietary intake is 600 mg this subject must manufacture 300 mg. Some persons can reduce dietary cholesterol to practically nothing, and their bodies continue to manufacture excessive amounts. Diet is of no help to them.

Individuals also differ in the kind of cholesterol they have in their blood. Cholesterol is carried in the blood by lipoproteins. We have heard of this substance before in this chapter. If cholesterol is transported by what we call high-density lipoproteins (HDL) the chances of its being deposited as plaque are much less than when it is carried by low-density lipoproteins (LDL) or very low-density lipoproteins (VLDL). (In early 1988 a VLDL form was isolated that may be the basic plaque-depositing agent). Thus a person whose cholesterol count is 230 (mg per 100 ml of blood) and who has a lot of HDL and very little LDL and VLDL might be at lower risk than one with a count of 180 mg and high levels of LDL and VLDL. A blood test is available today that measures the quantities of the respective lipoproteins so that people may know just how great their risk is.

Sugars raise the serum triglyceride (fat) levels of some persons, which is also a risk factor. Such individuals must reduce their intake of sugars. (Complex carbohydrates seem to make no difference, and lactose actually seems to help reduce cholesterol.)

Obesity can be a factor in cholesterol level. Obese persons often have high levels of triglyceride and cholesterol. Statistics show clearly that obese people have a higher incidence of heart attacks and strokes than persons of normal weight. In 1988 one medical authority made news when he announced that abdominal fat was a better indicator than body fat elsewhere in identifying persons at risk. This may support the old rule, "For every inch your waist is greater than your chest, take two years from your life." Deaths from heart attack and stroke are also far more common among diabetics than in the rest of the population.

Another individual factor is the way people react to salt (sodium) in their food. Some people can get 3000 mg of sodium a day or more and not be bothered by it, whereas others develop high blood pressure from that much or less. Some persons who have high blood pressure or heart disease have to restrict their intake of salt and foods containing sodium to avoid serious health problems. Again, heredity seems to play a part in high blood pressure. It runs along in families, and members of those families are more susceptible to problems caused by sodium than others.

What We Do Know

Some facts about CVD are well established. A high intake of saturated fat can raise the cholesterol level in many persons. Consuming too many calories seems to elevate serum cholesterol and triglyceride levels. Eating unsaturated fats, especially polyunsaturated ones, seems to reduce serum cholesterol. The consumption of some alcoholic beverage—not more than two drinks a day (say six ounces of wine or 24 ounces of beer or two ounces of 80-proof liquor)—seems to protect against heart attacks. Alcohol seems to increase HDL and lower LDL and VLDL, but alcohol in larger amounts can be harmful to health in other ways.

Some studies suggest that certain foods are helpful in reducing cholesterol and others are not. In some experiments eating oily fish such as salmon, mackerel, and trout was helpful. Shellfish, high in cholesterol, were not. Low-fat milk products and fermented milk products were good. Eggs were not. Eating plenty of fruits and vegetables, legumes, and rolled oats and other grains was beneficial. Vegetable oils were good, and cod liver and other fish oils were very good, because of their high polyunsaturated fat content. The saturated fat in highly hydrogenated vegetable oils raised cholesterol. Garlic has been touted as an effective agent for reducing high blood pressure but this was never proven; however, it seems to be effective in reducing cholesterol. Hot peppers do not reduce cholesterol but, like aspirin, they thin the blood and may help prevent embolisms. Ginseng may lower blood cholesterol.

A change in lifestyle (reducing stress, more moderate living, exercise, etc.) or environment also helps control weight and conditions the cardiovascular system. Smoking is very definitely associated with several cancers and with cardiovascular disease. Marijuana has been shown to raise serum cholesterol, as do contraceptives with an estrogen base. Taking an aspirin every other day is said to protect against thrombosis; it reduces the tendency of the blood to clot, which reduces the danger of a clot closing a narrowed artery. However, the FDA has asked aspirin manufacturers to go soft on this until there is absolute proof. Drugs containing ibuprofen also are supposed to do this. A new drug approved in 1988 is claimed to reduce blood cholesterol as much as 40%, whereas another approved about the same time increases HDL and reduces LDL and VLDL. There are other very promising experimental drugs.

What's the Answer?

There are no definitive answers yet, because the data are conflicting and we don't yet know enough about cholesterol. Nothing has worked for everyone, and we are still learning. However, we are gaining ground. Certainly it is possible to do more to prevent cardiovascular disease now than in the past. The fact that some new drugs show promise and that others of great promise are being tested is encouraging. Perhaps drugs will work for some people to control cholesterol and diet, for others.

Early attempts to treat high blood pressure, gout, arthritis, epilepsy, and other diseases used diet alone without much success, but when effective drugs were discovered, a combination of drugs and diet did the job. This may be how it will go with CVD. In the meantime, perhaps we should play safe and follow the advice of the Harvard Medical School and others. A prudent diet cannot do any harm and it might do some good and at least be insurance.

SUMMARY

Fats and oils belong to a family called lipids. A fat is made up of the same chemical elements and molecules as an oil. Both are triglycerides: each has a glycerol fraction to which are attached three fatty acids. The difference between fats and oils is only their physical state. A fat is solid at room temperature while an oil is liquid. Lipids have nine calories per gram.

The average American eats much more fat than the recommended 30% of total calories. Overweight people tend to have more health problems and die earlier than those whose weight is normal or slightly below normal. Only one fatty acid—linoleic acid—is known to be required in the diet.

Fats and oils may be saturated or unsaturated. A saturated fat is one that has all four of its available chemical bonds filled with an atom. An unsaturated fat has two of its bonds joined to another carbon atom; one of these bonds can easily break and bond to another substance. A monounsaturated fatty acid has only one double bond; a polyunsaturated one has two or more. The unsaturated bond can be filled with a hydrogen atom by a process called hydrogenation. Hydrogenation changes an unsaturated bond into a saturated one.

Fats and oils are absorbed from the intestines as triglycerides, diglycerides, monoglycerides, or as glycerol and fatty acids. They can go to the cells to be used there, or the liver can take them and convert them back into fat for storage in the body or use as energy. The breakdown of a fat is a complex process in which two-carbon units are broken off and then reduced to create energy. The fact that lipids have a lot of hydrogen in relation to oxygen means that the fat gives off more energy than carbohydrates or proteins, which have a higher proportion of oxygen. Sometimes the carbons produced by breakdown of lipids can join to form ketone bodies, which can be toxic. It is wise to consume some carbohydrate to help breakdown fats when a lot of fat is being metabolized as occurs sometimes in dieting.

Alcohol break down is also a very complex process, and overloading the liver can cause it to malfunction in metabolizing alcohol and, long-term, can cause permanent damage to the liver. Other effects of alcohol abuse are gout, cirrhosis of the liver, and kidney failure.

A number of substances related to fats and oils are important in the diet. Phospholipids help bring fats and oils together with water-based biological compounds. They are emulsifying agents. Lecithin is an important phospholipid in fatty substances and is an important part of the protoplasm of cells.

The sterols, including cholesterol, are related to fats and oils and are important in many hormones. They are products the body can make into substances such as vitamin D. Cholesterol is also important in making bile, a digestive fluid, and some sex hormones. Cholesterol is associated with arteriosclerosis, a disease in which the arteries gradually harden as fatty substances are included in their walls. High blood pressure, heart attacks, and other disorders can develop as the buildup progresses. The average daily diet contains about a half gram of cholesterol in foods, usually in fats. In addition, the body manufacturers about another half gram. Some people with cardiovascular disease may be put on a low-cholesterol diet, but it is not clear whether this does much good, since the body manufactures cholesterol whether or not it is provided in the diet. Men usually have a higher serum cholesterol level than women. A high level may be a risk factor for cardiovascular diseases.

To control the amount of fat in the diet the Basic Four Food Plan may be followed, which provides for about 1200 calories a day with a reasonable proportion of fats and oils. The *Dietary Goals for the United States* recommend that no more than 30% of our calories come from fat and this fat be divided equally between saturated, monounsaturated and polyunsaturated fats. Fat exchange lists provide reliable information on the fat content of food.

Foodservices personnel should know what kinds of fats are in foods, how to use them sparingly in menu planning, food selection, and preparation, and how to offer them to patrons.

Whether diet alone can control serum cholesterol enough to help reduce the risk of cardiovascular diseases is debatable. Reducing dietary cholesterol can do no harm, and until we know more about the effects of diet on cholesterol, it is prudent to limit its consumption.

Chapter Review

1. What is the chemical makeup of fat or oil? To what chemical family do fats and oils belong?
2. What are the benefits of dietary fats and oils? How can they be harmful?
3. How many calories does a gram of fat or oil contain?
4. What percentage of a dietary fat is stored as fat if used for stored energy?
5. What substances help transport lipids in the body?
6. Define saturated fat, monounsaturated fat, polyunsaturated fat, and triglycerides.
7. What is the difference between a fat and an oil?
8. What is hydrogenation? How can it make an unsaturated fat into a saturated fat?
9. What is a phospholipid? Lecithin? A lipoprotein?
10. What do HDL, LDL, and VLDL stand for? What is good about HDLs and bad about the other two?
11. What is cholesterol? What good does it do in the body? What harm can it do?
12. How does the body get cholesterol?

13. What is considered the upper safe level of serum cholesterol?
14. What do medical authorities recommend we do to lower serum cholesterol?
15. What does linoleic acid do in the body?
16. What percentage of total daily calories should come from fats and oils? How should this allowance be divided among saturated, monounsaturated, and polyunsaturated fats?
17. Is following the Four Food Groups Plan a safe way to avoid too much fat? Would it be if you followed it but then ate a lot of foods loaded with fats and oils to make up extra calories?
18. Why is glucose needed to burn fat?
19. What could you do to reduce the amount of fats and oils in foodservice dishes: In menu selections? In recipes? In preparation? In service?
20. In the Dietary Exchange Method, what two groups always contain fat?
21. Using the Dietary Exchange Method determine how many calories in these four dairy products represent fat: butter, 1 ounce (Fat List); from the Milk List, whole milk, 1 cup; low-fat (2%) milk, 1 cup; non-fat milk, 1 cup.
22. To see how well you are able to calculate the amounts of fat and calories in a food plan and a revision of it, use the following worksheet and see whether you come up with approximately 52 grams of fat and 468 calories less in the revised meal, or a 90% reduction in fat grams and in fat calories. (Your answer can vary with the table of food values you use. The grams and calories used in making up the answers given in the index came from Home and Garden Bulletin, No. 72, USDA, Washington, DC 1971.)

Worksheet

Food Selections	Grams of Fat	Calories
Chicken breast, fried, ½, skin and flesh only, 2.7 oz.	_____	_____
Change to		
Chicken flesh, broiled, 3 oz.	_____	_____
Change in fat grams	_____	
% change	_____	
Change in calories		_____
% change		_____
Potatoes, french-fried, 10 strips	_____	_____
Change to		
Mashed, no butter, 1 cup	_____	_____
Change in fat grams	_____	
% change	_____	
Change in calories		_____
% change		_____
Cole slaw, ½ c, 1 T mayonnaise	_____	_____
Change to		
Celery, 1 3-in. piece		
Carrots, 3 strips		
Cucumber, 4 slices		
Total	_____	_____
Change in fat grams	_____	
% change	_____	
Change in calories		_____
% change		_____
Biscuits, two, with 2 t butter	_____	_____
Change to		
Whole wheat bread, 2 slices, no butter, peach jam instead	_____	_____
Change in fat grams	_____	
% change	_____	
Change in calories		_____
% change		_____
Apple pie, 1/6 9" pie	_____	_____
Change to		
Apple	_____	_____
Change in fat grams	_____	
% change	_____	
Change in calories		_____
% change		_____
Total fat grams original	_____	
Total fat grams revised	_____	
Difference in fat grams	_____	
% difference	_____	
Total calories original		_____
Total calories revised		_____

Chapter 7
Controlling Calories

Chapter Goals

- *To indicate why people want to control their weight.*
- *To give some of the reasons why people become obese.*
- *To tell how to determine desirable body weight and how many calories are needed to maintain that weight.*
- *To list ways of setting up a program to control calorie intake.*
- *To detail important factors in reducing, maintaining or increasing weight.*
- *To summarize the steps to follow to attain a satisfactory calorie control program.*

CALORIE CONCERNS

When it comes to food and health, the number one concern of Americans is that food be good but not fattening (Fig. 7-1). Few want to be fat. There are several reasons why. First, overweight means a greater chance of health problems. Obese and overweight people have more health problems and die younger (Table 7-1). Today we not only diet to control weight but we jog or perform other exercise to encourage weight loss or maintenance by adjusting energy expenditure to calorie intake.

Secondly, there is strong social pressure to be thin, because the current populace esthetics hold that fat is unattractive. The epitomes of American beauty as portrayed in the media are a lithe, beautiful woman and a lean, well-muscled, handsome man. Overweight people are subject to prejudice because they look different. They often feel somewhat outside the mainstream. Being overweight is often uncomfortable: clothes, furniture, and other things don't fit well. It seems that practically everyone wants to be thinner.

TABLE 7-1
Percent of Deaths of Overweight Men and Women from 25 to 75 Years Over Normal Expectancies

Cause of Death	Men	Women
Cardiovascular disease	149	177
Organic heart disease	142	175
Cerebral hemorrhage	159	162
Chronic nephritis	191	212
Liver and gallbladder disease	168	211
Diabetes	383	372

(Data abstracted from Metropolitan Life Insurance tables)

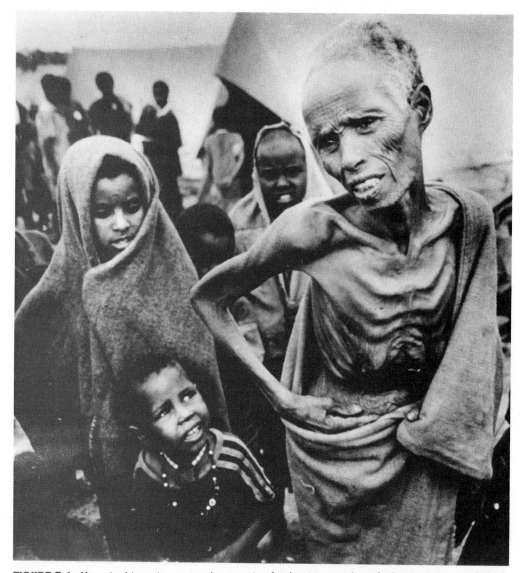

FIGURE 7-1 Many in this nation worry about getting fat, but in a number of other nations, people lack calories to the point of severe emaciation as shown here. The concern of such peoples is not avoiding calories but how to just get enough to survive. *(Miami Herald photo)*

Some people are so afraid of getting fat that they stop eating or limit their intake severely. They are pathologically terrified of gaining weight, even though they may not be a bit overweight in the first place. They diet successfully and lose weight, but when the goal is reached are not satisfied. They are afraid of losing control and re-gaining the lost pounds, so they continue dieting. This pattern can develop into *anorexia nervosa*, a serious disturbance that requires psychiatric care as well as nutritional support.

The typical patient is a teenage girl or young woman who thinks that being thinner would make her more popular or attractive or would otherwise fix what's wrong with her life. The muscles waste away and it is painful to be touched. Sexual development is retarded. The skin turns yellow and its texture is course. The hair is in poor condition. Anemia and low blood pressure and retarded metabolic rate can develop. There are severe sleep disturbances. If malnutrition has progressed too far, the patient can die. What started out as a goal can become a fatal obsession.

There is another equally disturbed and equally dangerous way people try to prevent weight gain, *bulimia nervosa*, or *bulimia*, and again the patients are most often young women. They go on eating binges and then, in remorse and frustration, force themselves to vomit or take large amounts of laxatives to eliminate the food before it can be absorbed. Such people get a special satisfaction from eating but are afraid of becoming fat, so when they eat they feel guilty. Bulimics are addicted to the experience of eating. They can spend a $100 a day on pastries, potato chips, ice cream, and other rich foods. Bulimics become secretive and reclusive, trying to hide their problem. They need psychiatric care, and often the recovery is difficult and prolonged. There may be relapses, when the cycle starts all over, and this upward and downward teeter-totter continues until some patients die. Those who recover can become quite normal adults.

HEREDITY OR ENVIRONMENT?

Some people seem to be able to eat all they want and never gain a pound, whereas others cut back, try to eat less fattening foods, and still gain weight, or at least fail to lose weight. How can this be so? Let us take a quick look at some of the theories about this apparent paradox. The reader can decide which to accept, because no definitive answer exists. When one does, it may be easier to prevent overweight.

Heredity

There is an old saying that fat women have fat babies. There is some truth in this. Studies of families find that overweight often can be traced back generations and that many in the family were fat. Studies of thin families find that that characteristic goes way back, too. A recent study of many sets of siblings who were separated and raised in different families pointed to heredity as a factor in body weight. A significant number of the babies whose biological parents were overweight grew up to be fat themselves, no matter what the eating habits of their foster or adoptive parents, and children of lean natural parents tended to grow up lean.

Environment

Conventional wisdom has it that people gain weight because they do not control their appetite. They eat more than they need. The excess calories become fat. Hence, the remark, "The way to lose weight is to exercise: exercise by pushing yourself away from the table." No doubt some of this is true.

Another theory is that as babies everyone develops fat cells that "learn" to be fat and that the cells, all the rest of that baby's life, exert a demand to be maintained, making the person eat almost compulsively until the fat cells are "satisfied." This theory is supported by some fairly convincing statistics. When babies are overfed and become fat babies, the tendency seems to persist.

Some people think it is good to be fat. They are not numerous in the United States, however. In some less-developed countries fat is a badge of affluence; it proves that this person never wants for food as the emaciated underprivileged people do. They wear fat the way the wealthy in some countries wear jewelry; it reflects their status in life. We also are learning that it is not good to be too thin. For a long time insurance companies' "ideal weight" tables were slanted toward people who were too thin. Now, these tables have been revised, because the studies had sampling defects. It is also considered undesirable today for elderly people to be too thin. If they get ill or must have surgery, they may lack enough energy reserve to see them through (Fig. 7-2).

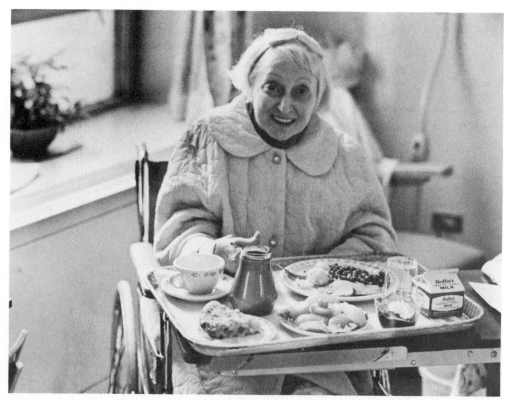

FIGURE 7-2 It is extremely important that the elderly receive adequate food to maintain weight. An elderly person who is allowed to become too lean has no reserves to call upon if a critical illness strikes.

Some people overeat because of anxiety, stress, or social pressure. The satiety and nurturing quality of food is sought. A person who is upset about something and eats a lot is seeking comfort in a full belly.

Other reasons why so many are overweight is because of changes in our eating patterns and the kinds of food available today. We are a snacking nation, and much of this food is high-calorie and low in nutrients. A 10 ounce bowl of chili con carne with six saltines is almost 500 calories, a fourth of what many of us need a day. Have corned-beef hash with a poached egg for breakfast and you've had almost the same number of calories. Much of the food in fast food operations is high in calories.

Another factor in life styles is that we have become less active. Instead of pitching hay, we operate a computer or machinery. We work shorter hours at much less physical work and, so, need fewer calories. We often ride several blocks instead of walking as we used to do and to compensate for this inactivity we jog or take other exercise. We have available many conveniences that save energy, yet we still have the same appetites and want about the same quantity of food.

There are powerful factors at work to stabilize weight. Some people are underweight no matter what they do. Others get fat on very little. Some go up and down. Often the factors causing this are very difficult to control. Some may be hereditary and others, environmental.

If a person is strongwilled enough and wants to change his or her weight, it can be done. It takes stamina, determination, and control, but the rewards are great: better health, improved appearance and attitude.

BODY COMPOSITION

Some people have large frames that carry a lot of muscle (Table 7-2 and Fig. 7-3). Such a person is *not* necessarily fat but may weigh a fair amount. Thus, we often evaluate body composition (proportion of muscle and fat) to see whether a person is overweight. There are several ways to gauge body composition. Sometimes it is obvious that a person has far too much fat by his or her appearance. An overweight person and a lean, muscular person of the same weight will not be the same sizes, because fat takes up more space than muscle per pound.

An easy test is to measure the chest, abdomen, buttocks, and other areas, then look up on a reference chart how the average of these measures compares in lean-to-fat ratio with others of the same height-weight range and sex. We can also perform a "pinch test" using special calipers to pinch a fold of flesh. The calipers exert a standard pressure and give a reading determined from the pressure—fat exerts less pressure than muscle—that tells how much fat the subject has in proportion to muscle. The pinch test is usually done at the midpoint of the back of the upper arm or at the bottom of the angle of the right shoulder blade with the shoulder. A fairly good impression can be gotten using the thumb and index finger to pinch. A soft feel indicates a lot of fat; muscle feels harder. You can get the feel of this by pinching your own body over the abdomen or hips and then over a muscle.

IDEAL WEIGHT AND ENERGY NEEDS

Body size, shape, composition, age, and sex and other factors influence whether a given person meets desirable weight standards. Most Americans exceed it. A few approach it, and far fewer are below ideal weight.

One of the simplest ways to estimate ideal weight is to use height-weight tables (Tables 7-2 and 7-3). Often such tables add five pounds for people with large frames and deduct five pounds for people with small ones. It is said that a person normally reaches ideal weight between the ages of 20 and 25 and that that weight should then be maintained throughout life. In fact, on average, Americans gain about 30 pounds between age 25 and 65.

Women (on average) weigh less than men, because they are generally shorter and usually have smaller frames and because they naturally have a greater proportion of fat than men, and fat weighs less than muscle.

In any weight control program, the name of the game is *calories*. More accurately, the game is *energy balance*. A person who consumes more calories than are needed gains weight; one who consumes less than are needed loses weight. If calorie intake equals energy expenditure, weight remains stable. It sounds simple, but for many people controlling weight takes a lot of will power and knowledge. While some people say that they get fat because they must work around food all the time or they have a glandular problem, 99.9% of the time they simply consume too many calories.

TABLE 7-2
Height-Weight Tables

MEN* Height Feet	Inches	Small Frame	Medium Frame	Large Frame	WOMEN* Height Feet	Inches	Small Frame	Medium Frame	Large Frame
5	2	128-134	131-141	138-150	4	10	102-111	109-121	118-131
5	3	130-136	133-143	140-153	4	11	103-113	111-123	120-134
5	4	132-138	135-145	142-156	5	0	104-115	113-126	122-137
5	5	134-140	137-148	144-160	5	1	106-118	115-129	125-140
5	6	136-142	139-151	146-164	5	2	108-121	118-132	128-143
5	7	138-145	142-154	149-168	5	3	111-124	121-135	131-147
5	8	140-148	145-157	152-172	5	4	114-127	124-138	134-151
5	9	142-151	148-160	155-176	5	5	117-130	127-141	137-155
5	10	144-154	151-163	158-180	5	6	120-133	130-144	140-159
5	11	146-157	154-166	161-184	5	7	123-136	133-147	143-163
6	0	149-160	157-170	164-188	5	8	126-139	136-150	146-167
6	1	152-164	160-174	168-192	5	9	129-142	139-153	149-170
6	2	155-168	164-178	172-197	5	10	132-145	142-156	152-173
6	3	158-172	167-182	176-202	5	11	135-148	145-159	155-176
6	4	162-176	171-187	181-207	6	0	138-151	148-162	158-179

*Measurements assume clothes: height in 1-inch heels, weight of clothes for men, 5 lb.; for women, 3lb.
(Source: Reproduced with permission of Metropolitan Life Insurance Company. Source of basic data: 1979 Build Study, Society of Actuaries and Association of Life Insurance Medical Directors of America, 1980)

TABLE 7-3
Mean Heights and Weights and Recommended Energy Intake[a]

Category	Age (years)	Weight (kg)	(lb)	Height (cm)	(in)	Energy Needs (with range) (kcal)	(kcal range)	(MJ)
Infants	0.0—0.5	6	13	60	24	kg × 115	(95—145)	kg × 0.48
	0.5—1.0	9	20	71	28	kg × 105	(80—135)	kg × 0.44
Children	1—3	13	29	90	35	1300	(900—1800)	5.5
	4—6	20	44	112	44	1700	(1300—2300)	7.1
	7—10	28	62	132	52	2400	(1650—3300)	10.1
Males	11—14	45	99	157	62	2700	(2000—3700)	11.3
	15—18	66	145	176	69	2800	(2500—3300)	12.2
	19—22	70	154	177	70	2900	(2500—3300)	12.2
	23—50	70	154	178	70	2700	(2300—3100)	11.3
	51—75	70	154	178	70	2400	(2000—2800)	10.1
	76+	70	154	178	70	2050	(1500—3000)	9.2
Females	11—14	46	101	157	62	2200	(1500—3000)	9.2
	15—18	55	120	163	64	2100	(1200—3000)	8.8
	19—22	55	120	163	64	2100	(1700—2500)	8.8
	23—50	55	120	163	64	2000	(1600—2400)	8.4
	51—75	55	120	163	64	1800	(1400—2200)	7.6
	76+	55	120	163	64	1600	(1200—2000)	6.7
Pregnancy						+300		
Lactation						+500		

[a] The energy allowance for the young adults are for men and women doing light work. The allowances for the two older age groups represent mean energy needs over these age spans, allowing for a 2-percent decrease in basal (resting) metabolic rate per decade and a reduction in activity of 200 kcal/day for men and women between 51 and 75 years, 500 kcal for men over 75 years, and 400 kcal for women over 75 years. The customary range of daily output is shown in parentheses for adults and is based on a variation in energy needs of ±400 kcal at any one age, emphasizing the wide range of energy intakes appropriate for any group of people.

Energy allowances for children through age 18 are based on median energy intakes of children of these ages followed in longitudinal growth studies. The values in parentheses are 10th and 90th percentiles of energy intake, to indicate the range of energy consumption among children of these ages.

(Source: Recommended Dietary Allowances, 9th ed., Washington, D.C.: National Academy of Sciences—National Research Council, 1980)

Height and body type are important factors (Fig. 7-3). The body of an endomorph is compact and short, the mesomorph has an athletic body, and the ectomorph has a tall, thin body. A body that is compact and short loses fewer calories in body heat than a tall, thin one, which has more exposed body surface. The compact, short body conserves energy.

The number of calories needed varies with age. Babies have the highest demand per kilogram of weight or square meter surface because they grow extremely fast. Table 7-4 shows how the need for calories drops from age three to age 75. The need for calories varies also according to body composition. Women need fewer calories per square meter of body surface, because they have a greater proportion of fat. Women also seem to be more efficient users of calories.

Another important factor in deciding how many calories we need is activity. A person working at a sedentary job needs fewer calories than one working at digging

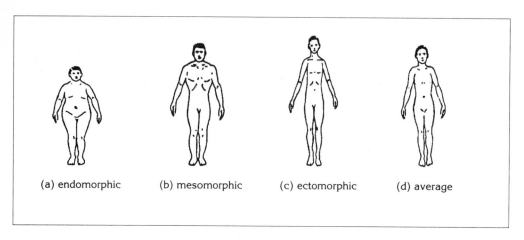

(a) endomorphic   (b) mesomorphic   (c) ectomorphic   (d) average

FIGURE 7-3 The four figures above show typical body types.

ditches (Table 7-5). An athlete during an athletic event can burn up a tremendous amount of energy. This has to be supplied in the diet (Fig. 7-4).

Some hormones affect how many calories a person needs. The hormone thyroxine, made in the thyroid gland, governs the speed at which body cells work. If

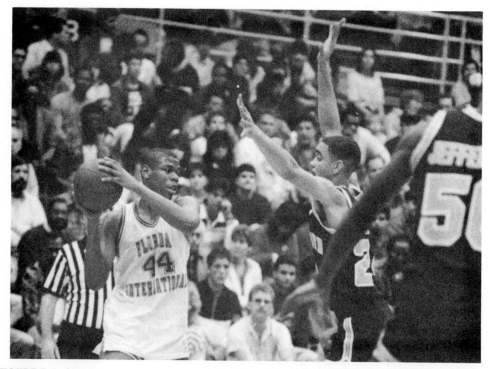

FIGURE 7-4 Strenuous exercise such as basketball takes a lot of calories. It is very important that the right kind of food and the right amounts be consumed to meet the demands of such strenuous exercise. (Courtesy Florida International University)

a person has a high level of thyroxine, the body works faster and uses up energy. Epinephrine, made in the adrenal glands, also governs the speed with which we use energy. If the body produces a lot, the energy need is increased. The amount of thyroxine and epinephrine the body secretes can affect personality. People with a good supply are more active, alert, and aggressive. Often the "hyper" person is one who burns up a great deal of energy.

Body temperature can influence caloric need. A person with a high temperature (fever) uses more

TABLE 7-4
Calorie Needs of Various Ages

Age (years)	Calories per hour per square meter of body surface	
	Males	Females
3	60	54½
8	51	48
16	42	37
20	40	35½
27	38	35
34	37	35
45	36	33¾
55	35	32¾
65	33½	31½
75	32	31

calories. If the room or the weather is cold, more energy is burned to keep the body warm. Finally health or special state in life makes a difference in calorie requirement. Pregnant and lactating women need more calories, as do many patients recovering from surgery, trauma, or illness.

ESTIMATING CALORIE NEED

Laboratory Tests

There are a number of ways to estimate calorie requirements. A complex one is to collect all the carbon dioxide exhaled while a person performs some activity or exercise. From that it is possible to calculate the number of calories burned during such exercise.

Tables

Another way to calculate caloric need is to use tables. Recommended Dietary Allowances (RDA) tables indicate what people of different ages, sexes, and stages of life need. Table 7-3 is a table of this sort.

Mathematical Estimation

A very simple calculation of calorie requirement is to multiply *desired* weight by 18 (for men) or 16 (for women). A man who wants to maintain his weight at 172 pounds would need 3096 calories per day (172 x 18). Reducing that intake by 500 calories a day would result in an average weight loss of approximately one pound per week, since 3500 calories are about equal to a pound of body fat. A 110-pound woman needs 1760 (110 x 16) calories a day to maintain weight. She would have to reduce her calories to 1260 per day to average a pound loss a week. Many physicians feel it is healthiest to lose no more than a pound per week.

Basic Metabolic Rate and Specific Dynamic Action

Several methods of calculating calorie needs fairly accurately are available. Two commonly used methods require that three variables first be determined: basic metabolic rate (BMR), activity need, and specific dynamic action or effect (SDA or SDE).

BMR tells how many calories it takes just to maintain the body at complete rest with no digestion going on. This energy is used to maintain body temperature and keep organs and cells functioning. Typically, BMR is about 1200 calories or more. It is the single greatest calorie need for most persons.

Activity need refers to calories needed for daily activities. It takes calories to walk, sit, run, wash dishes, wait tables, sit and read, and sweep floors. This energy must be supplied by calories. (See Tables 7-5 and 7-6.)

SDA represents the energy expended in digesting and absorbing food. It varies somewhat with the composition of the foods eaten as it takes more energy to utilize fat and protein than carbohydrate. Table 7-7 shows one way of making a BMR-activity-SDA calculation for a 110-pound woman 20 years of age.

Another way to get BMR and SDA is to record time spent in different activities. Multiply the energy cost of the specific activity times the length of time spent in the activity times the body weight of the person participating in the activity. Tables 7-5 and 7-6 show the energy needs of various activities. Thus, if washing dishes for one

TABLE 7-5
Hourly Calorie Expenditure* of Various Activities

Bicycling, 5½ mph	1.4	Paring potatoes	0.3
Bowling	2.0	Personal toilet	0.5
Canoeing, 4 mph	2.8	Playing football	6.0
Classroom work	0.7	Playing piano, moderate	1.4
Crocheting	0.2	Rowing, race	7.3
Cross-country running	4.4	Running, 8½ mph	7.0
Dancing, moderately	1.7	Sawing or chopping wood	2.7
Dancing, vigorously	2.3	Showering	1.1
Dishwashing	1.0	Singing	0.5
Domestic work	1.2	Sitting quietly	0.4
Dressing/undressing	0.9	Skiing, 10 mph (cross-country)	4.0
Driving car	1.0	Sleeping	0.4
Driving motorcycle	1.5	Standing relaxed	0.4
Eating	0.7	Swimming, crawl, 45 yd/min	3.5
Exercise, light	1.0	Tennis	4.5
Exercise, heavy	3.5	Typing	1.0
Gardening	1.5	Volleyball	1.4
Golf	1.7	Walking, 3 mph	1.5
Horseback, walk	0.9	Walking upstairs	6.9
Horseback, trot	1.2	Walking downstairs	2.7
Laundry, light	1.3	Watching TV	0.4
Lying awake	0.4		

* Per pound of body weight data adapted variously from Taylor and Pye: *Foundations of Nutrition*, ed 6. New York, 1967, Macmillan. Consalazio, CF, Johnson, RE, and Pecora, LJ: *Physiological Measurements of Metabolic Functions in Man*, and *USDA/USPHS Dietary Guidelines*.

TABLE 7-6
Estimated Daily Calorie Requirement Based on Activities*

Activity	Cal/lb/hr	Time in Hours	Calorie Requirement
Dressing/undressing	0.9	1	99
Walking (3 mph)	1.5	1½	248
Eating	0.7	1¼	96
Studying and class	0.7	6½	500
Driving car	1.0	1	110
Running (8½ mph)	7.0	1	770
Washing dishes	1.0	½	55
Watching TV	0.4	1	44
Playing piano	1.4	½	77
Typing	1.0	1	110
Light laundry and ironing	1.3	¾	107
Sleeping	0.4	8	352
Total caloric need		24	2568

* Includes BMR and SDA needs, so the result is total caloric need of a 110-lb person.

hour costs 1.0 calories per pound, the energy need for a woman weighing 110 pounds is 1/2 hour x 110 lbs x 1.0 calorie = 55 calories. The values stated in most energy-activity tables, as in Tables 7-5 and 7-6, include both BMR and SDA; otherwise, each must be calculated and the results added together.

PANACEAS FOR WEIGHT LOSS

Many remedies are offered for weight control. Some promise results from wearing a certain kind of amulet or girdle. Many prescribe bizarre diets combined with "medications." Most claims that sound too good to be true are false. You just can't get away from the fact that the best way to control weight is to balance calorie consumption and activity.

Some physicians prescribe amphetamines such as dexedrine and benzedrine. They temporarily curb appetite and may help increase metabolic rate. They perform for a while, but the dieter usually gains back the weight when the appetite returns. Sometimes diuretics ("water pills") are recommended. They rid the body of excess water temporarily, but often there is no excess. And water is not the cause of overweight; fat is. Some so-called diet drugs can be harmful. Starch blockers inhibit the enzymes that digest carbohydrates. The Food and Drug Administration (FDA) banned their sale because they caused nausea, vomiting, diarrhea, and stomach pains and did very little to block the digestion of carbohydrates. Thyroxine can be taken but it is not very effective and can be downright dangerous. Human Chorionic Gonadotropin (HCG) made from a hormone in the urine of pregnant women, has been prescribed by doctors, but the consensus is that it has little effect on weight loss and does not suppress hunger.

TABLE 7-7
One Method to Calculate Calorie Need

Step I: Calculate BMR

Formula: (24 hours × body weight in pounds) ÷ 2.2 lbs = BMR

Example: $\dfrac{24 \text{ hours} \times \text{lb body weight}}{2.2 \text{ lbs}} = \dfrac{24 \times 110 \text{ lb}}{2.2} = 1200$ calories

Step II: Calculate Activity Need

Formula: (a) sedentary activity: if under 76 years) .30 × BMR;
           (if over 76 years); .20 × BMR
       (b) moderate activity: .40 × BMR
       (c) strenuous activity: .50 × BMR

Example: .40 × 1200 =   480 calories

Step III: Calculate SDA

Formula: .10 × BMR

Example .10 × 1200 =   120 calories

Total Calorie Need (1200 + 480 + 120)   1800 calories

Some desperate people have their stomachs made smaller surgically so they feel full after eating less. Another surgical strategy is to bypass a large portion of the small intestine to reduce absorption of food. Some resort to surgical removal of fat, a sort of body facelift. Others have their jaws wired so they can take only a liquid diet. Most such measures are not too successful in the long run, and some are dangerous. Obviously, any surgery carries risks.

Then there is the endless variety of fad diets so widely publicized and promoted (see Chapter 2). Few are effective and trying one after another leads to frustration and despair. Some things show promise. A few drugs work, but they can be dangerous and should be taken only under medical supervision and monitoring. A new fat substitute acts like fat in foods (so it can be used for baking, for example) but lacks fats' calories. In 1988 a news release said the product—a sucrose polyester, more closely related to carbohydrates than fats—was nearing the end of testing and would be marketed in a short time. The Japanese for centuries have used a product called glucomannan, a substance from the konjac tuber, to cause weight loss, though it is now believed that it does little. The search continues because the rewards can be great. So many people want to control calories that an effective and safe product would earn tremendous financial rewards.

FOLLOWING THROUGH

Knowing how many calories should be consumed to gain, lose, or maintain weight is a big step in calorie control, but the hardest part is setting up a program and following it.

Some admonitions about reducing calories to lose weight should be noted. The wrong diet can cause the wrong kind of weight loss because weight is lost from muscle, not fat. This occurs if the diet does not contain enough carbohydrate or enough total energy (calories), and the body utilizes muscle for energy. Carbohydrate is important in a weight reduction diet not only to help burn fat and avoid ketosis but also to spare muscle (protein). Very severe dietary restrictions can cause loss of heart muscle and, in the extreme case, heart arrest.

Another caution is to stay with the diet until the goal is reached and then maintain the new weight. In a weight reduction diet the body tends to "defend itself" by reducing the BMR to compensate for the loss. The result is a point where caloric intake and expenditure are equal and the dieter reaches a plateau in weight loss. Often this BMR slowdown tends to be long-lasting, especially with the frequent dieter, so on any subsequent weight reduction program the calorie reduction must be even more drastic. Such a BMR adjustment can persist until it is extremely difficult to lose weight because the BMR just won't permit it.

Daily Food Plan

A daily food plan is a list of everything a person is going to eat, the sizes of portions and the calorie yield (Table 7-8). It is easy to keep, and many tables are available that indicate the number of calories in a portion.

Diary Method Plan

A Daily Calorie Management Diary is constructed after the fact (Fig. 7-5). It indicates the daily calorie need, the calorie intake plan, what actually was taken in, and the calorie saving. A weight column records original weight, present weight, and desired weight. (Weight should be taken at the same time every day, and about the same kind of clothing, if any, should be worn.) The desired weight is given and then what is still left to be lost. Naturally the date should be noted. Below all this is the foods consumed that day, in this case (Fig. 7-5) by a 28-year old, 5-foot 10-inch male, who leads a sedentary life.

The diary in Figure 7-5 shows that the objective was achieved. Actually, calories might have been underestimated. The potatoes and cabbage were boiled in the corned beef stock and each could have easily picked up a teaspoon of beef fat as it was being dished out. This would add 90 calories. Skimming the fat from the stock before boiling the potatoes and cabbage would eliminate this problem. If a woman were to follow this diet who needed, say, only 1900 calories per day, the milkshake would have to be replaced with a glass of skim milk, no sugar could be added to the iced tea, and the butter might have to go. This would save about 500 calories.

Basic Four Food Plan

Another way to control calories is to follow the Basic Four Food Plan. Table 7-9 gives food selections and information on how they are used. One drawback of the Basic Four Food Plan is that it does not provide calorie counts, so one must estimate. Following the minimum diet with no extras gives about 1200 to 1400 calories a day.

Exchange Method Plan

For reasonable accuracy and simplicity the Exchange Method plan seems to be most desirable. Table 7-10 lists day's intake of approximately 1,200 calories; the intake is based on the Exchange Method. Table 7-11 shows food plans that provide from approximately 1000 to 2000 calories a day along with the number of food exchanges one selects under each. Table 7-12 is a day's menus using 1500 calories. (See also the discussion in Chapter 3.)

ADDING WEIGHT

To add weight requires taking in more calories than one needs, including using fewer calories. Activity usually should not be reduced unless it is causing problems.

TABLE 7-8
Preset Menu for One Day

Food Item	Portion	Calories
Breakfast		
Sliced banana	1 medium	100
Bran flakes	1 cup	105
Milk, skim	½ cup	40
French toast	2 slices	270
Syrup	2 tbsp	120
Coffee, ad lib	—	—
Calories		635
Lunch		
Large tossed salad with one medium tomato	2 cups	45
Low-calorie French dressing	2 tbsp	30
Roll	1	65
Milk, skim	1 cup	80
Cantaloupe	½	60
Calories		280
Dinner		
Tomato juice	½ cup	22
Broiled salmon with lemon wedge	5 ounces	200
Steamed rice	½ cup	112
Carrot, celery, and green pepper strips	10 strips	40
Roll		65
Butter, whipped	1 tsp	25
Fresh pineapple, diced	1 cup	75
Calories		539
Total calories		1454

This points to increasing food consumption, and perhaps, selecting different foods. Fruits and vegetables are low in calories but are vital to good health and nutrition. Increasing fat intake adds calories, but this must be done carefully lest too much fat or the wrong kinds are consumed.

Knowing how many calories various foods contribute can help a person add calories. Often a fairly high-carbohydrate diet with some added fats and other foods to complement them is recommended for weight gain. Adding 500 calories per day over and above those needed should produce a weight gain of a pound a week. As in reducing, there will be plateaus. Sometimes appetite is a limiting factor, so concentrated calories (fats), an extended time-frame, and strength-building exercises need to be part of the program to gain weight.

Daily Calorie Management

Calories/Day
Need _2,200_
Planned _1,700_
Consumed _1,699_
Reduced _501_

Weight
Original _172_
Present _168_
Desired _155_
To go _13_

Date _Mar. 17, 1988_

Foods Consumed Today

Breakfast			Lunch			Dinner		
Item	portion	calories	Item	portion	calories	Item	portion	calories
Orange Juice	½ c	55	Hamburger with condiments and lettuce & tomato		260	Bouillon	1 c.	4
Wheat Flakes	1 c.	105	vanilla shake	2 c.	350	w/spinach noodles	½ c.	50
Milk, skim	½ c.	40	apple	1 med.	80	* Cornbeef, boiled	3 & 3	250
English Muffin	1	65				Potatoes, boiled	1 m.	90
Butter, whipped	1 t.	25				cabbage, boiled	1 c.	30
Jam	1 t.	55				lettuce salad	1 med.	15
Coffee						low cal fr. dressing	1 t.	15
						Raisin Bread	1 sl.	65
						Butter, whipped	1 t.	25
						Pistachio Ice Milk	½ c.	90
						Ice Tea, lemon		
						Sugar	2 t.	30
						* St. Patricks Day Dinner		
		345			690			664

FIGURE 7-5 Daily calorie intake.

TABLE 7-9
One Day's Selection of Foods Meeting the Basic Four Food Plan*

Breakfast	Lunch	Dinner
6 ounces orange juice	Large bowl cream of	Grilled chicken,
¼ cup oatmeal with ½	tomato soup	4 ounce
cup whole milk	Toasted cheese sandwich	Boiled potato with ½
3-ounce slice grilled ham	Coca-cola, 8 ounces	cup sauerkraut
1 slice whole-wheat		Pear Waldorf salad
toast, buttered		2 baking-powder bis-
Black coffee		cuits, 2 pats butter
		Iced tea, lemon slice
		Apple betty

Plan Tabulation

Milk group: ½ cup milk, cream of tomato soup, cheese, and milk in the baking-powder biscuits meet this requirement

Meat group: The ham and the chicken more than meet the requirement

Vegetable-fruit group: Orange juice, tomatoes in the soup, sauerkraut, pear salad, and apple betty more than meet requirements for this group. Vitamin C needs are more than met with the orange juice, tomato soup, and sauerkraut. The diet needs a better source of vitamin A the next day than was obtained in this day's milk and cream of tomato soup.

Cereal group: The oatmeal, toast, sandwich with 2 slices of bread, 2 baking powder biscuits, and crumbs in the apple betty more than meet this requirement.

* Source: Kotschevar, L. H: Quantity Food Production, ed. 4. New York, Van Nostrand Reinhold, 1988.

MAINTAINING WEIGHT

There is no magic formula for maintaining desirable weight. It is merely a matter of matching caloric intake to caloric expenditure by balancing diet and exercise. Monitoring weight daily or at least weekly allows steps to be taken when a change is noted in order to compensate accordingly with diet and activity.

When the desired goal is reached, the old food consumption patterns must be changed permanently. This often is done by behavior modification and following a good dietary maintenance program.

Most people seem to achieve a level of food intake and exercise that maintains weight satisfactorily, and they seldom think about it. Even those who have trouble maintaining a desired weight cultivate habits and patterns that promote calorie control.

TABLE 7-10
Menu Based on the Food Exchange Plan

	Carbohydrate (grams)	Calories
Breakfast		
½ grapefruit	15	60
Poached egg on	7	75
whole-wheat toast,	15	80
with butter, 1 tsp	0	45
Milk, skim, 8 ounces	12	90
Totals	49	350
Lunch		
¼ cup low-fat cottage cheese	12	120
Sliced tomatoes	5	25
6 saltines	15	80
with 1 tsp butter	0	45
½ banana	15	60
Totals	47	280
Dinner		
Chicken fricassee (4-ounce leg, no skin)	28	220
Dumpling	15	80
Green beans, steamed	5	25
Sliced cucumbers in vinegar	5	25
Plain roll	15	80
Strawberries, ¾ cup	15	60
with light cream, 4 tbsp	10	90
Skim milk	12	90
Totals	105	650
Totals for all day	201	1,280

STEPS TO A SUCCESSFUL PROGRAM

Today, with nutrition labeling and other information on food packages it is easier to know the caloric content of foods. Figure 7-6 shows how one large baking company indicates how to control calories by slicing its pound cake to a specific size.

In any food program for managing calories, certain steps must be taken:

1. Know your weight, height, body frame, and your body composition. Know your activity rate and the kind of person you are—whether your metabolism is fast or slow. "Hyper," constantly active people burn calories faster than quieter, more placid ones. Get an idea of your personal calorie needs.

TABLE 7-11
Food Exchanges to Meet Specific Calorie Needs

Exchange Group	Calories per Exchange	Calories per Day									
		1000		1200		1500		1800		2000	
		No. Exch.	No. Cal.	No. Exch.	No. Cal.	No. Exch.	No. Cal.	No. Exch.	No. Cal.	No. Exch.	No. Cal.
Milk, skim	90	2	180	2	180	2	180	2	180	2	180
Vegetable	25	3	75	5	125	6	150	6	150	6	150
Fruit	60	2	120	3	180	4	240	4	240	4	240
Bread, low-fat	80	3	240	4	320	5	400	7	560	8	640
Meat, lean	55	6	330	7	385	8	440	9	495	10	550
Fat	45	2	90	3	135	3	135	5	225	7	315

2. Set up a program, using a method that is easy for you to follow and that will produce results. Several reliable ones have been mentioned here, and there are others. Don't make it such hard work that it becomes onerous and distasteful. Be flexible. Ups and downs, peaks and valleys, are normal, and almost inevitably there will be plateaus, even though you meet your consumption goals. Don't get discouraged. Continue on a steady, even pace. And plan to make changes in your eating habits as plateaus are reached and your body adjusts to reduced food intake.

3. Finally, after reaching the desired goal, remember that you are not through with the program. Food consumption patterns and exercise levels usually must be altered permanently. (The young man of 28 could easily have lost weight by following a much less rigid food plan but increasing activity. A person of that age should not live such a sedentary life that he needs only 2200 calories per day. Just 45 minutes' jogging would burn up 500 calories more.) The best

TABLE 7-12
Food Exchange Selections for a Day
(approximately 1500 calories)

Breakfast	Lunch	Dinner
Baked apple Dry cereal, 1 cup Milk, skim, ½ cup Egg, boiled Toast, 2 slices Butter, 2 tsp Coffee	BLT sandwich Mayonnaise, 1 tbsp Vegetable soup, 1 cup Cottage cheese, low-fat, ½ cup Milk, skim, 1 cup	Broiled grapefruit Broiled salmon, lemon wedge Parsleyed potato Steamed broccoli, ½ cup Roll Butter, 1 tsp Mixed green salad, no-cal dressing Pineapple snow pudding, ½ cup Iced tea, unsweetened

strategy is to develop a program of sensible eating that can be followed routinely and to include a reasonable level of exercise. It enhances physical and mental health. It's worthwhile and so very, very much better than going on a crash diet that might take off weight the wrong way, without changing eating habits.

SUMMARY

People want to control their weight for medical and personal reasons. Sometimes such motivation is healthy, as when it compels a person to choose a sensible weight-control program. Neurotic compulsion to overeat or to lose weight can bring on life-threatening physical disorders.

Difficulty controlling weight may arise from hereditary or environmental factors or a combination of both. Certainly we know that people who have good self-control can reach desired goals by following a good weight control program.

It is advisable in any weight reduction eating plan, to be sure to eat enough carbohydrates (to dispose of the fractions of fat broken off as the body tries to use fat for energy) to avoid developing ketosis, a potentially dangerous condition. Carbohydrate in the diet also obviates the body's breaking down valuable muscle to get the glucose needed to burn fat.

Knowing one's body size, composition, and height help determine ideal weight. There are simple ways to calculate ideal weights, but many weight tables are also available.

Individual calorie need is influenced by body frame size, body composition, age, sex, activity level, endocrine status, and other factors. An assessment of these should be made before it can be determined how many calories a given person must consume to maintain, reduce, or increase weight. There are simple and complex ways to do this. Using simple calculations and consulting tables are probably the most practical methods for most people.

There are also several good, practical, and relatively simple ways to set up a program for controlling calories.

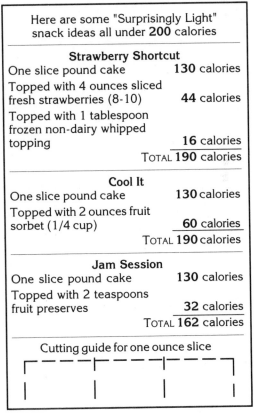

Here are some "Surprisingly Light" snack ideas all under **200** calories

Strawberry Shortcut

One slice pound cake	**130** calories
Topped with 4 ounces sliced fresh strawberries (8-10)	**44** calories
Topped with 1 tablespoon frozen non-dairy whipped topping	**16** calories
TOTAL	**190** calories

Cool It

One slice pound cake	**130** calories
Topped with 2 ounces fruit sorbet (1/4 cup)	**60** calories
TOTAL	**190** calories

Jam Session

One slice pound cake	**130** calories
Topped with 2 teaspoons fruit preserves	**32** calories
TOTAL	**162** calories

Cutting guide for one ounce slice

FIGURE 7-6 Manufacturers of food, aware of a desire of many to hold down calories, are putting more information onto packages. Here, several ways of serving pound cake are given along with a cutting guide to gauge the thickness of a slice of cake that yields 130 calories.

Following the Basic Four Food Plan, or the Exchange Method Plan, or keeping a food diary seem to be the most popular methods.

Someone who needs to gain weight can do so only by increasing calorie intake above what the body needs. Maintaining weight is primarily a matter of balancing calorie consumption and expenditure by adjusting diet, activity level, or preferably both.

The basics of a calorie control program are:

- Know how many calories you should consume.
- Set up a good program and follow it.
- After the goal is reached, maintain it.

Chapter Review

1. Give some of the reasons that people want to control calories and weight.
2. What do *you think* are the causes of overweight?
3. Do you think a person can really control calories to attain a certain weight objective? If so, what is it helpful to know in order to begin a successful weight control program?
4. How can body composition be determined?
5. If you had a 10-pound cube of adipose tissue (fat) and a 10-pound cube of muscle, which would be larger?
6. What is the ideal weight for your height and body frame size?
7. Are you an endomorph, a mesomorph, an ectomorph, or a combination of these? Which is called average?
8. What two hormones affect how many calories we need?
9. Define BMR and SDA.
10. What three types of energy uses make up our total energy need?
11. Which plan would *you* use to set up a weight control program?
12. Set up a three-day reducing program of 1500 calories per day. Show the foods consumed, the approximate number of calories from each, and total calories for each meal and for each day. Does each day's list meet the Basic Four Food Group recommendations?

Chapter 8
Vitamins

Chapter Goals

- To define "vitamin."
- To indicate the nature and importance of vitamins in the diet.
- To discuss the different vitamins, how they contribute to health, and the symptoms of vitamin deficiencies.
- To identify the best food sources of vitamins.

In 1912, a Dr. Casimir Funk found an amine substance that had a remarkable effect in promoting life. He called it a vital amine, or "vitamin" for short. The word became a general term for a group of protein substances that regulate body functions and are essential to good health and the preservation of life.

Today at least 13 vitamins are known and more may yet be discovered. The vitamin family includes fat-soluble ones (A, D, E, and K) and water-soluble ones (thiamine, or B_1, riboflavin, or B_2, niacin, pyridoxine, or B_6, folic acid, or folacin, pantothenic acid, biotin, cobalamin, or B_{12}, and C). As they were discovered, the letters of the alphabet were used to name them, but soon after vitamin B was named, it was discovered to be not one but a group of complex substances with discrete functions. They were named B_1, B_2, and so forth. Some substances first identified as B vitamins were discovered not be vitamins or to be identical to others that already had names. Thus, there are gaps in the vitamin B numbers. Vitamins B_4, and B_8, for instance, do not exist. Most vitamins have a variety of names (Table 8-1), which can make it hard sometimes to recognize a familiar one (e.g., *retinol* is vitamin A). Some are referred to by the disease they prevent or cure (e.g., the *beri-beri vitamin* is thiamine).

A vitamin is an organic substance that is necessary for the normal metabolic functions of the body. To be specific, a vitamin must possess the following characteristics: it must be present in food and be needed in minute amounts. The body cannot manufacture vitamins. Vitamin C is needed in the greatest quantity, 60 milligrams (mg) a day. A milligram is one thousandth of a gram; some vitamins are measured in micrograms (μg), millionths of a gram. In pure form, the complete daily supply of all 13 vitamins is less than one eighth teaspoon. Vitamins are essential in regulating the body; if the body can make enough of it, it is not essential. Thus, it has to come in the diet or from outside the body.

Vitamins work together in various combinations to produce energy. When a vitamin combines with an enzyme, it forms a coenzyme, which acts as a catalyst for reactions in the body. Coenzyme catalysts promote a process but are not involved in the chemical reaction. One can visualize them as spaceships in the body, each designed to attract only specific satellites. When they join onto two or more of the satellites they are designed to attract, they change them, locking them together or breaking them apart. In protein synthesis, the coenzyme may grab onto a carbohydrate chain and tack on a nitrogen atom. Or, they may bring in a phosphate substance and break up a carbohydrate chain into water and carbon dioxide, releasing energy. Vitamins are necessary to metabolism; our bodies would not function without them.

Not all vitamins in food are in usable form; some are present in an inactive form (precursor or provitamin) and must be converted into the active vitamin. Ergosterol is converted to vitamin D when sunlight strikes it in the skin. Carotene in food is converted in the body into Vitamin A. An *antivitamin* is a substance that can take the place of a vitamin in an atom, blocking its action. A substance in egg white neutralizes the action of biotin. Sometimes substances are touted as vitamins that are not. Lipoic acid is a substance in food used to help promote energy, but since the body can make all the lipoic acid it needs, it fails to satisfy the definition of a vitamin (i.e., that the body cannot produce it). Inositol and choline are sometimes called vitamins, but it is not clear whether they are essential, another criterion for being a vitamin. Pegamic acid (B_{15}) and laetrile (B_{17}) have never been proven effective and are not considered vitamins.

Vitamin deficiency is not an uncommon condition in the United States. Vitamins A and C and folic acid are most frequently lacking. Certain metabolic disorders and

TABLE 8-1
Principal and Alternate Names of Vitamins

Water-Soluble Vitamins

B Vitamins	
Thiamine	Vitamin B_1
Riboflavin	Vitamin B_2, lactoflavin
Niacin	Nicotinic acid, nicotinamide, niacinamide
Vitamin B_6	Pyridoxine, pyridoxal, pyridoxamine
Folic acid	Folate, folacin
Vitamin B_{12}	Cobalamin, hydroxocobalamin
Pantothenic acid	Pantoyal-B-alanine
Biotin	None
Vitamin C	Ascorbic acid, antiscorbutic vitamin

Fat-Soluble Vitamins

Vitamin A	Retinol, carotene, dehydroretinol, retinoic acid
Vitamin D	Cholecalciferol, ergocalciferol
Vitamin E	Alpha-tocopherol
Vitamin K	Menaquionone

some drugs cause vitamin deficiency, no matter how much of a vitamin is consumed in foods. Nonbiological causes of vitamin deficiencies could include apathy, unavailability of money with which to buy adequate foods, ignorance of the importance and the food sources of vitamins; and, as people get dependent on foodservices for more of their meals, unavailability of convenient, appealing, vitamin-rich menu choices.

In the discussion below some vitamin deficiency diseases are described, because they illustrate vividly the importance of getting the minuscule required amounts of these substances. While the dramatic symptoms of extreme deficiencies are seldom seen in the U.S., milder deficiency conditions can occur even among the affluent if they eat carelessly. Symptoms of mild deficit may be undiagnosable but may manifest instead as lifelong subtle physical and mental low-optimal health.

FAT-SOLUBLE VITAMINS

Vitamins A, D, E, and K are soluble in fat, and they or their precursors often are present in animal or vegetable fats. As each may have several chemical forms, they might be thought of as several vitamins within a vitamin.

Unlike water-soluble vitamins, which are easily dissolved and excreted from the body, fat-soluble ones can be stored, usually in the liver and adipose tissue. This means that they may not have to be consumed in foods every day if storage supplies are adequate. It is also possible to store too much, which can have toxic effects. Deaths have resulted from overdoses of fat-soluble vitamins taken as supplements.

Vitamin A

Vitamin A comes in two forms. The first is retinol, vitamin A from animal sources. It is found in cream, butterfat, egg yolk, and ocean-fish oils. Authorities recommend that half our intake come from some animal sources and the other half from carotenes, yellow pigments found in fruits such as oranges, cantaloupes, and peaches and in vegetables such as carrots, yellow squash, and leafy green vegetables such as spinach or broccoli. (The green in the green plants hides the yellow or orange carotene.) Carotene is not absorbed or utilized as efficiently as retinol, but it is an important source. We need to take in five units of carotene to equal one unit of retinol. Vitamin A as retinol is essential for maintaining cell health in our eyes. It also produces a substance that helps us see in dim light. An early symptom of vitamin A deficiency is nightblindness. If the deficiency continues too long, permanent damage can occur. Vitamin A also helps us see in regular light. A continued insufficiency finally causes eye inflammation and then a condition called dry-eye—the tear ducts lose their ability to produce moisture, the eye cells begin to harden and an opaque covering called Bitot's spots begins to form over the eyeball. The last stage is blindness. This disease, called *xerophthalmia*, afflicts millions in Third World countries, especially children. The condition of *keratomalacia*, or eye ulcerations, is also related to lack of vitamin A together with a lack of protein.

Vitamin A is involved in bone and tooth development. Vitamin A insufficiency can cause tooth deterioration as well as retarding physical growth and slowing tissue repair. In extreme deficiency states growth of bones is sacrificed to allow growth of body tissues to continue. This may cause the skull and spinal column to stop growing while the brain, teeth, and nerves continue to grow crowding the brain in the skull and the teeth in the jaws and pinching the nerves in the spinal column. The result can be lifelong skeletal and neurologic disorders.

Vitamin A keeps the tissue linings of the respiratory, digestive, and urogenital tracts healthy. Without it, epithelial cells in the linings of these passages are vulnerable to infection. Some think the common cold is partially caused by a lack of the vitamin or a problem in its use.

Vitamin A is also necessary for healthy skin. The skin becomes hard and coarse textured in deficiency states, looking much like permanent goose pimples. These epithelial tissue and skin problems are thought to arise because vitamin A is associated with the production of carbohydrate products that keep the mucous membranes moist and fight off infections. Mucous tissues can deteriorate to the point where severe diarrhea occurs, probably because the intestinal lining has broken down.

If there is not enough vitamin A in the epithelial tissues, the testicles may fail to produce sperm. Vitamin A deficiency in pregnancy may cause miscarriage. Vitamin A is also involved in the manufacture of glycogen and in how the body handles cholesterol.

How Much Vitamin A? A normal adult male who eats a balanced diet of plant and animal foods needs 1000 retinol equivalents (REs) of vitamin A (or 5,000 IUs) per day and a normal woman 800. During pregnancy a woman should add 200 REs, and during lactation, 400 RE. Rapid growth in infants, children, and teenagers can increase the need for vitamin A, but the total need per day is related to body size. An infant under six months needs 420 REs and from six months to three years, 400 REs.

Vitamin A is stored in the liver. Some people can store enough to last a year. The American Medical Association has warned that taking much over 1000 REs a day from animal sources over an extended period can be dangerous. Too much can cause a loss of appetite, drowsiness, diarrhea, dry skin, and hair loss. Too much at one time can be very toxic. Some people take massive doses attempting to overcome colds, acne, sinusitis, or influenza, even to reduce the effects of sunburn, but this can be dangerous without medical monitoring. Following the Basic Four Foods Plan, thus having a good source of the vitamin at least every other day, should satisfy needs.

Food Sources of Vitamin A. Most good sources of vitamin A were listed above. Unfortified skim milk products have little or none, but if they and other low-fat milk products are fortified with vitamin A they can be equivalent to whole milk products. Most vegetable margarines are fortified, and so are common foods such as cereals. Vitamin supplements and diet preparations should be taken judiciously to avoid overdosing on vitamin A.

Vitamin D

Vitamin D is called often the "sunshine vitamin," because it can be made from ergosterol or cholesterol in the skin when ultraviolet rays from sunlight strike them. It is a fat-soluble vitamin sometimes referred to as calciferol, ergocalciferol, or the antirachitic vitamin (because it cures rickets). Active vitamin D is available from some food sources, such as cod liver oil (Fig. 8-1).

Vitamin D's Functions. Mobilizing calcium and phosphorus to build bones and teeth is vitamin D's principal function. Another is to affect the absorption of calcium through the intestinal walls; a lack of vitamin D can cause precious calcium to be excreted in the feces. Vitamin D guards calcium stores in the bones, adding to stores as needed and allowing only so much to be taken out.

Maintaining the blood calcium level is a top priority, because all cells need calcium and the blood carries it. Vitamin D acts as a monitor for each of the three areas in the body from which calcium may be available for the blood: the skeleton, the kidneys, and food in the digestive tract. Vitamin D works to ensure that enough calcium is supplied to the blood, even if it must withdraw it from bones.

A lack of vitamin D causes rickets, a disease of children in which bones fail to calcify, or harden. For this reason, a prominent sign of rickets is bow legs. The child shows a lack of vitality, growth stops, and there is general loss of muscle tone

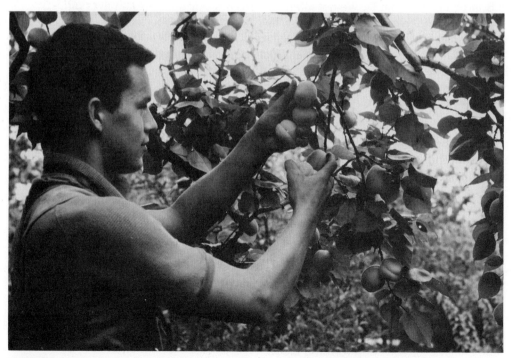

FIGURE 8-1 Any yellow or orange fruit or vegetable or any leafy green vegetable is usually a good source of vitamin A. These apricots provide about 2700 IU per 100 grams (about 3 1/2 ounces). *(USDA photo)*

evidenced by a pot-belly. Tooth decay is rampant. Osteomalacia is adult rickets. Calcium may be withdrawn from the bones, but without enough vitamin D, it is not able to perform, so still more calcium is withdrawn. Meanwhile calcium and phosphorus are not stored effectively and may simply be excreted. Some persons actually shrink in stature and become stoop-shouldered from mineral loss and bone deterioration. The bones become porous and weak and fracture readily. Hearing problems can result as the tiny bones in the inner ear degenerate.

How Much Vitamin D? The Recommended Daily Allowance (RDA) for vitamin D is closely correlated with growth. Infants, children, and adolescents need 10 µg (400 IU) a day. When skeletal growth stops, the need is 7.5 µg (300 IU). The need increases during pregnancy and lactation. An excess can drive up the blood levels of minerals, especially calcium and phosphorus, possibly forcing the body to mine its own bones for these minerals. Symptoms of vitamin D toxicity are intense thirst, vomiting, diarrhea, weight loss, irritability, loss of appetite, high blood calcium, and deposition of calcium in the muscles and even in blood vessel walls or in the body's major artery, the aorta. Eventually death occurs. An overdose from exposure to ultraviolet rays is not possible. Overdose results from abuse of supplements or fortified diet preparations. Certain people who live in an area that has little sun may need to take supplemental vitamin D. Blacks and other dark-skinned people may also benefit by careful food choices, because the sun cannot penetrate the skin readily to make the vitamin.

Food Sources of Vitamin D. We get vitamin D from foods such as fish liver oil, butterfat, egg yolks, and liver. Foods fortified with vitamin D are good sources. Most forms of milk are fortified with 10 µg per quart. Plant foods are such poor sources of vitamin D that fortified milk or soy products are highly recommended for vegetarians and children. Because there is some question as to whether too much vitamin D is being added to foods, the government sets standards and limits.

Vitamin E

The name tocopherol was given to vitamin E because it was once thought to be associated with human fertility. The Greek words "tokos" and "pherin" combined mean "to bear a child." It is important to fertility in rats, but not in humans. The complete role of this vitamin is still not understood, and there is much controversy about what it does. Claims are made for it, from cleaning out the lungs of smokers to enhancing sex drive.

Vitamin E's Functions. Vitamin E is an "antioxidant." It joins easily with oxygen, and in the body picks up stray oxygen that might be harmful. It can prevent oxygen from bonding with (oxidizing) other substances, thus preserving those substances. Vitamin E helps maintain cell membranes, especially those of red blood cells and those in the lung lining, both of which are constantly exposed to oxygen. Some evidence supports the claim that the antioxidant action of vitamin E may offer limited protection against air pollutants in the lungs. Vitamin E is also thought to assist in making some enzymes involved in forming blood.

We have no proof that vitamin E prevents heart attacks or aging. Dr. A. Tappel, professor of nutrition science at the University of California at Davis, who has published over 200 papers on the vitamin, states that although people are "wasting" over $100 million a year on this vitamin as a supplement, it is useless beyond normal intake for curing any of the many disorders that quacks claim it does. A physician with the National Institute of Arthritis, Metabolism, and Digestive Diseases says bluntly, "The evidence is that vitamin E supplements won't do anything for normal people." Still people continue to buy vitamin E supplements and many forms that are applied to the body, such as deodorants, skin creams, hair conditioners, and cosmetics. Claims it cures muscular dystrophy are unproven. It is true that rats fed a diet deficient in vitamin E did develop symptoms similar to those of muscular dystrophy, but no creditable research has linked this to the human disease.

The single proven deficiency condition afflicts premature infants. Most of the vitamin E transfer from the mother takes place in the last few weeks of a normal pregnancy. Premature infants may not have enough vitamin E and can become anemic (deficient in red blood cells) because the unprotected red blood cells rupture. Vitamin E therapy prevents this.

How Much Vitamin E? The RDA for vitamin E increases with body size, with a need of 8 mg for females and 10 mg for males by the mid teens. Another 2 mg should be added during pregnancy and 3 mg for lactation. The need for vitamin E goes up as one's intake of unsaturated oils increases, to prevent their oxidation. The need may also increase where there is considerable air pollution. Because vitamin E is so widespread in foods, deficiency is unlikely. Supplements are recommended only under medical supervision—for premature infants, leg cramps, certain breast lumps, and several nervous system and blood disorders.

Food Sources. Although there are four kinds of vitamin E with varying activity, the one found in vegetable oils seems to be the most useful. Many processed foods containing fats or oils can help supply the vitamin, as can pure vegetable oils. (On some labels it may be called tocopherol.) Vegetable oils contain from 60 to 100 mg per 100 grams. Mayonnaise or margarine made from these oils contains from one half to two thirds the quantity of vitamin E that the pure oils do. Other good sources are green leafy vegetables, butter, liver, fish, whole grain cereals, and eggs. A tablespoon of almost any kind of vegetable oil daily can give us all the vitamin E we need. Usually we get this easily in the foods we eat.

Vitamin K

Without vitamin K, the blood would not clot, so wounds would not heal. Bacteria in our intestines manufacture some vitamin K. It is fat-soluble, but researchers have developed several water-soluble forms that are easier to absorb. These are used in medicines.

Vitamin K's Functions. The main job of vitamin K is to catalyze (cause, aid, or speed up) the formation of at least two proteins required to make the blood thicken and clot when necessary. The liver is thought to take the vitamin and join it to calcium to make the protein prothrombin. Then, after a series of reactions, the prothrombin is turned into fibrin, the key substance in blood clotting. Without this action, hemorrhage or uncontrolled bleeding results that can be fatal. Whether bleeding is external or internal, the blood must first clot to stop bleeding; only then can the healing process begin. Vitamin K is not involved with hemophilia, a genetic condition in which blood fails to clot because other chemical factors are missing. This condition is hereditary rather than a vitamin deficiency.

Sources of Vitamin K. No specific daily requirement has been established for vitamin K. It is plentiful in green, leafy vegetables, egg yolks, liver, and alfalfa sprouts. With what we get in the diet and through manufacture in our digestive tract, a deficiency is rare. Babies at birth may show a lack of vitamin K, in which case it would be administered. Mothers may receive it before birth to prevent hemorrhage. Accident victims who are losing a lot of blood may receive it as therapy. Vitamin K is fat soluble and can be toxic if stored in excess. In fact, as a vitamin supplement, it is available only by prescription.

WATER-SOLUBLE VITAMINS

The nine water-soluble vitamins perform much of their service as coenzymes: like the second key in a double lock, they are absolutely essential for enzyme action. Being water-soluble, they can be absorbed directly from the digestive tract. Each performs its job many times over and then is excreted. Also because they are water-soluble, they are rarely stored for long. The body will pull what it needs from an available pool and use it. Increasing the amounts of water-soluble vitamins into the system through supplementing does not cause the body to use more than needed, but it may upset delicate balances by crowding out nutrients the body needs. Thus, the idea that "taking a lot of vitamins cannot hurt" is faulty. The way some people guzzle supplements has prompted the observation that Americans have the most expensive urine in the world. Water-soluble vitamins should be replenished daily through selecting and consuming a wide variety of foods (Table 8-2).

The B Vitamins

Eight of the 13 known vitamins belong to the vitamin B complex. Collectively, several things can be stated about them: They are fragile, sensitive to high heat (light in some cases), and leach into water easily during cleaning, cooking, or storing. They participate in reactions that make other nutrients available to each of our millions of cells and are essential in the breakdown of the three energy nutrients—carbohydrates, proteins, and fats. They are necessary for the synthesis of proteins. They often are found together in foods and absence of one often means absence of others, causing symptoms of a general deficiency. Traditional foods such as milk, meats, legumes, fresh vegetables, and whole grains are equally good or better sources than products such as desiccated liver pills, brewer's yeast, and bran concoctions. Stress, such as an illness, and certain medicines such as sulfa drugs and hormone preparations, among others, can affect B vitamin production or absorption; these medications should be taken only on medical advice.

TABLE 8-2
Good Sources of Various Water-Soluble Vitamins

Food*	Portion Size	Amount (mg)	Food*	Portion Size	Amount (mg)
Ascorbic Acid			**Riboflavin**		
Orange juice	½ cup	62	Liver, beef, fried	2 ounces	2.35
Grapefruit	½	44	Egg	1	.13
Lemon juice	1 tbsp	4	Hamburger, broiled	3 ounces	.18
Strawberries	1 cup	88	Beef heart, braised	3 ounces	1.04
Cantaloupe	½	63	Lamb roast	3 ounces	.25
Brussels sprouts	½ cup	67	Oysters, raw	½ cup	.17
Spinach	½ cup	25	Milk, whole	1 cup	.41
Cabbage	½ cup	48	Cheddar cheese	1 ounce	.13
Potatoes, baked	1	20	Cottage cheese	½ cup	.30
Broccoli	½ cup	70	Ice cream	½ cup	.14
			White bread, enriched	1 slice	.06
Thiamine			Whole wheat bread	1 slice	.03
Pork roast, lean	2.4 ounces	.24			
Oysters, raw	½ cup	.33			
Liver, beef, fried	2 ounces	2.37	**Niacin**		
Almonds, shelled	½ cup	.17	Beef liver, fried	2 ounces	9.4
Peanuts, shelled	½ cup	.27	Tuna, canned	3½ ounces	12.0
Peas, green	½ cup	.22	Peanut butter	2 tbsp	2.4
Sirloin steak, cooked	6 ounces	.15	Green peas	½ cup	1.9
Lamb roast	4 ounces	.17	Pork roast	3 ounces	4.7
Orange	1 medium	.13	Chicken, broiled	3 ounces	3.7
Whole bread, enriched	1 slice		Whole wheat bread	1 slice	.8
White bread, enriched	1 slice	.06	Bran flakes	1 cup	2.7
Oatmeal, cooked	1 cup	.19	White bread, enriched	1 slice	.6
Rice, cooked, enriched	1 cup	.81			

For the first three B vitamins—B₁, B₂, and niacin—grain products labeled as "enriched" are sources. Grain products, after enrichment, have levels of iron, riboflavin, and niacin that would be equal to levels expected in whole grain products and twice the amount of thiamine.

Thiamine. Thiamine must be available in order for the cells to be supplied with energy. Much of the body's thiamine is in the muscles, where it works with other nutrients, enzymes, and coenzymes to furnish fuel and oxygen to cells. It also helps convert the amino acid tryptophan into niacin. With pyridoxine (B₆), thiamine is thought to help change amino acids into energy.

Thiamine helps make ribose, a five-carbon sugar needed to make ribonucleic acid (RNA) and deoxyribonucleic acid (DNA), two of the substances that direct cell functions and cell replication (division). Thiamine combines with at least 24 enzymes, but what each product does we are still learning. It contributes to good appetite, good muscle tone, and a balanced mental attitude.

Beriberi is the result of thiamine deficiency. The disease is evidenced first by loss of ankle and knee-jerk reflexes. Then muscle pains begin, and there is loss of energy and vitality. Mental problems start, and the deterioration of muscle and nerve functions continue until death occurs. As the disease progresses, acidity of the stomach decreases, in turn reducing the ability to digest thiamine, so the problem gets worse. The cure for beriberi was found when it was observed that Japanese sailors did not get the disease when they consumed whole grains, but did if they ate only polished rice. Decades later it was learned that polishing removed the bran layer from the rice, and the bran contained thiamine, the key to preventing beriberi. Thiamine has been administered to help increase the appetite of patients with anorexia.

How Much Thiamine? The need for thiamine is determined by how much energy is used, so intake should not fall *below* the RDA (.5 mg for every 1000 calories for adults), regardless of calorie intake. Older people use thiamine less efficiently and should maintain an intake of at least one mg per day even if they burn few calories. Alcoholics, pregnant and lactating women, and active persons need more thiamine. It is not stored in appreciable amounts and, so, should be consumed daily. In some cases of fasting, a thiamine supplement may be advisable. There is no evidence of benefit or toxicity from an excess.

Food Sources of Thiamine. Thiamine is found in small amounts in many foods. Pork is relatively high, but all flesh foods contain some. The daily diet should be varied, about 10 servings composed of animal foods, legumes (especially soybeans and peanuts), nuts, whole grain or enriched flour products, cereals, dairy products, leafy greens, and fresh peas and green beans provide enough (Fig. 8-2).

Riboflavin (B_2). Riboflavin was discovered when a fluorescent, yellowish-green film was noticed on the top of whey left from cheese making. It turned out to be a substance that promoted growth. First called vitamin G, it was found to be related to vitamin B and, since vitamin B_1 (thiamine) had been isolated from the B group, it was called vitamin B_2. Later its chemical structure was determined, and it was named riboflavin.

Riboflavin has many jobs joining with enzymes and coenzymes. It helps join hydrogen to oxygen to make water when energy is made. It joins with niacin and thiamine also in making energy, works with pyridoxine (B_6) and thiamine in making niacin from tryptophan, and assists in using amino acids from protein for repair, maintenance, and growth.

How Much Riboflavin? The RDA for riboflavin is 1.2 mg for adult females and 1.6 milligrams for adult males. Pregnant and lactating women need more, and adolescents and infants need more per kg of body weight, because they are growing. Deficiency is uncommon but sometimes occurs in alcoholics. Some riboflavin can be made by intestinal bacteria, which may explain the low incidence of deficiency. Some authorities predict that decreasing consumption of milk and its products may put Americans at risk for riboflavin deficiency.

Food Sources of Riboflavin. Food sources of riboflavin are somewhat limited. Milk and its products are rich sources, but many people consume little or none of these. Meat and eggs, fish, poultry, and other flesh products, especially organ meats, contribute some riboflavin. Leafy, deep green vegetables are a fair source; people who avoid milk and its products and/or meat should eat a lot of these vegetables. Whole grain products are only fair sources, but since several servings often are consumed daily, they can be a significant contribution. Sources include whole grain or enriched rice, hot or cold cereals, pasta products, enriched flours, crackers, and bread products. Some cereals are fortified to provide 100% of the RDA.

Niacin. Niacin is active in three forms: niacin, nicotinic acid (*not* related to the nicotine in tobacco products), and niacinamide. Niacin is unique because it can be consumed preformed as niacin, or it can be made in the body from the essential amino acid tryptophan. It takes 60 mg of tryptophan to make one mg of niacin. Of course, once converted, tryptophan is unavailable as a protein. Though consuming enough tryptophan from protein foods will ensure an adequate supply of niacin, it is recommended that some preformed niacin be consumed as well. Typically, niacin helps form coenzymes which are necessary for releasing energy. It also helps fatty acid production and cell and tissue respiration. The work of one coenzyme as a vasodilator (blood vessel enlarger and relaxer) may counteract high blood pressure. A low niacin level is usually accompanied by low levels of other B vitamins in the

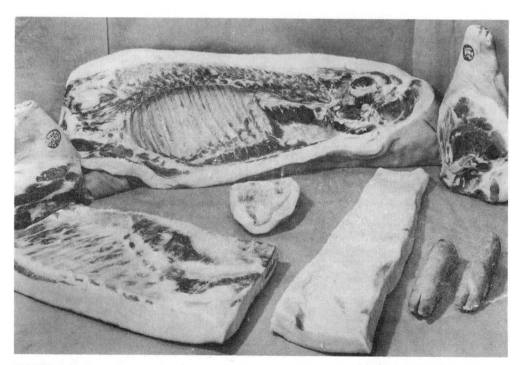

FIGURE 8-2 Meat is an excellent source of B-complex vitamins. Pork is especially high in thiamine. (*USDA photo*)

blood. Amino acid levels may also be low. When niacin is absent, the body cells cannot receive enough energy. That is why the niacin deficiency disease, pellagra, manifests itself in such dramatic and distressing symptoms.

Pellagra often afflicts people whose diet contain little lean meat. At one time in history people ate a diet that consisted largely of salt pork and corn, and many developed pellagra. It was also referred to as the 4 Ds disease for the symptoms— dermatitis (skin inflammation), diarrhea, and dementia (loss of mental powers) and, if untreated, death. Pellagra became widespread during the early part of the 20th century in the American South, because many people ate a diet that consisted largely of the 3 Ms—molasses, maize (corn), and "meat" (really salt pork, which is mostly fat).

Abundant claims have been made that niacin calms the nerves, helps reduce stress reactions, and even cures insanity. None of this has been proven. When niacin was found to reverse the dementia of pellagra, studies were conducted to see whether it benefited persons with other mental disorders, but even megadoses had no effect. The research continues.

How Much Niacin? The RDA for niacin is a generous 13 to 18 mg daily for adults. How much niacin is needed is related to how much energy is generated, since it is so involved in the production of energy. Usually 6.6 mg of niacin is needed for every 1000 calories expended. Although niacin is water soluble, megadoses can be toxic, causing liver damage and peptic ulcers.

Food Sources of Niacin. Recommended sources of niacin are foods that contain it or a goodly amount of tryptophan. Good sources of the vitamin are organ meats and others, tuna, poultry, peanuts, and enriched or whole grain products. While milk and its products contain only a little niacin, they are good sources of tryptophan. Both fresh and dry legumes also contain tryptophan. Because plants provide relatively small amounts of niacin, strict vegetarians should consume abundant quantities of legumes. Ordinary brewed coffee has about 0.1 mg of niacin per six-ounce cup; instant coffee contains about half that. This could be a significant source for persons who drink a lot of coffee.

Pyridoxine (B_6). The principal function of vitamin B_6 when combined with phosphate, is to split apart and put together (metabolize) amino acids. An offshoot of its protein role is as a precursor of the red blood cell protein, heme, a molecule essential for oxygen delivery by the blood. Vitamin B_6 also breaks down glucose to produce energy and is thought to be involved in metabolism of fats, especially unsaturated ones. In another role, it is concerned with the formation of enzymes used in the nervous system and brain. Histamine, a powerful blood vessel dilator and the principal agent in allergic reactions is formed with the aid of B_6. So is serotonin, which is important in transmitting messages along nerves to the brain and stimulates the release of some hormones, B_6 is important in converting tryptophan into niacin. B_6 deficiency is sometimes mistaken for niacin deficiency, since the symptoms are similar.

How Much B_6? The amount of protein metabolized determines how much B_6 is needed. The RDA is from 0.3 mg per day for infants and to 2.0 to 2.2 mg for normal adults. Deficiency may result in the underproduction of blood and of antibodies, which fight off infections.

Food Sources of B_6. Avocados, bananas, and liver are good sources of pyridoxine. Fair sources are meats, fish, poultry, and whole grain cereals. A wide range of vegetables provide a fair supply. There should be no lack with a good diet.

Vitamin B_6 is easily dissolved in water and is sensitive to light, alkalis, and oxygen. Many food processing and preparation procedures destroy it; indeed, half may easily be lost during food processing. People who abuse alcohol or consume a large proportion of their foods in highly processed, or empty calorie, foods can become deficient in vitamin B_6. Enrichment of foods does not supply or replenish this nutrient.

Folic Acid (Folacin). The words folic acid and folacin are related to the word "foliage," because the vitamin is commonly found in the chlorophyll (green pigment) of plants. It may also be called folate or folinic acid. The diets of many Americans do not include adequate amounts of green plant foods and are deficient in folic acid.

Folic acid plays a coenzyme role in supplying the building blocks for nucleic acids, and so is vital for cell division and maintenance. Its job is to ensure constant cell repair and regeneration, a tremendously important function. Folic acid breaks down amino acids and assists in converting them to others: phenylalanine to tyrosine or glycine to serine, for instance. It also can be involved in forming choline, sometimes considered a B vitamin. With vitamin C, folic acid helps make red and white blood cells. Several kinds of anemia (too few red blood cells) are associated with a deficiency of folacin.

How Much Folic Acid? In the 1930s it was learned that folic acid deficiency was associated with anemia, but an RDA was not published until 1968. The normal adult should have 400 μg a day. Newborn babies need only about 30 μg a day, and children, from 100 to 400 μg depending on their age. The RDA increases to 500 a day during lactation but doubles with pregnancy (800 μg) because folic acid is involved in growth.

Pernicious anemia is an anemia evidenced by the production of large red blood cells that is caused by a deficiency or malabsorption of vitamin B_{12} or its cofactor. A high intake of folic acid can mask the early symptoms of pernicious anemia; that is, the telltale large red blood cells may not develop owing to the presence of folic acid though the underlying disease process progresses. This can be a problem for strict vegetarians, who get a great deal of folic acid in vegetables but may get no B_{12} unless they consume animal products.

Most anemias caused by a lack of folic acid are evidenced by an inflamed tongue and intestinal distress with diarrhea. The intestinal malfunction reduces the ability to absorb folic acid, which makes the problem worse. Many categories of over-the-counter and prescription medications interfere with the functioning of folic acid.

Food Sources of Folic Acid. Organ meats, such as liver, are principal sources of this vitamin. Green, leafy vegetables are also an excellent source. Fair sources include the starch vegetables, such as potatoes and lima beans, as well as milk products, eggs, and whole wheat bread. One reason that the Basic Four Foods Plan recommends green leafy vegetables is to ensure enough carotene (vitamin A precursor) and folic acid in the diet. The vulnerability of folic acid to heat underlines the need to consume some fruits and vegetables raw.

Cobalamin (B$_{12}$). The term "cobalamin" is coined from the words "cobalt" and "amine," because it contains both. The fact that raw liver was found to cure pernicious anemia led to the identification of cobalamin. Vitamin B$_{12}$ depends on the cooperation of two components called, respectively, "intrinsic factor" (IF) and extrinsic factor" (EF). IF is a substance normally found in the small intestine. Cobalamin coming into the body in food is EF. They join together in the digestive system and make the "antipernicious anemia factor." Once IF and EF join, they are pulled through the intestinal wall, where the new substance is available to make DNA and RNA, the units that tell cells how to function. If the factor is not absorbed by the gut, the cells don't receive instructions and one of the effects is pernicious (unrelenting) anemia, a condition that was a death sentence until early in this century.

Of the many other functions of cobalamin, two more well-studied ones are its work with folic acid in assisting in the manufacture of healthy red blood cells and its part in maintaining the sheaths (protective coverings) surrounding nerves. A shortage of vitamin B$_{12}$ can result from a dietary lack of EF or from a lack of IF. Defective IF can be inherited, or the body may stop secreting IF adequately in adulthood. When IF is deficient, improving the diet does no good, because the body cannot absorb the cobalamin consumed. Such persons must get B$_{12}$ by injection for the rest of their lives, since they are unable to get it in the intestine.

How Much Cobalamin? The quantity of vitamin B$_{12}$ required daily is minuscule: the three μg RDA for adults would weigh about as much as the ink dotting this "i." Children require slightly less, and pregnant and lactating women an additional microgram. Yet, even this tiny amount is needed to keep us alive. Poor absorption of vitamin B$_{12}$ caused by megadoses of vitamin C, low iron or vitamin B$_6$ intake, and age, etc. can cause failure to absorb cobalamin. Persons whose bodies are secreting IF properly should get adequate B$_{12}$ from one or two portions of animal products per day (which may include milk and eggs).

Food Sources of Cobalamin. No plant food contains cobalamin. Good sources are meats, eggs, and milk and milk products. Some fermented products seem to supply "animal" products in the form of bacteria, including yeast, brewer's yeast, some fermented soy (soy milk) products, and according to some, bacteria in the air. Some whole grain or enriched cereals may be fortified with it. A vegan (strict vegetarian) should plan to use these foods and possibly to take B$_{12}$ supplements to avoid pernicious anemia, particularly pregnant women.

Pantothenic Acid. The word "pantothenic" means "from all sides," indicating that the vitamin is widely available in foods. For this reason, deficiency is unlikely. It is an important constituent of a hard-working coenzyme, coenzyme A, needed to produce energy. Coenzyme A also works to manufacture cholesterol, choline, red blood cells, and steroid hormones, among other tasks, and deficiency is associated with lower levels of vitamin C and cholesterol in the blood. Pantothenic acid is needed for growth, normal skin, tissue health, and good functioning of the nervous system.

How Much Pantothenic Acid? No requirement has been established for the vitamin. A normal adult diet contains about 10 to 15 mg per day.

Food Sources of Pantothenic Acid. Organ meats are rich in the vitamin; whole grain cereals and egg yolks are also good sources. A pint of milk provides 1.6 mg. About 50% of the pantothenic acid in grain is estimated to be lost in milling. Freezing and canning take a toll, because it is heat sensitive. In a varied diet, especially one including unprocessed foods, no shortages seem evident.

Biotin. The intestines can make enough biotin to satisfy the needs of most individuals, so deficiency is unusual. The word "biotin" comes from the Greek word "bios," life. Like several other B vitamins, biotin helps change fats, carbohydrates, and proteins into energy. It also forms a coenzyme that can add carbon dioxide to a carbon chain, especially fatty acid chains, or take it away. In addition, it appears able to change amino acid forms and to aid in making niacin from tryptophan.

How Much Biotin? There is no recommended level of intake for biotin. Deficiency is rare, because it is made in the body and is readily available in many foods. The average diet provides 150 to 300 mg, and 150 mg is considered enough for an adult. Antibiotic therapy can kill the intestinal bacteria that manufactures biotin and cause a temporary disruption in the supply. Raw egg white contains a substance called avidin that renders biotin unabsorbable, but few people eat much raw egg white. Heating egg white destroys avidin.

Food Sources of Biotin. Good food sources include organ meats, legumes, nuts, yeast, egg yolks, and tomatoes. Milk, meat, grains, and many vegetables and fruits contain it as well.

Vitamin C

Vitamin C is also called ascorbic acid, "ascorbic" meaning "without scurvy," the dreaded vitamin C deficiency disease that killed thousands of people as late as the 1700s. Vitamin C is also called the "antiscorbutic vitamin." It is water soluble, but is not a member of the vitamin B group.

Ascorbic acid helps form collagen, the substance that binds together tissues such as skin, bones, and muscles. Collagen is first deposited to build supporting structures for calcium and phosphorus that form bones and teeth. Collagen is needed for wounds to heal; old wounds can break apart if both vitamin C and protein are lacking. Collagen is sometimes called the intercellular cement because of its strengthening and binding role. It prevents rupturing or bruising of capillary walls, helps build strong bones, and aids in healing broken bones. In a similar way, vitamin C works with minerals to maintain strong and disease-resistant teeth and gums.

Scurvy was a common disease during winter months in medieval Europe, when fruits and vegetables were in short supply. Several terrible plagues took place that wiped out large numbers of people. During hard winters, cereals, too, were in short supply, and the poor had to eat bread made from moldy rye, which contains coumarin, a substance that destroys the ability of vitamin K to clot blood. In scurvy the blood vessels are brittle from lack of collagen, and they rupture easily, causing bleeding. The combination of fragile blood vessels and blood that would not clot killed thousands. Scurvy is often called the "sailor's disease," because on long voyages, half or more of the sailors might die from it. The accounts of explorers of the time are filled with the terrible hardships and death brought on by the disease. Scurvy manifests as generalized weakness, easy bruising, shortness of breath, loss of appetite, tenderness in the legs, infection and bleeding in the gums, and swelling of the tissues. Later, nosebleeds are common, along with loosening of the teeth and then internal hemorrhaging. Death usually results from cardiac failure. As little as five to 10 mg per day of ascorbic acid can prevent scurvy.

Because scurvy was such a handicap to British naval power, James Lind, a ship's surgeon, set about to find a cure. In 1747 he discovered that eating citrus fruit not only prevented scurvy but cured it. It took a long time for British brass to understand the importance of his discovery, but in 1789 all ships of His Majesty's Navy were ordered to issue daily rations of citrus fruit, often limes. This not only got rid of the dreaded malady, but earned British sailors the nickname, "limey." Although it was known that something in certain foods cured scurvy, it was not until 1933 that Drs. King and Waugh in Pittsburgh, and Dr. Szent-Gyorgyi of Hungary discovered the actual vitamin. Szent-Gyorgyi described it in more detail, winning the Nobel prize for chemistry that year.

Like vitamin E, vitamin C is an antioxidant. It protects water-soluble substances from being destroyed by oxygen. We can see the effect of this when we sprinkle lemon juice over cut apple or banana slices: they are protected temporarily from oxidation, which would ordinarily cause them to turn brown. Vitamin C also activates folic acid, so without vitamin C, folic acid would not be able to do its work. Vitamin C is necessary to convert iron in food into a form the body can absorb; ascorbic acid influences the formation of hemoglobin, the iron-binding protein in red blood cells, and aids in maintaining iron supplies. Thus, a shortage of iron or folic acid may actually be caused by vitamin C deficiency. Other vitamins with which vitamin C is involved include A, B, and E. Researchers call this relationship a "sparing effect," meaning that the availability of sufficient vitamin C may allow the body to use less of the others. Vitamin C is involved in many metabolic reactions in changing amino acids to different substances. Although we do not know the mechanism, vitamin C also may function to protect us against infections and bacterial poisons.

How Much Vitamin C? If one listens to some authorities, any amount from 45 to 10,000 mg per day is a requirement. The RDA is 60 mg for adults, 80 for pregnant women, and 100 for lactating women. Five to 10 mg per day prevents scurvy. Burn and surgical patients may need quite high doses because a great deal of collagen is needed to promote healing. More vitamin C may be needed by persons under stress.

Interestingly, although it is water soluble, taking megadoses of vitamin C has had negative effects, one of which seems to be lowered resistance to infection. Other claims made for vitamin C are that it aids in reducing the effects of allergies, rheumatism, and aging, and that it may help alleviate schizophrenia and help cure ulcers. These claims have meager support.

It has been claimed that megadoses of vitamin C can cure the common cold or help prevent it and can even help ward off cancer. Claims for other benefits have also been made. Some studies seem to give partial qualified support to some claims about colds but not for cancer. However, some evidence exists to indicate heavy doses can result in adverse reactions, some of them serious. The FDA has said that "The best answer seems to be wait and see." Better studies must be completed before anything authoritative can be said for megadoses of vitamin C.

Food Sources of Vitamin C. Good sources of vitamin C are citrus fruits, tomatoes, cantaloupes, berries, leafy greens, green peppers, cabbage and sauerkraut, potatoes and fleshy tropical fruits (but not bananas). Little or no ascorbic acid is found in dry legumes, meat, fish, poultry, eggs, cheese, cereals, fats and oils, and sugar. Milk has only a small amount, but it is well utilized by the body (Fig. 8-3).

SUMMARY

Vitamins are substances in food that the body needs to function but needs only in tiny quantities, which maintain health, promote growth, and are critical in supplying energy to cells although they themselves do not supply energy. Without vitamins, these functions could not take place; life could not go on, even in the presence of plenty of calories from the energy nutrients. Vitamins do not become a part of the processes they facilitate. Thus, vitamins perform or catalyze countless functions that keep the body operating. Once a biochemical reaction takes place, the vitamins move on to work on another. Soon they are exhausted, however, requiring the body to get more from foods. Although some vitamins are converted within the body from vitamin precursors, by definition, they are essential in that the body cannot create them but must obtain them, or their precursors, from food.

Most vitamins do not work alone but together with minerals, enzymes, or other body substances. There are 13 known vitamins, and scientists continue to search for more. We do not yet know all the functions vitamins perform and assist in.

Vitamins are classified as fat soluble and water soluble. The fat-soluble group includes vitamins A, D, E, and K. Because they can be stored by the body to some extent, it is sufficient to get them from food sources every second day. The water-soluble vitamins include vitamins C, and eight B vitamins: thiamine (B_1), riboflavin (B_2, niacin (B_3), pyridoxine (B_6), folacin, cobalamin (B_{12}), pantothenic acid, and biotin. Because they dissolve readily in liquids, two matters are particularly important: it is recommended that many be consumed daily, and food sources must be conscientiously stored and handled to preserve the vitamins. Table 8-3 provides a summary of the vitamins, featuring the principal food sources of each, RDAs, main functions, and consequences of deficiency.

The term enriched, as defined by law, means specifically that processed grain products so labeled contain supplemental riboflavin, niacin, and iron equal to the levels expected in whole grain products and that thiamine has been added at twice its expected original level.

Evidence does not support theories that taking megadoses of different vitamins benefits healthy persons. The body takes only as much as it needs from any available vitamin. Excess intake of fat-soluble vitamins (and surprisingly, also for certain water-soluble vitamins) from supplements or dietary preparations can have toxic effects.

TABLE 8-3
Vitamin Summary

Vitamin Name	Selected Food Sources	Adult RDA	Selected Functions	Effects of Deficiency
Vitamin A	Vitamin A-fortified products, liver, egg yolk,	Males: 1000 RE or 5000 IU Females: 800 RE or 4000 IU	Dim light vision, maintain epithelial tissues Promotes growth	Night blindness, xerophthalmia, keratinization of eyes, stunted growth
Carotenes (alpha, beta, gamma)	Provitamin A in sweet potatoes, carrots, winter squash, cantaloupe, dark leafy greens	Low levels are not uncommon in U.S.		
Vitamin D	Vitamin D-fortified products, Fish (liver oil), Milkfat products, Egg yolk, Liver	Males: 5 ug Female: 5 ug Excess can cause mineral loss	Make calcium and phosphorous available to cells and facilitate their absorption; assists in regulating level of calcium stores in bones	Rickets in children, osteomalacia in adults in combination with other dietary deficiencies
Vitamin E Tocopherol (alpha, beta, gamma)	Vegetable oils (except coconut), dark green leafy vegetables, some sea fish	Males: 10 mg Females: 8 mg	Acts as an antioxidant for unsaturated fats and for vitamins A and C	There is seldom a lack in adult diets
Vitamin K	Dark green leafy vegetables, alfalfa sprouts, egg yolks, liver	None set; deficiency unlikely	Necessary for clotting of blood	None in healthy adults
Vitamin B_1 (Thiamine)	Meat, whole and enriched grains, legumes, milk and its products	Males: 1.4 mg Females: 1.0 mg (or 0.5 mg per 1000 calories) Seniors: 1 mg	Assists in energy release for cell use Helps change tryptophan to niacin Essential in nucleic acid functions (genes)	Beri-beri
Vitamin B_2 (Riboflavin)	Milk products, deep greens (leafy vegetables), meat (esp. liver), whole and enriched grains	Males: 1.6 mg Females: 1.2 mg	Assists in energy release for cell action Joins in changing tryptophan to niacin	Ariboflavinosis
Niacin	Meat (esp. liver), poultry, greens (broccoli, peas), whole and enriched grain products, peanuts	Males: 18 mg Females: 13 mg Need 60:1 ratio of plant form, tryptophan	Assist in energy release Vital to tissue respiration Joins in amino acid synthesis	Pellegra

TABLE 8-3 (continued)
Vitamin Summary

Vitamin Name	Selected Food Sources	Adult RDA	Selected Functions	Effects of Deficiency
Vitamin B$_6$	Organ meats and others, avocados, bananas, whole grains	Males: 2.2 mg Females: 2.0 mg	Active in amino acid and gluose metabolism Involved in forming hemoglobin and hormones Helps convert tryptophan to niacin	
Folic acid (Folacin)	Organ meats, deep green leafy vegetables, mushrooms, starchy vegetables, milk	Males: 400 ug Females: 400 ug RDA doubles in pregnancy	A nucleic acid building block Builds cell strength Active in amino acid metabolism	Anemias (can mask Vitamin B$_{12}$ deficiency)
Vitamin B$_{12}$ (Cobalamin)	Animal foods, some fermented soy products (soy milk)	Males: 3 ug Females: 3 ug Vegetarians may need supplementation	With folic acid, builds cell strength Helps protect nerve fibers Involved in building nucleic acids	Pernicious anemia
Pantothenic Acid	Organ meats, whole grains, egg yolks, (widely available)	None established	Required in energy cycle Helps form cholesterol and some hormones Active in manufacture of hemoglobin	Uncommon
Biotin	Organ meats and others, egg yolks, legumes, yeast, whole grains, many fruits and vegetables	None established	Assists in energy release Involved in fatty acid and amino acid metabolism Helps convert tryptophan to niacin	Uncommon
Vitamin C (Ascorbic acid)	Citrus fruits, tomatoes, berries, cantaloupe and fleshy tropical fruits, cabbage-family vegetables, potatoes	Males: 60 mg Females: 60 mg	Helps form collagen (intracellular cement) Forms durable capillaries Promotes mineral use in building strong teeth and bones Serves as antitoxidant Functions against infections	Scurvy

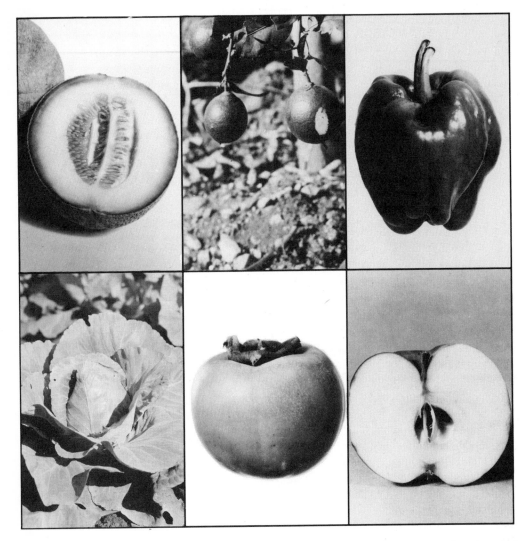

FIGURE 8-3 Which of the following: cabbage, lime, cantaloupe, green pepper, tomato and apple would be a good source of vitamin C and which would not? *(USDA photos)*

Chapter Review

1. What is a vitamin? Why are they considered *essential*?
2. On what basis are vitamins named? On what basis are RDA values stated?
3. What is a provitamin or precursor? What is an antivitamin?
4. Why doesn't everyone require the same amounts of vitamins? Check an RDA table to get a clue to the answer.
5. Can there be any harm in taking an excess of vitamins "just to be sure"?

6. List the fat-soluble vitamins and indicate their functions. Check this and add any main function you omitted.
7. Indicate how much of each of the fat-soluble vitamins normal adults need.
8. How are bones and teeth formed? What is osteomalacia?
9. List some good sources of fat-soluble vitamins.
10. Give some history of the discovery of the B vitamins.
11. What does thiamine do? How much is needed in relation to the number of calories in the diet?
12. What are some good sources of thiamine?

13. What functions does riboflavin perform in the body? How much does an adult need daily? What are some good sources?
14. Niacin can be made from what amino acid? What is the ratio used to calculate how much niacin is produced? How much niacin does an adult need daily?
15. What does niacin do in the body? What are some good sources?
16. What are the jobs of pyridoxine? In what foods is it found?
17. Folic acid is important for what reason? In what foods is it found?
18. Biotin performs what jobs in the body?
19. Cobalamin must be produced from an intrinsic and an extrinsic factor. Explain how this works.
20. What is the meaning of the name "ascorbic acid"?
21. What functions does vitamin C perform?
22. Give the pros and cons in the debate over whether megadoses of vitamin C can cure or prevent colds and other infections.
23. What are some good sources of vitamin C?
24. How much ascorbic acid does the average adult need per day?
25. How does vitamin C function in wound healing? In making bones and teeth?
26. Vitamins A and C and folic acid frequently are lacking in the diets of Americans. What foods alone supply two or all three of these vitamins? Describe an appealing entree, side dish, and salad each of which contains all three.
27. What is the definition of the term "enriched" when used on a food label? What types of foods are enriched? Why?

Chapter 9
Water and Minerals

Chapter Goals

- To discuss the importance of water in the diet and how the body uses it.
- To describe sources of water and how it is lost from the body.
- To describe the problems of ensuring safe, potable water.
- To indicate the body's need for water.
- To specify what minerals the body needs, in what amounts and the best sources.
- To present the basic concepts of how minerals build and regulate the body.
- To describe how minerals become electrolytes and how electrolytes function in the body.
- To list the benefits and toxicities of minerals.

WATER

Water is absolutely essential to life. A person can survive weeks without food but no more than a few days without water. It is no wonder that civilizations flourish around the world's sources of pure, plentiful water.

Our bodies are about 60% water by weight. The loss of 10% of this water (dehydration) can cause illness. A 20% loss is usually fatal. About 3 to 6% of the body water is replaced each day. The body can generate about 6% of what it needs every day, so 94% must be taken in in food and beverages.

Water seldom works alone; usually it facilitates physiological functions. It regulates body temperature: Perspiring and the evaporation of perspiration from the skin cool the body by taking heat to evaporate the moisture. Water is the medium of many body processes. The regulatory functions depend on surrounding fluid to carry nutrients to the cells, and the water in joint fluid allows smooth, low-friction movement. Water transports other substances in the body—nutrients and oxygen to the cells and wastes to be eliminated. Water gives uniform strength, shape, and cushioning to the cells. A dehydrated cell collapses for lack of such support, so, in one way, water may be considered the skeleton of the cell. Water-based body fluids cushion vital organs and the spinal cord and cradle a developing fetus. Some water contains needed minerals, especially fluorine, chlorine, calcium, magnesium, and sodium (depending on geographic area and water treatment practices). It can also contain contaminants.

Water in the Body

Intake and excretion of water must remain balanced. The average adult must have the equivalent of six to 10 cups of water per day (about two liters). The kidneys can conserve or eliminate water to achieve a balance. Water is also lost by evaporation of sweat, exhalation of breath from the lungs, and sometimes from diarrhea, vomiting, or fever. A built-in mechanism signals thirst and regulates the sodium balance (Fig. 9-1). In some older people this thirst mechanism is faulty, so they must be reminded to drink water and doctors often advise ill patients, "Get plenty of rest and fluids." Sweating profusely increases the need to drink water.

Salty foods cause the body to hold onto water; when salts are lacking in the body, fluid is lost. The hormone aldosterone regulates this fluid balance. Some substances can trigger a fluid loss. We call them diuretics. Caffeine in coffee is one (Fig. 9-1).

FLUID SODIUM STATUS	ALDERESTERONE BALANCING SODIUM
This Situation ⟶ ⟶ ⟶	*Needs this to Restore Balance*
Too much sodium	Trigger thirst; we become thirsty
Relatively low	
amount of water	Do not conserve sodium
Not enough sodium	Not thirsty
Relatively high	
amount of water	Conserve sodium

FIGURE 9-1 The levels of body fluid and of sodium are tied to one another. If the level of sodium is low, the fluid volume is too; if the level of sodium is high, so is fluid volume. The adrenal gland hormone aldosterone regulates the sodium level. When salt and fluid are not in balance, excess fluid leaks from the blood vessels and cells producing puffiness, or swelling, of tissues engorged with water. Some foods contain considerable salt such as bouillon, and the kidneys may have to use much water to get rid of this extra salt. Coffee, for instance, also acts as a diuretic, causing the body to expel more fluid.

In measuring fluid intake, soup, tea, coffee, milk, and dishes that are quite moist are considered, as well as plain drinking water. Even solid foods contain water (see Table 9-1). Burning energy in the body produces water—which is used in various bodily processes.

Minerals and Our Water Supply

Modern population concentration patterns and huge industrial centers make it harder to keep water resources safe. Chemical herbicides, pesticides, and fertilizers add to pollution. Some of our water requires triple recycling (cleaning and sanitizing) to be potable. In some places like the Ohio and Mississippi River drainage areas, community after community takes water from the rivers and dumps in its waste, which the next community downriver picks up and reuses. The lowest part of the Colorado River now contains water that has such high levels of dissolved salts of one kind or another that it is hardly fit for drinking and cannot be used for irrigation. Unless steps are taken to lessen the buildup of mineral and other substances in our water, we may find ourselves with a national crisis (Fig. 9-2).

TABLE 9-1
Water Content of a Variety of Foods and Beverages

Food	Percent Water	Food	Percent Water
Meat, Poultry, Seafood		Bread, whole wheat or white	36
Chicken, skinned, broiled	71	Corn flakes, plain (no milk)	4
Swordfish, broiled	65	Fruits and Vegetables	
Tuna, canned in oil, drained	61	Broccoli, cooked	91
Chicken with skin, broiled	58	Soup, minestrone	90
Beef, lean roast, cooked	57	Orange, peeled, raw	86
Beef, lean and fat roast,		Potato, baked	80
cooked	40	Raisins, seedless	18
Dairy Products		Fats and Oils	
Milk, fluid, lowfat (2%)	87	Margarine or butter, soft,	
Cheese, cottage, uncreamed	79	whipped, or stick	16
Cheese, cheddar	37	Vegetable oil	0
Other Protein Foods		Other Beverages	
Eggs, whole (shelled)	74	Beer, regular	92
Beans, dried, cooked	69	Cola, regular	90
Peanut butter	2	Spirits, 80-proof, (gin, run,	
Grain and Grain Products		vodka, whiskey)	67
Macaroni, spaghetti or rice,			
cooked tender	72		

In some areas the water is described as "hard" or "soft" because of the minerals it does or does not contain. Some water is slightly tinged by organic matter, but usually it is potable. Water may contain beneficial substances such as fluorine and calcium.

The delicate nature of water and the water content of foods suggest some guidelines for quality inspection, storage, handling, cooking, and service of foods. Water evaporates readily during open storage and cooking. Appropriate wrapping or covering can maintain food quality. Evaporation in cooking can also cause shrinkage and loss of nutrient quality. Maintaining moisture in food during cooking often is a must if the product is to be good. Water expands in freezing and ice crystals in food can rupture cell walls causing loss of moisture, flavor, and texture. Refreezing or poor freezer temperature control can compound such losses.

Chlorine is often added to municipal water to kill harmful microbes. Though concentrated chlorine gas is a poison, the body needs it to operate. Hydrochloric acid is secreted in the stomach.

Fluorine is also added to some municipal water supplies because it strengthens tooth enamel and prevents tooth decay. Some persons inveigh against adding fluorine and chlorine to drinking water, feeling that they are harmful. The scientific evidence seems to support the assertion that fluorine in the amounts added does much good. The argument against the addition of chlorine is a little stronger: there is some evidence that it may be harmful in the amounts added to some water supplies, though the destruction of harmful bacteria far outweighs what is presently known of the undesirable effects, so it continues to be used in the smallest amounts that are practical. Efforts to protect the water supply from harmful bacteria and other pollutants must be redoubled so that less chlorination is necessary.

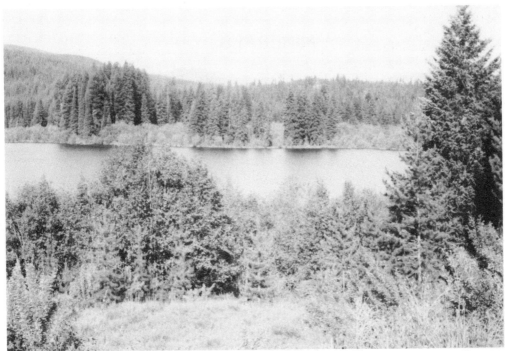

FIGURE 9-2 A remote mountain reservoir such as this one can provide a vast amount of potable water for a large urban area. It is important that it be protected and that its water not be contaminated after it leaves the reservoir.

Sodium often occurs naturally in water in the form of carbonates, sodium chloride (table salt), and others. Soft water can be high in sodium, whereas hard water contains greater levels of calcium and magnesium. Washing with soft water takes less soap or detergent because hard water salts combine chemically with soap or detergent, rendering them useless for cleaning. Soft water seems to clean better; hard water can leave a gray cast to linens and a build-up of crusty crystalline deposits around tubs and faucets and in cookware. However, studies support the claim that persons who consume hard water over a long period have a better health record, probably because of the beneficial chemicals they get from water. Soft water can leach toxic metals such as cadmium and lead from water pipes.

Water Softening

In foodservice work, hard water can be hard to work with. It can give a bad taste to products, produce poor cleaning, and damage equipment, so many foodservices use various treatments to overcome these problems.

For dishwashing, water can be softened by circulating it through sodium chloride (table salt) a process that replaces the hard water minerals with those that produce soft water, at the same time adding sodium to the water. Such water should not be used by persons who need to reduce sodium intake. Offering such drinks as mineral water, spring water, and seltzer, which guests perceive to be more healthful or pleasant, may be well accepted. In Europe many operations routinely serve mineral water.

TABLE 9-2
Percentages of Some Minerals in the Human Body

Mineral	Percent of Body Weight
Macrominerals	
Calcium (Ca)	1.5 to 2.2
Phosphorous (P)	0.8 to 1.2
Potassium (K)	0.35
Sulfur (S)	0.25
Chlorine (Ch)	0.15
Magnesium (Mg)	0.05
Microminerals	
Iron (Fe)	0.004
Manganese (Mn)	0.0003
Copper (Cu)	0.00015
Iodine (I)	0.00004
Trace Minerals	
Cobalt (Co)	Trace
Zinc (Zn)	Trace
Fluorine	Trace
Chromium	Trace
Strontium	Trace
Miscellaneous Trace Minerals	
Nickel (Ni)	Trace
Selenium (Se)	Trace
Tin (Sn)	Trace
Lead (Pb)	Trace
Silicon (Si)	Trace
Mercury (Hg)	Trace
Aluminum (Al)	Trace
Cadmium (Cd)	Trace
Titanium (Ti)	Trace
Others	Trace

MINERALS

Essential minerals together comprise about 4% of body weight. Selected minerals are plotted in Table 9-2 to show the amounts of each in the body, and the quantity contrasts, from thousands of grams to thousandths (milligrams - mg). The commercial value of those in an adult's body is slightly under $2, but without these minerals, we could not live.

Minerals are the part of food that remains as ash or residue after food is burned. Unlike vitamins and the energy nutrients, minerals are not destroyed in nature, they simply cycle as elemental atoms or chemical compounds through water and soil to plants and animals, and the food chain cycle continues. Although minerals do not disappear from the face of the earth, they can be lost from our diet by careless handling of foods, such as discarding cooking liquids or trimming and carving foods in wasteful ways.

Table 9-3 lists the macro and trace minerals in human beings and what we know about their bodily levels. Macrominerals are ones of which we require more than 100 mg daily; each also occurs in the body in amounts greater than 5 grams (1 teaspoon). Elements of which we need less than 100 mg daily are called trace minerals, trace elements, or sometimes microminerals. Though, taken together, the microminerals in the body would total less than a teaspoon, they are just as crucial as the major minerals. Over twenty minerals are believed to be essential, and human requirements for additional minerals are uncertain. Researchers are unsure whether these other minerals are necessary to body functions, or whether they just happen to get into the body from the environment. Table 9-3 also points out that six minerals are listed on the regular RDA chart and nine more have "estimated safe and adequate daily dietary intakes" listed as ranges on the supplemental table.

The Functions of Minerals

Major roles of minerals are outlined in Table 9-4. Some minerals work together in combination, but each has its own jobs to do as well. Minerals are integrally involved in body metabolism.

TABLE 9-3
Major Minerals and Trace Minerals of Interest in Food for Humans

Intake Status	Major Minerals	Trace Minerals	
Have "Recommended Dietary Allowance" (RDA)	Calcium Magnesium Phosphorus	Iodine Iron Zinc	
Have "Estimated Safe and Adequate Intake" as daily range guide	Chlorine Potassium Sodium	Chromium Copper Fluorine	Manganese Molybdenum Selenium
Believed to be essential: no recommendations	Sulfur	Cobalt Nickel Silicon	Tin Vanadium
Always or sometimes present in humans; health roles and requirements unclear		Aluminum Arsenic Barium Boron	Cadmium Lead Mercury Silver

Building. Minerals are involved in building body cells. Bones and teeth are largely calcium and phosphorus. Soft tissues (blood, muscle, organs, and glands) contain minerals, as do hormones, enzymes, and other substances that help regulate the body. DNA and RNA, the genetic material, depend on minerals for their structure. The body stores minerals in bones, eyes, muscles and other areas so they are available when the body needs them.

Regulating. Minerals often regulate the pace and processes of tissue development and upkeep as well as the rate of metabolism. The mineral iodine is a very significant part of the hormone thyroxine, which regulates the speed at which body processes occur. Minerals also help maintain the body's acid-base balance. Calcium is required to help release energy to contract muscles; cobalt is a part of vitamin B_{12} (cobalamin), which helps produce blood cells; with potassium, sodium transmits

TABLE 9-4
Major Functions of Minerals

Regulating Functions: e.g., electrolyte and other chemical reactions	Building Functions: e.g., maintain, repair, develop (including during growth and pregnancy)
Governing hormones, e.g., thyroid activity	Bones and teeth
Activating and stimulating, e.g., clotting of blood	Soft tissues, blood, organs, glands
Nerve responses, and muscle control, e.g., maintaining regular heartbeat	Mineral bank (stores in bones, eyes, etc.)
Acid-base balance of body fluids, and fluid electrolyte balance, e.g., osmosis, diffusion, absorption	Certain regulating substances (hormones, enzymes, etc.)
Transporting, e.g., carrying oxygen from lungs to tissues	Genetic material (DNA, RNA)

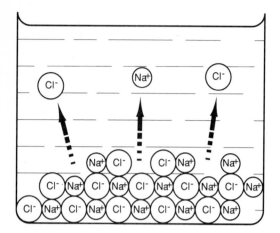

FIGURE 9-3 As salt dissolves in water it dissociates (separates) into sodium (NA+) and chloride (Cl-) ions. Each positive and negative ion is now capable of being chemically active.

signals for muscle responses; minerals control shifts in body fluid levels and foster nutrient absorption; iron enables the blood to transport oxygen.

Electrolytes. Mineral elements have electrical charges that cause them to bond to others to form compounds. Thus, table salt—sodium chloride—is made up of a sodium atom (Na+) with a positive charge and a chloride atom that is negatively charged (Cl-). The positive and negative charges attract each other creating a chemical bond. When table salt is added to water, the sodium and chloride split apart and regain their positive or negative electrical charges (Figure 9-3). Atoms with electrical charges are called ions. The principal ions that participate in multiple chemical reactions in the body are known as electrolytes; their electrical charges control those reactions. Either ion is free to bond with the electrolytes of other substances to make new compounds. Thus, a hydrogen ion (H+) joins with a chloride ion (Cl-) to make hydrochloric acid, a component of gastric juice. An amino acid is made up of a negative amino unit (NH_2) and a positive, long chain of carbon, hydrogen, and oxygen atoms. Soap is the product of bonding a fatty acid and sodium. Compounds that have a positive charge are called acids and those with a negative charge are alkalies, or bases. The strength of an acidic or basic electrolyte has much to do with how chemically active it is. It all depends on how much of a compound dissociates (separates into electrolytes) in water. Sodium chloride separates readily and is quite active chemically. In the body sodium is a strong base. When hydrochloric acid (H+ and Cl-) dissociates, there are always equal numbers of negative and positive charges. Also, some elements or compounds acting as electrolytes can carry one, two or more electrical charges of the same kind. Thus, oxygen which has two negative electrical charges joins with two positive hydrogen charges to make water (H_2O). Sulfur with four positive charges (++++) joins with two oxygen, each with two negative charges (--), to make sulfur dioxide SO_2.

Some elements can increase or decrease their electrical charge. By doing so, iron

A $\begin{matrix} H+ \\ H+ \end{matrix}$ with O = H_2O (water)

B S++++ with $\begin{matrix} O-- \\ O-- \end{matrix}$ = SO_2 (sulfur dioxide)

C Fe$\begin{matrix} O \\ O \end{matrix}$ with O = Fe—O $\begin{matrix} O \\ O \end{matrix}$ (ferrous oxide to ferric oxide)

FIGURE 9-4 (A), Two hydrogen ions join with one atom of oxygen to make water (B), Two oxygen atoms join with one sulfur to make sulfur dioxide (C), Ferrous dioxide changes its electrical charge to become ferric oxide, picking up one oxygen atom in the lungs.

helps to pick up oxygen in the lungs and carry it to the body where it is used for energy or other purposes. The electrolyte change in iron is from its ferrous state ($Fe++$) to its ferric state ($Fe+++$). Thus, when the blood reaches the lungs, iron changes from ++ to +++ state and this enables it to pick up an extra oxygen going from FeO_2 to FeO_3. When the blood is ready to give up its oxygen in the body, it changes FeO_3 to FeO_2 and the oxygen is deposited where it is needed. The FeO_2 is then free to repeat the process. Other important shifts occur in the body so we can function. Figure 9-4 shows some of these electrolyte changes.

Minerals use their electrical charges to maintain a proper acid-base balance in the body, which is crucial, for instance, in maintaining the proper balance of water inside and outside cells (Table 9-5). If too much acid forms in the body, alkaline electrolytes can be called upon to neutralize them and vice versa. Proteins help to do this because they are amphoteric (i.e., they can act as an acid or as a base).

Electrolytes also work to pull substances with the opposite charge into or out of a cell. Thus, potassium (+) pulls in negative charges like chloride that the cell needs. Negatively charged waste products are pulled out then by sodium (+). This is the way cells are able to function, or respire. The process of pulling things through the cell wall is *osmosis*. Figure 9-5 shows how increasing the concentration of potassium inside the cell pulls negatively charged ions away from sodium, but how sodium increases its concentration outside the cell and pulls negative particles through the cell wall so they can be carried away.

TABLE 9-5
Activities and Teamwork of Three Balancing Minerals

	Sodium	Chloride	Potassium
Where They Work	Outside the body cells in intracellular fluid	Both inside and outside the cells: cross cell membranes	Inside all body cells
Main Teammate	Chloride as sodium chloride (salt)	Both sodium and potassium (also alone)	Chloride, as potassium chloride
Acid or Base?	Base for fluids outside cells	Acid for blood and body fluids (chlorine shift)	Base for interior of cells. Works with kidneys
Water Pressure (Osmosis) Balance	For fluids outside cells	Balances fluid pressure on both sides of cell wall	For interior of all cells
Neuromuscular Signals	Works with potassium; relaxes muscles		Works with sodium (e.g., regulate heartbeat)
Using Nutrients	Aids absorption of sugar and protein	Component of stomach's hydrochloric acid; co-digests starch	Helps store glycogen and proteins' nitrogen

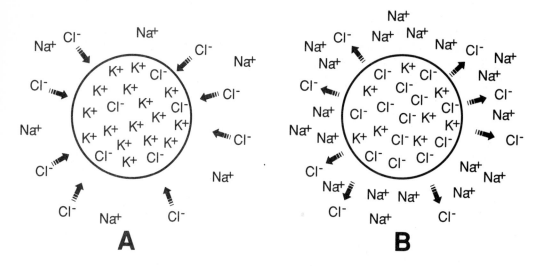

FIGURE 9-5 (A) Concentrated potassium (K+) *within* the cell has more power to pull the chlorine ions away from than the fewer sodium (Na+) electrolytes outside the cell. (B) The greater number of sodium (NA+) ions outside the cell overpower the potassium (K+) ions inside the cell so the sodium ions win this one. The movement of electrolytes through the cell walls is called *osmosis*.

Mineral ions (electrolytes) have the ability to pick up and pass on electrical charges, which capacity makes it possible for them to transmit nerve impulses at lightning speed in nerves and brain and to flex or relax muscles, impulses that are triggered by electricity.

MACROMINERALS

Calcium

The body has as much calcium by weight as it has of all the other minerals combined. An adult has two to three pounds of it, about 2% of body weight. Of this amount nearly 98% is in the bones, another 1% is in the teeth, and 1% more is in the soft tissues, including body fluids.

Functions of Calcium. The main job of calcium is to build bones and teeth. An earth metal, calcium is only a bit harder than lead, but when it combines with other minerals, it becomes very hard and strong. This provides us with a solid skeleton, and strong teeth with which we can chew tough foods.

The body uses the bones as storage depots for calcium required by the blood and soft tissues. The blood has first rights to the calcium. If too much calcium is withdrawn, the bones become porous, fragile, and liable to fracture. One such condition is *osteoporosis*.

In osteoporosis, weakened, calcium-poor bones fracture and vertebrae collapse, making the spine—and the person—shorter. Persons with severe osteoporosis can break a bone while lying in bed. Vitamin, mineral, and hormone treatments can sometimes strengthen the terribly fragile bones. While osteoporosis and other conditions of bone weakness such as *osteomalacia* (soft bones) and rickets do not appear to be *caused* solely by calcium deficiency, they seem to be linked with inadequate storage of calcium with other nutrients during the years of bone development.

The osmotic pull of calcium (a base) moves fluids in and out of cells. It also works constantly to contract muscles. Potassium, magnesium, and sodium team up to stimulate the nerve impulses that relax muscles. Calcium deficiency can cause muscle spasms, or even convulsions. Because the heart is a muscle, its functioning relies on calcium. If it lacks calcium, it may beat irregularly, which is a serious problem. The diaphragm, which controls breathing, may also malfunction if calcium is lacking.

Calcium combines in cell membranes with lecithin to permit substances to pass in and out. Blood that lacks calcium can fail to clot. Through a series of reactions involving calcium and vitamin K, blood turns from a liquid to a gel: actually a substance called thromboplastin changes to fibrin.

Calcium participates in a process that forms milk into curds in the stomach with the enzyme renin. This helps keep the milk in the stomach so it can be partially digested.

The Utilization of Calcium. The RDAs for calcium are 360 to 540 mg for infants; 800 mg for children; 1200 mg for fast-growing adolescents; and 800 mg for adults. A woman's need increases by 50% during pregnancy or lactation to 1200 mg. Normally the body absorbs only 30% of the calcium in foods, but it can absorb as much as 60% when it needs more and there is not much calcium in the digestive juices. Even though the diet is high in calcium, absorption may be poor. Vitamins C and D must be present for good absorption of calcium, as must protein and phosphorus. Available fluorine promotes the use of calcium in building strong bones and teeth. Children and adolescents who get adequate amounts of fluorine seem able to retain calcium and phosphorus better in bones and teeth and to build stronger cells. The tendency to develop osteoporosis and related problems in old age is reduced if fluorine is present in the growth years of life.

The ratio of calcium to phosphorus in the digestive juices also affects calcium utilization. A ratio of 1:1 is desirable, but up to 1:2 is all right. Too much phosphorus in the diet can cause a loss of calcium, especially in older people. Some researchers are concerned that our liberal intake of phosphorus in soft drinks may be contributing to early calcium loss. By taking in large amounts of phosphorus in the absence of calcium, the body may attempt to balance this phosphorus with hard-won calcium, causing the body then to excrete both because fluid levels are too high, resulting in undesirable calcium loss. A high protein diet is also associated with a greater requirement for calcium, as it is excreted during protein digestion. Persons who eat few animal products need less calcium.

Calcium Sources. Milk and its products, such as cheese, yogurt, and ice cream, are good calcium sources. An 8-ounce glass of milk provides 290 mg of calcium. Two glasses, as called for in the Four Food Groups Plan, gives 580, about three fourths of a day's requirement of 800 mg. Molasses and canned fish with bones soft enough to eat (e.g., salmon) are good sources. Leafy green vegetables, broccoli, citrus fruit, legumes, meats, and whole or enriched grains are fair sources. Many dishes made with milk or its products are fair sources (Fig. 9-6), and hard water may contain calcium. (See also Table 9-6.) Sources for trace minerals can be found in Table 9-12.

There is calcium in food additives such as calcium propionate, a bread dough conditioner, and in some leavening agents. Soybean curd (tofu) is precipitated by adding calcium chloride (plaster of Paris). Hominy is produced by soaking corn in calcium hydroxide (lye).

Foodservices can find many ways to use milk or milk products in menu offerings. Instead of diluting a cream soup or hot chocolate with water, dilute with milk. Half and half contains more calcium than artificial whitener products. Real cheese can replace filled products since the latter often provide less calcium.

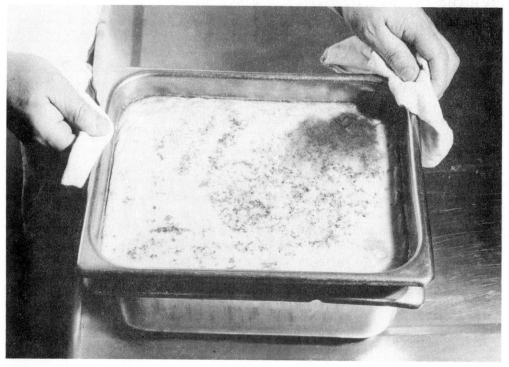

FIGURE 9-6 This custard, which is rich in milk, is a good source of calcium. The eggs help to bind the milk to make a firm clabber and provide iron and other valuable nutrients.

Phosphorus

A Greek word meaning "light bearer" gave phosphorus its name. The mineral fluoresces with a greenish glow. This can be seen on a bright moonlit night when the phosphorus in the ocean waves gives them an eerie sparkle as they crash ashore. About 1% of total body weight is phosphorus, and around 90% is in bones and teeth. Most of the remainder is in the muscles. A tiny amount remains to conduct a wide array of tasks in the cells.

The Functions of Phosphorus. Sometimes phosphorus is called the metabolic twin of calcium, since the two minerals work so closely together. Both also are found in many of the same food sources; and their RDAs are virtually the same. Each is regulated by parathyroid hormone in association with vitamin D, and both must be present at once to build bones and teeth.

Phosphorus alone performs several tasks. It combines with fat to form *phospholipids*, in which fat is transported in the body. It is involved in metabolic reactions as part of DNA and RNA molecules and as part of the energy storage molecules known as ADP and ATP. It helps break down fat to allow absorption and better use of glucose. Finally, it contributes to the body's buffer system in the form of phosphoric acid and phosphate (a base).

The Utilization and Sources of Phosphorus. Only about 10% of the phosphorus in the diet is absorbed. Antacid medications can cause the bones to lose considerable amounts of phosphorus, and taking high doses of supplemental calcium, aluminum, or iron, easily can block absorption of phosphorus.

TABLE 9-6
Food Sources of Essential Minerals

Major Minerals	Meat, Poultry and Fish	Eggs	Milk and Milk Products	Whole Grains	Leafy Vegetables	Fruits, Nonleafy Vegetables and Legumes	Other Products
Calcium	In fish eaten with bones	Yolk	Yes	Yes	Yes	Nuts, citrus, fruit, legumes	Hard water, food additives
Chlorine	Some	Some	Some	Some	Some	Some	Table salt (sodium chloride)
Magnesium	Yes	Some	Yes	Yes	Yes (raw)	Bananas, legumes, nuts, seeds	Medicines, chocolate, cocoa
Phosphorus	Yes	Yolk	Yes	Yes	—	Legumes, nuts	Cola, processed foods
Potassium	Yes	Some	Some	Yes	—	Oranges, bananas, legumes, potatoes	Coffee, tea, cocoa
Sodium	Some	Some	Some	—	Spinach	Beets, celery, carrots, artichokes	Table salt, sodium additives
Sulfur	Yes, especially beef and clams	—	—	Wheat germ	—	—	Legumes

Meat, fish, poultry, milk, eggs, and cheese are good phosphorus sources, as are grains and legumes. Most fruits and vegetables are not good sources, but because they may be a substantial part of the diet, collectively they may contribute significant amounts. All plant and animal foods supply some phosphorus: in plants, it tends to be in the seeds, whereas calcium is available from the leaves.

It is not difficult to get enough phosphorus if milk is consumed as recommended in the Four Food Groups Plan. A glass of milk contains about the same amount of phosphorus as calcium, and the meats and cereals recommended in this plan, along with the vegetables, contribute the rest. A diet that contains enough protein or calcium usually has enough phosphorus.

Potassium

The third most plentiful mineral in the body is potassium: it represents less than 0.5% of total body weight. The name derives from potash, to which it is related. Like its close relative sodium, potassium is a good electrical conductor, which makes it a good electrolyte, furnishing electrical charges.

Potassium teams up with the mineral chlorine inside the cell. It is found throughout the body in the intracellular (inside) fluid and in lean body tissue. In the common form of potassium chloride, it functions inside cells to exert osmotic pressure, balancing the pressure from sodium chloride outside the cell wall in the extracellular fluid. The body cells use potassium to pull in fluids and nutrients, whereas sodium pulls moisture and wastes out. The potassium content of the healthy body is fairly stable, since so much is locked in cells. Potassium also works with the kidneys to maintain the acid-base balance.

Along with sodium and calcium, potassium helps complete the circuit for neuromuscular transmission, or the sending of nerve signals from the nerves to muscles. This function is particularly crucial in heart rhythm. Even small changes in the serum potassium level can lead to serious heartbeat irregularities. Potassium is even at work in the digestive process. It is essential to the storage of glycogen and of nitrogen in the protein of muscle and other cells.

No RDA has been established for potassium, but the "safe and adequate" range is 1875 to 5625 mg. It is so plentiful in foods that there is little chance of deficiency. A condition of too little serum potassium is called hypokalemia, which can result from prolonged vomiting and diarrhea, which cause loss of electrolytes. Severe hypokalemia can be fatal. Abusers of diuretics or laxatives (e.g., bulimics) are at risk, as are those with anorexia nervosa. Diuretics, which stimulate secretion of large volumes of urine, may cause the body to excrete too much potassium. If the sodium-potassium ratio is unbalanced, muscle may harden. The result can be an increase in blood pressure because arteries also harden.

Potassium is found in a broad range of foods. Good sources are legumes, fruits such as oranges, bananas, and dried fruits, potatoes, avocados, meats, peanuts, bran, and whole grain cereals. Fair sources are molasses, tea, cocoa, coffee, and other fruits and vegetables. There is rarely a shortage in a diet that includes a wide variety of foods.

Sulfur

Sulfur is a nonmetallic mineral present in all protein as a constituent of three amino acids: cystine, cysteine, and methionine. An adult male has about six ounces of sulfur in his body. Sulfur in the amino acid molecule considerably changes the nature of the amino acid. Whether serving as a spiral of DNA, as a hard thumbnail substance or as a complex enzyme, sulfur's ability to form sturdy protein units makes possible durable structures, such as hair and nails. Amino acids lacking sulfur lack such hardiness. No deficiencies are known, so there is no recommended intake. Sulfur is found widely in animal and plant foods.

Sodium

Many years ago the Chinese knew that when the pulse intensified, health problems often followed. They also knew salt was involved; they said, "Salt makes the pulse hard." Wise in the knowledge of medicinal herbs, they concocted a brew from plant leaves that reduced the "hardness." Centuries later western medicine rediscovered high blood pressure, or *hypertension*, and formulated drugs to reduce it. They contain the same substances as the ancient Chinese folk medicine!

For centuries civilization has valued salt. Once it was so scarce and valued that it was used as money. The words "salary" and "sale" derive from "salarius," Latin for "salt." Salt was valued because it heightened the flavor of foods and—more important—could be used to preserve food. The salt mines of Salzburg ("City of Salt"), Germany made it an important trading center in the Middle Ages.

Like so many things in life, too much salt is harmful to most people. It can be a factor in causing high blood pressure, or hypertension. This can lead to heart attacks, strokes, and kidney disease.

What Is Hypertension? Hypertension is another word we use for high blood pressure. "Hyper" means an excess and "tension" means pressure. About 20% of Americans have hypertension—45% of those 45 to 55 years of age. This high rate correlates well with salt intake. In Japan in areas where people consume a lot of sodium in fish, seafood, and sea vegetables, 80% of adult men have high blood pressure. We can similarly go around the world and find such correlation; a high intake of sodium usually means a high incidence of hypertension and a low intake means few, if any, have it.

How Much Sodium? A lot of dietary sodium comes from table salt, which is 40% sodium. (Chlorine makes up the other 60%.) Thus, if we consume a teaspoon of salt a day, or five grams, we are getting two grams of sodium ($5 \times .40 = 2$). A taste for salt is an acquired one. Many people are "hooked" on salt; as the habit grows, some develop an almost insatiable craving. No food as served contains enough and they salt food liberally even before tasting it.

A normal adult readily tolerates about 2000 mg of sodium (2 grams) per day, which is 1 teaspoon of table salt, although the actual need is 400 mg, the extra being there for food palatability. Table 9-7 lists the sodium in some foods that are unprocessed and unsalted. The sodium is absorbed naturally as the food grows.

TABLE 9-7
The Amount of Sodium Found Naturally in Foods

Food	Portion	Sodium (mg)
Artichoke	1	43
Avocado	1	11
Beans, white, cooked	1 cup	18
Beef, broiled	3 1/2 oz	60
Beets, cooked	1 c	43
Bluefish, broiled	3 1/2 oz	104
Broccoli, cooked	1 c	28
Cabbage, cooked	1 c	20
Cantaloupe	1/2	47
Carrots, cooked	1 c	48
Cauliflower, cooked	1 c	11
Celery, cooked	1 c	177
Chard, raw	1 c	245
Chicken, roasted	3 1/2 oz	64
Clams, raw	3 1/2 oz	115
Cocoa	1 oz	77
Cod, broiled	3 1/2 oz	110
Cream, coffee	1 tbsp	7
Cucumber	1 med	17
Flounder, baked	3 1/2 oz	237
Haddock, fried	3 1/2 oz	177
Halibut, broiled	3 1/2 oz	134
Kale, cooked	1 c	48
Lamb, roasted	3 1/2 oz	70
Lettuce, iceberg	1 head	41
Liver, beef, fried	3 1/2 oz	184
Mango	1 small	10
Milk, whole	1 c	122
Onion, raw	1 med	11
Oysters, raw	1 c	176
Peas, fresh, cooked	1 c	2
Pike, walleye, raw	3 1/2 oz	51
Pork, roasted	3 1/2 oz	65
Potatoes, raw	1 med	5
Raisins, pressed down	1 c	45
Salmon, Chinook, raw	3 1/2 oz	45
Scallops, steamed	3 1/2 oz	265
Shrimp, raw	3 1/2 oz	140
Snapper, raw	3 1/2 oz	67
Spinach, cooked	1 c	91
Spinach, raw	1 c	40
Turkey, roasted	3 1/2 oz	90
Turnips, raw	1 c	72
Veal, broiled	3 1/2 oz	80

Source: Eat Smart, Random House, Inc., New York, 1984.

Some authorities say that the average person gets about one third of dietary sodium from salt added to foods in cooking and at the table, one third from salt added to foods in processing, and one third from sodium that is part of natural foods. Table 9-8 lists the amount of sodium in some foods, both prepared and natural. Not all sodium comes from food. There are many other sources: *monosodium* glutamate, carbonated beverages (sodas), common antacids and related remedies, baking soda and baking powder, effervescent headache remedies, and a host of others. Drinking water can contain sodium, especially water softened by using the sodium in common table salt to replace hard water salts in our drinking water. The American Heart Association recommends that the amount of sodium in public water supplies be limited to 20 mg per liter; that level now is exceeded in the water supplied to over half the U.S. population.

Hypertension Causes. It bears emphasizing that sodium is not the only believed *cause* of hypertension. It is often a factor and an influential one. Some people are believed to inherit a sensitivity to sodium, but it also can develop over time if there is too much sodium in the diet. Such sensitivity increases blood pressure. Some people who get plenty of sodium suffer no harm.

Obese people are more susceptible to the effects of sodium. If they lose weight, they often lose their sensitivity and also their hypertension. Obese persons tend to have great aldosterone activity; aldosterone is a hormone that regulates sodium excretion and fluid intake by stimulating thirst. In obese people this increased hormone activity can tend to retain sodium in their bodies (Fig. 9-1).

TABLE 9-8
Sodium Countdown

Food item	Measure	Sodium (mg)
Common Fast food Recipes		
Chicken, fried	3-piece dinner	2285
Hamburger	1 large	1500
English muffin, fried egg, cheese, bacon	1 sandwich	914
Pie, apple,	1 piece	382
Milkshake, chocolate	1 medium	306
Potato chips	14 (1 ounce)	230
Mustard	1 tbsp	212
Ketchup	1 tbsp	154
French fries	Medium portion	113
Other Food and Beverage Products		
Salt, table	1 tsp	2000
Dill pickle	1 large	1450
Soy sauce	1 tbsp	1000
Monosodium glutamate ("Accent")	1 tsp	315
Salad dressing, Italian	1 tbsp	315
Drinking water	1 cup	0—75
Beer	12 ounces	200
Animal Products, (Except Milk)		
Sausage or lunchmeat	3 ounces	1100
Crab, steamed	3 ounces	840
Ham, boneless	3 ounces	840
Tuna, salmon, or sardines, canned	3 ounces	800
Bacon	2 strips	250
Flounder, cooked	3 ounces	200
Beef, fish, or poultry; fresh, cooked	3 ounces	75
Egg, chicken	1 large	54
Grain and Legume Products		
Beans, baked, recipe, canned	3/4 cup	600
Saltines	10 each	430
Quick bread (muffin) baking soda	1 medium	400
Corn flakes, plain	1 ounce	282
Bread, white, yeast	1 slice	150
Hot cereal, rice, pasta	1 cup	10
Legumes, cooked	3/4 cup	0
Puffed cereal (wheat, rice)	1 ounce	0
Bread, white, yeast, low-sodium	1 slice	0
Vegetables and Fruit		
Sauerkraut	1/2 cup	550
Olives, green, pickled	5 large	463
Peas, canned	3/4 cup	450
Banana, fresh	1 medium	405
Celery, fresh	1 cup, diced	151
Apple, fresh	1 medium	95
Potato, boiled, or baked	3 ounces	2
Peas, green, fresh	3/4 cup	0
Dairy Products		
Cheese, American, processed	1 ounce	400
Milk, cows, whole	1 cup	120
Butter or margarine	1 tsp	50

One of every three blacks over 18 in the U.S. has high blood pressure. There may be several reasons. Blacks as a group tend to live under more stress; they often face disadvantages economically, socially, politically, and otherwise. An interesting fact is that the blacker the skin, the greater the susceptibility to hypertension. Predisposition to hypertension may be an inherited characteristic. One theory holds that black peoples evolved in interior areas where there was little or no salt and, over eons, their kidneys learned to conserve it. Salt-sparing was also necessary because in such hot climates much was lost in sweat. Today though this function is now detrimental, the kidneys still work to retain sodium. As is often said, we are living in a modern world in millions-of-years'-old bodies. We also know that as people age, many tend to develop high blood pressure.

Certain dietary factors besides sodium can influence blood pressure. Insulin, the hormone that helps the body use carbohydrate, can affect how the kidneys excrete sodium; a high level of insulin in the blood reduces sodium loss. Therefore, a high intake of simple carbohydrate which produces a sharp rise in insulin, can increase sodium in the blood and elevate blood pressure. Linoleic acid produces the opposite effect, encouraging the kidneys to eliminate sodium in the urine. Linoleic acid is a polyunsaturated fatty acid found in many vegetable oils. (see Chapter 6).

Sweating causes loss of sodium and of other minerals and water. Taking salt tablets can be a poor way to restore salt lost in profuse sweating; usually this can be achieved by consuming regular foods along with plenty of fluid. The World Health Organization of the United Nations feels it is safe for a worker to lose five quarts of sweat in an eight-hour shift without needing extra salt but that, beyond this, perhaps some salt should be added. Salt depletion may cause weakness, dizziness, and nausea due to dehydration. Salt depletion is a component of heat exhaustion.

Stress is associated with hypertension, and alcohol even in moderate amounts raises blood pressure. Coffee and tobacco are also pressure raisers but the effects are not lasting unless a great deal is used over a long time. Exercise counteracts the effects of high blood pressure on the heart by strengthening it, lowering the pulse rate and reducing arterial resistance.

Thus, to sum it up, sodium is not the only cause of high blood pressure; other things can cause it, but sodium and these other things coupled together make it sure for some. It depends upon the individual and how he or she reacts to sodium and these other factors. Some are not bothered by any of them; others are. Some at one stage of life are more susceptible. Young people are much less apt to have hypertension than older ones. Pregnant women are susceptible and women after menopause likewise. The contraceptive pill for some women may cause hypertension, especially if accompanied by smoking, drinking alcohol, some kidney disfunction or other health problem. As with blacks, the elderly and obese people tend to be at greater risk of hypertension than others.

The Dietary Control of Sodium. The average person gets between six and 18 grams of sodium per day, even though a normal adult needs only about 1 gram of salt a day (or about 400 mg of sodium). This easily can come from natural foods if a varied diet is consumed.

Reduced Sodium Condensed
VEGETABLE SOUP (Vegetarian)
The delicious flavor comes from light, nutritious vegetables, delicately seasoned and with natural cut appearance that looks like homemade.

NUTRITION INFORMATION PER SERVING
Serving Size . . . . 3 oz condensed
(6 oz as prepared—170 g)
Servings per Container 17
Calories 60
Protein (grams) 1
Carbohydrates (grams) 11
Fat (grams) . . . . contains less than 1 gram
Sodium (milligrams) 140
Potassium (milligrams) 190
Percent of U.S. Recommended Daily Allowances (U.S. RDA)

Protein	2	Riboflavin	2
Vitamin A	8	Niacin	2
Vitamin C	40	Calcium	2
Thiamine	2	Iron	4

FIGURE 9-7 Sodium and potassium content of reduced-sodium soup is given on the label and suggests consumer awareness of the need to balance potassium and sodium. In this soup the proportions are good.

It is often very difficult to know how much sodium one is getting from prepared or processed foods. Canned peas and some other legumes are high in sodium because of their salt-brine treatment. Canned soups, TV dinners, cured meats, and many other processed foods are very high in salt. Pickles, olives, catsup, Worcestershire sauce, mayonnaise, soy sauce, mustard, and almost all similar condiments contain large amounts of salt. Crackers, potato chips, corn chips, salted nuts, pretzels, and other snacks are packed with salt. A cup of canned chicken with noodle soup—even after dilution with water—contains 1110 mg of sodium, and all regular canned soups are similarly salty. Because of a rising demand for foods low in sodium, some food manufacturers are producing low-sodium foods (Fig. 9-7). Table 9-9 compares the sodium content of regular and low-sodium canned soups. A frozen TV chicken dinner has 1500 mg of sodium. With cocktails before dinner, one half ounce of Roquefort cheese, an ounce of smoked oysters, and a slice of dry salami, this would add 670 mg of sodium without the crackers, puff balls, salted nuts, and other "nibblers" often served with drinks. There is also a lot of salt in some convenience foods:

8-ounce frozen beef pot pie	1100 mg of sodium
1 cup chow mein with vegetables	1300 mg of sodium
1 frankfurter	640 mg of sodium
1 wedge pizza with sausage	546 mg of sodium
1 cup popcorn	177 mg of sodium
1 cup chili con carne	860 mg of sodium
1 cup vegetable soup	978 mg of sodium
1 piece devil's food cake, iced	300 mg of sodium

Labels provide some information on sodium content. The government requires that most packaged foods list the ingredients in the product in decreasing order of amount. Thus, if a soup base starts out with "salt, monosodium glutamate, beef fat, beef essence," there is a lot of sodium there both in the salt and in the MSG. Also, the amount of sodium per serving must be listed when nutrition labeling is included.

TABLE 9-9
A Comparison of the Sodium Content of Regular
and Low-sodium Canned Soups

| Soup Type | Sodium per 6 ounce serving* | |
	Low-sodium soup (mg)	Regular soup (mg)
Tomato	150	590
Tomato rice	160	650
Vegetarian vegetable	140	580
Chicken vegetable	160	640

*3 ounces condensed and 3 ounces water

It is important to remember that, in any program to manage sodium it may be advisable to monitor the intake of potassium so they remain in proper ratio. In discussing electrolytes, we indicated how sodium and potassium worked in opposition to pull substances in and out through cell walls, and in a later discussion how an excess of sodium can cause a hardening of body cells which in the arteries results in high blood pressure.

Chlorine

Chlorine is a halogen gas whose name means "green gas." It is poisonous in large quantities and has even been used in chemical warfare. Chlorine compounds are added to drinking water to destroy disease-producing bacteria. One danger in using such substances in drinking water is that chlorine is a highly active chemical and might combine with other substances to form poisonous chemicals. Health authorities believe that pollution management, not chlorine restriction, is the proper solution to this problem. Chlorine exists in the body in nearly the same quantity as sodium (about three ounces).

The chloride ion (chlorine with a negative charge) has the unusual ability to move freely back and forth across cell membranes (Fig. 9-5). When outside the cell, chloride most often pairs with sodium to make sodium chloride which participates importantly in maintaining acid-base, fluid, and osmotic pressure balances. Chloride ions *in* cells bond with potassium. Chloride is an important part of gastric juices, making up hydrochloric acid. The chloride shift is a very important reaction. This occurs when a chloride shifts from the red blood cells into the plasma, thus enabling the blood to carry large amounts of carbon dioxide to the lungs. In addition, chloride activates the salivary glands to produce the substance that begins digesting starch in the mouth. The body can be depleted of chloride by severe diarrhea or vomiting that results in a serious electrolyte imbalance. For an adult, the RDA estimated safe and adequate daily intake range is 1700 to 5100 mg in the form of chloride. It comes largely from table salt (sodium chloride), but milk, meat, and eggs also supply it.

Magnesium

An average adult's magnesium supply is less than two ounces, the least of the seven major minerals. It is a strong, hard-working metal, most of which is stockpiled in bones. It is a part of the enzyme that creates energy. It is also needed to transfer nerve impulses and to relax muscles after they have contracted. It is used in building bones and teeth and helps harden tooth enamel. The rate at which the body functions is controlled by the hormone thyroxine; magnesium may trigger the activation of thyroxine to speed up body functioning, for instance, in response to cold. A lack of magnesium can cause nervous disorders or convulsions, calcification of soft tissues, or tetany (involuntary muscle spasms). Its lack may also show up in faulty cardiac function.

Need and Sources of Magnesium. The magnesium RDA varies from 50 mg for newborn infants, 350 for adult males, 300 mg for normal women, and 450 for pregnant and lactating women. Except in chronic alcoholics, magnesium deficiency that produces physical symptoms is rare. Yet some nutritional survey data suggest that RDA levels for magnesium are not being met.

All green plants contain magnesium in their chlorophyll. Dark leafy greens are particularly good sources; a half cup of spinach yields 57 mg. The same measure of legumes gives about 40 mg. An ounce of most nuts averages 50 to 70 mg of magnesium, and about 30 mg is provided respectively, by a 3 1/2-ounce portion of most meats, a medium banana, a cup of milk, or two slices of whole wheat bread. Chocolate and cocoa also contain this mineral. It is not unusual for some persons to consume large amounts of magnesium in the form of Epsom salts or laxative formulations such as milk of magnesia or in antacids containing magnesium hydroxide. This appears to cause no harm.

TRACE ELEMENTS

At least fourteen trace minerals are known to be essential (see Tables 9-2 and 9-3). Nine have established intake recommendations, but the need for the remaining five seems so minute that need levels remain under study. Essentiality measurement is painstaking; using laboratory animals, attempts are made to test the results of completely eliminating a substance from the diet. Yet minute but life-sustaining quantities of some minerals might even be carried by dust in the air or on laboratory tools. It is little wonder that disagreement exists about whether some minerals are "required for life" or only "beneficial for health." We do not discuss all the trace elements here; rather we point out their collective importance and discuss those of special interest: iron, iodine, and zinc, and, in more abbreviated profiles, copper, manganese, fluorine, chromium, selenium, and cobalt. The featured minerals are those that are likely to have the greatest impact on health through diet choices and those that figure prominently in advertising and in research updates.

Iron

The average adult male has less than three grams of iron in his body, 70 to 80% of it in the blood. A woman has about one half gram less. Iron is in nearly every part of the body and is stored in the spleen, liver, and bone marrow. A tough, hard metal, iron is quite active with other body substances. Lack of iron is probably the most prevalent nutrient deficiency in the U.S. today.

Iron is a crucial substance in blood and in its formation. The body produces red blood cells in the bone marrow, where an iron-bearing substance aids the process. In the first of two steps in producing blood, the mineral iron combines with the amino acid glycine, making heme; this then links with globin, making hemoglobin, the compound that is responsible for carrying oxygen and carbon dioxide into and out of cells. To produce blood, the body must have adequate copper, pyridoxine (B_6), vitamin C, and protein, in addition to iron.

A young person makes about 100 new red blood cells every minute in the bone marrow. Blood cells do not reproduce themselves, and they have only about a four-month life cycle before they are broken down in the spleen, where most of the iron is salvaged and recycled back to the bone marrow. About 20 to 25 mg of iron per day are conserved this way. Still more must be replaced constantly from outside sources, namely food.

Blood in the veins going to the lungs is dark red, because it is full of carbon dioxide, but when it reaches the lungs and takes on oxygen, it turns bright red. This oxygen-rich blood travels to the muscles, where the oxygen is picked up by the protein myoglobin, which also contains iron and which makes the oxygen available to the cells. Iron is the vital component that allows these oxygen transfers to occur. Without iron, the cells would suffocate and die.

Iron deficiency anemia, a shortage of hemaglobin within red blood cells, can be caused by a lack of iron: because the blood lacks hemoglobin (and therefore oxygen) the person feels tired and is hard put to work or exercise. Anemic persons may have very pale skin because of the lack of red cells. Gastric problems can occur, and some people become more susceptible to infections. A lack of glycine and other protein substances, pyridoxine, or copper can also cause anemia. Extensive hemorrhaging is another route to anemia, as are parasites that attach themselves to intestinal walls, sucking blood, and as are bleeding ulcers. A woman in a menstrual period can lose enough blood to deplete iron stores. Pregnant and lactating women and women and children in low income groups are most prone to have iron-deficiency anemia.

The RDA of iron is particularly important in view of the widespread problem of low iron intake, even in the U.S. Adult males need 10 mg per day, and females from age 11 should have 18 mg, a quantity that requires making wise food choices if she is trying to control calories as well. The need for iron increases during pregnancy to such an extent that supplements are often prescribed; even the RDA chart, in a rare gesture, suggests supplements of 30 to 60 mg. Such quantities simply cannot be obtained in a typical American diet.

Full-term infants are born with sufficient iron to last them four to six months, provided that the mother had adequate supplies before and during pregnancy. If not, the offspring can develop iron-deficiency anemia. Milk other than human milk is low in iron, so, long before the child is weaned its iron stores can run out, and the diet must provide the needed quantity. Infants should have from six to ten mg per day for the first half year. Between the ages of six months and three years, growing youngsters have an iron RDA—15 mg—that surpasses that of an adult male. The RDA increases to 18 mg for adolescents: teenaged girls, particularly, may experience a "triple threat" to iron supplies—fast growth, menstruation, and a teenager's diet.

Iron supplementation can be overdone. Excess iron (over 100 mg per day) can be stored in the liver causing a condition called siderosis, which can spread to the pancreas, heart, and other organs. Only about 10% of the iron in food is absorbed, but if body iron stores are low, more is absorbed. The body tends to balance utilization to loss as long as iron is available to utilize.

Sources of Iron. Good iron sources include organ meats, especially liver, molasses, red meats, egg yolks, bivalves such as clams and oysters, and leafy greens (Table 9-10). Legumes, nuts, dried fruits, and enriched or whole grain cereals supply significant amounts as well. Even potatoes have iron in them which is efficiently utilized. If eaten in good quantity, they can furnish a useful amount. Although they are little used in foodservices operations, cast iron skillets and utensils can contribute iron to foods cooked in them.

A high fiber diet can interfere with iron absorption, increasing the dietary need. A diet made up of predominately plant foods has less total iron and its iron is less well absorbed than the iron in a diet that includes a normal proportion of meat. Iron absorption is reduced to a small extent by the phytates in whole grains and bran, cellulose in vegetables, and tannic acid in tea, among others. Strict vegetarians may find it difficult to obtain and to absorb a healthful quantity of iron. Meat usually is a good source of iron so those who eat meat may not find it as difficult. In addition, meats seem to enhance absorption of iron from other foods eaten with them. Normally a balanced diet of sufficient calories that contains some meat, whole or enriched grains, and leafy green vegetables provides enough iron. Sugar aids iron absorption, while starch seems to inhibit it. Acidic foods, and vitamin C itself, assist in absorption of iron. To maximize the iron value of a particular menu, it should contain good vitamin C sources to aid in iron absorption. Some authorities advocate iron fortification of foods over and above the enrichment of processed grains now in place. Some even advocate iron-fortified soft drinks! While this could benefit many persons, particularly women and children, it could provide too much iron for adult males and for the many persons who consume copious quantities of soft drinks.

Iodine

Iodine is used within the thyroid gland as a vital constituent in the synthesis of the hormone thyroxine. Thyroxine is responsible for regulating growth and development of children, and regulating the basal metabolic rate (BMR) at all ages, the rate at which the body uses energy for fuel. We have only a tiny amount of iodine in our bodies—20 to 30 mg—but the *i* in iodine could stand for "important." Most is stored

TABLE 9-10
Sources of Iron

Item Description	Item Measure	Iron (grams)
Meat, Poultry, Fish and Eggs		
Liver, beef, cooked	85 grams	7.5
Clams, raw	3 medium	3.0
Beef, ground, cooked	85 grams	2.7
Oysters, eastern, raw	3 average	2.4
Ham, smoked, no bone	85 grams	2.2
Lamb, leg, no bone, fat trimmed	85 grams	1.9
Flounder fillet	85 grams	1.2
Egg, chicken, white	1 large	1.1
Egg, substitute (Fleischmann's)	1/4 cup	1.1
Chicken, 1/2 breast w/o skin	85 grams	.9
Grains		
Corn Total cereal (Gen. Mills)	1 ounce (1 cup)	18
Cream of Wheat (Nabisco)	1 cup, prepared	8.1
Cheerios cereal (Gen Mills)	1 ounce (1 1/4 cup)	4.5
Wheat germ	1/4 cup (1 oz)	2.7
Biscuit mix	1 cup	2.2
Rice, white, enriched, long gr.	1/2 cup	.9
Bun, hamburger	1 medium	.8
Bread, Italian	1 slice	.7
Bread, enriched, white	1 slice	.6
Macaroni, enriched, cooked	1/2 cup	.6
Pancake (Aunt Jemima)	1 at 4"x1/2"	.5
Bread, cracked wheat, raisin	1 slice	.3
Legumes, Nuts		
Pinto beans	1/2 cup	3.7
Pork and white beans (tom. sauce)	3/4 cup	3.2
Black-eye peas	1/2 cup	2.1
Imitation breakfast links, (Morning Star Farms)	2 strips	1.8
Cashews	1/4 cup	1.3
Celery seed	1 teaspoon	1.0
Fruits and Vegetables		
Lima beans, baby, frozen	1/2 cup	2.3
Asparagus, canned, drained	1/2 cup	2.2
Spinach, fresh, cooked, drained	1/2 cup	2.0
Cucumber, raw, not peeled	1 average	1.9
Mushrooms, fresh, sauteed	6 medium	1.3
Prunes, dry	3 average	1.2
Potato, in jacket, baked	1 average	1.1
Nectarine, fresh	1 average	.8
Carrot, raw	1 average	.6
Corn, sweet, fresh, cob	1/2 cup	.5
Dairy Products		
Cheddar cheese	1 ounce	.2
Cottage cheese	1/2 cup	.2
Milk, cow, 2 percent	1 cup	.1
Other		
McDonalds' hamburger	1 regular	2.9
Molasses	1 tbsp	1.2
Fat or oil	1 tbsp	0.0

in the thyroid gland (in front of the throat) where the body can bank about a two-month supply. In large amounts, iodine is a potent poison. Painted on cuts it kills bacteria.

Iodine is thought to be involved in the utilization of carbohydrates and in the production of both protein and cholesterol, if we include the latter as a lipid. (Notice this involves all three energy-nutrient groups.) In addition, iodine may be required for the conversion of vitamin A precursors into vitamin A.

The RDA for healthy persons over the age of 10 is 150 micrograms per day. The greatest need for iodine is during pregnancy and lactation; 25 μg are added for pregnancy and 50 should be added by nursing mothers. Ordinarily, the tiny amount needed at each age level is supplied easily by consuming a variety of foods, and iodine supplementation requires no special attention. Consuming seafood once or twice a week can supply what is required.

Goiter—enlargement of the thyroid gland—can result from lack of iodine. In the early 1900s the condition was so prevalent in the north-central U.S. that the area became known as the "goiter belt." When the body lacks sufficient iodine, the thyroid is unable to make thyroxine. It reacts by enlarging as part of a desperate attempt to obtain every available trace of iodine so thyroxine production can continue. Persons with goiter tend to become sluggish and to gain weight without thyroxine to control BMR. The eyes may protrude, and choking or suffocation can result from pressure by the grossly enlarged thyroid.

A lack of iodine during pregnancy can have horrible consequences; fetal development is threatened, and the infant can be born with cretinism, a severe, irreversible physical stunting and mental retardation. It is possible to correct the mother's iodine deficiency during the pregnancy and to avoid much of the retardation. Without correction, however, the offspring may be dwarflike, with an I.Q. as low as 20, and a vacant expression. Those that avoid the full sentence of cretinism may be born deaf or mentally retarded but of nearly normal stature.

It is estimated that millions of persons worldwide suffer from goiter today, and goiter and cretinism are reappearing in the interior regions of the U.S. even though as early as the 1930s, iodine deficiency was recognized as the cause and iodine-fortified foods as a solution. This unnecessary suffering is back with us because of improper eating. Many who do not remember the 1930s are ignorant of the consequences of not having enough iodine, and better public education is needed to inform citizens of the danger.

Some drugs, such as sulfa and other antibiotics, can interfere with thyroid function. Also, members of the cabbage and turnip families contain a substance called goitrogen, which inhibits formation of the thyroid hormones. If large quantities are eaten raw, the interference can be significant.

The effect on the thyroid gland of taking in too much iodine is similar to that of not taking in enough. The gland enlarges. The Japanese sometimes report this swelling because they consume so much iodine from their seafood-rich diets. It is estimated that 2000 ug per day could be toxic; with too much food fortification this limit could be exceeded. From 1960 to 1974, daily iodine consumption in the U.S. rocketed from 150 ug to 800 ug, an increase of over 500% in less than 15 years. Iodine is getting into food in many ways. An iodide used to clean cows' teats and to sanitize milking equipment has caused high levels of iodine in some milk products. Foodservices and many food processors also use iodides to sanitize equipment and utensils. Iodates are added to condition yeast-bread dough. Consumers may come to seek alternate food or bring public pressure to eliminate or reduce amounts of iodides in foods.

Food from the sea is a very reliable source of iodine (Fig. 9-8). (Fresh-water fish have little; fish that migrate between the two have an intermediate amount.) The iodine content of the soil in areas near the ocean usually is sufficient to provide plant and animal foods that supply enough iodine. Wide distribution of foods from such areas makes it possible for more people to get a greater variety of these healthful foods.

The fortification of salt with potassium iodide (1/2 to 1 part per 10,000 of salt) began in the 1930s to combat goiter, and the practice continues today, but both iodized and noniodized salt are available. The label may state: "This salt supplies iodine, a necessary nutrient." Sea salt, sometimes sold in health-food stores, loses most of its iodine in the drying process.

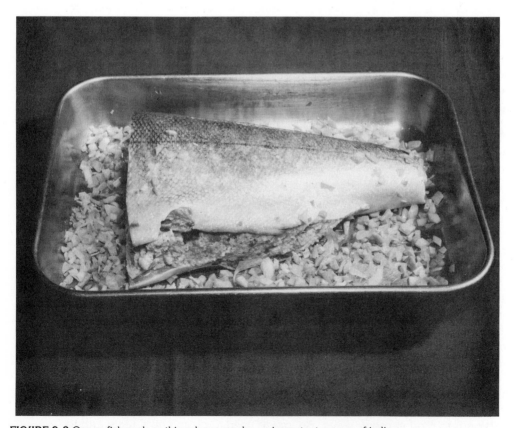

FIGURE 9-8 Ocean fish such as this salmon can be an important source of iodine.

Zinc

Zinc is in demand among fitness-conscious people. Most people do not get enough. The tiny amount of zinc in our bodies is in every tissue, but most is stored in the eyes. Other main zinc harbors are the liver, muscles, bones, and the male sex glands and their secretions.

Zinc is a co-factor for dozens of enzymes with which it performs functions such as cell production and release of carbon dioxide, structuring of bone, and utilization of vitamin A. Zinc is essential in protein synthesis and is involved in the immune response, in DNA production and cell replication, in the action of insulin, in wound healing, and in the development of sperm and of developing fetuses. Zinc also facilitates our perception of taste via the tongue.

From age 11, our zinc RDA is 15 mg. The average zinc intake in the U.S. is probably close to 10 mg. Most persons who consume sufficient protein get enough zinc in these foods to avoid deficiency signs, but zinc deficiency has been identified in the U.S. and in other developed countries, and concern is growing that it may pose a health threat to vulnerable Americans. A deficiency of zinc can result in stunted growth, deformed bones, poor healing, and loss or change in the sense of taste. Male adolescents may have retarded development of secondary sex characteristics (e.g., a deep voice, facial hair) and of sex organs. Night blindness can also occur, as zinc is necessary to activate vitamin A.

Some of the many possible causes of zinc deficiency are a diet lacking meat; alcoholism; and a steady diet of substantial amounts of low-nutrient density foods. Zinc is toxic only when consumed in large quantities. High levels can cause a lack of muscle coordination, vomiting, fever, and even death. Misuse of zinc supplements is the most likely way to obtain too much zinc. Over time, the body seems able to flush an excess from the system.

Zinc is available in the highest concentrations in meat and eggs, oysters, and liver. Good sources include dairy products and legumes, including peanuts. Whole grains bring with them some zinc, but it is not as well absorbed as that from animal foods. Combining the two seems to make plant zinc more available. A simple example would be a sandwich of sliced turkey on whole wheat bread.

Galvanized containers—iron or steel clad with a coat of zinc such as cans and buckets—are sometimes used in foodservices. Highly acid food or beverages can break down the zinc and form poisonous compounds. A health inspector would not quarrel with the presence of a galvanized bucket in the dishroom or one to be used for cleaning, but the same bucket would be considered unsafe if it were used to hold fruit punch, because it could taint the punch with too much zinc.

Copper

An adult may have a mere one-tenth gram of copper distributed in the blood, bone marrow, brain, liver, kidneys, and even the hair. It is vital to the formation of hemoglobin. Copper is also present in certain enzymes, helping break down glucose and other food substances into energy. Still other enzymes use copper to produce melanin, a pigment that darkens skin and hair. Copper also participates in the formation of phospholipids, which protect nerve fibers. With vitamin C, copper assists in building connective tissue; the connective tissue called elastin gives stretch and durability to the heart muscle and arteries. It is also an important part of the muscle structure.

True deficiencies of copper are rare. Average intake is two to three mg per day. A deficiency of copper can cause anemia and perhaps bring about other blood changes. About a third of the copper a person consumes is absorbed; absorption is aided by the presence of protein and other team nutrients in the intestinal tract.

Copper is available in most foods with the exception of dairy foods, which contain little copper. Good sources are whole grains, organ meats, shellfish, legumes, grapes, wine, and nuts. Some other fair sources are vegetables, dried and fresh fruits, and egg yolks. Meat is a fair copper source. Some water supplies contain a significant amount. Copper is a part of arsenic, a poison. In the presence of a strong food acid, a copper utensil can leach enough copper to form arsenic. Copper utensils used in foodservices should be tinned inside to prevent copper's contact with food acids.

Manganese

A mere three-fourths of an ounce of the metal manganese in the body functions as a necessary co-factor in both energy metabolism and in protein processes with amino acids. Manganese must be present for the production of fatty acids, cholesterol, urea, and bile. Two more tasks of manganese are to aid in the normal development of bone and to enhance the body's ability to hold on to thiamine.

Manganese deficiency is yet to be documented. The estimated safe and adequate adult intake ranges from 2.5 to 5 mg. Most normal diets provide this amount, although it is not widespread in foods. Superior sources are whole grain cereals, nuts, organ meats, legumes, coffee, cocoa, and some teas. Other plant foods are modest sources, whereas animal foods offer little manganese.

Fluorine

Fluorine is a gas, but it occurs in food and water in the form of fluoride ions. Only a trace is found in the body, the highest concentrations being in calcified tissues such as bones and tooth enamel, though some fluoride also is in soft tissues. Fluorine has no known required metabolic roles, although its presence may be beneficial for activating or inactivating certain enzymes. Fluorine does help the body build larger and stronger bone and teeth crystals. It actually replaces a substance that makes weaker bones and teeth, making teeth resistant to decay. Thus, many communities supplement drinking water with 0.8 to l.2 parts per million of fluoride. Fluoridation of water plus the use of toothpaste with 0.1% fluoride have reduced the incidence of tooth decay in certain segments of the U.S. population, and an adequate supply of fluoride during childhood also seems to confer protection later in life from osteoporosis.

Human beings can live without fluorine, but it is needed for optimal health. For this reason, it has a provisional estimated safe and adequate adult range of 1.5 to 4.0 mg per day. At even moderate levels, fluorine is very toxic. If fluorine is present in drinking water, whether naturally or as a supplement, there is no need for it elsewhere in the diet, but the average diet without this cannot supply the suggested quantities in many areas. Food sources of fluorine include certain teas and some fish products with which the bones are eaten, such as sardines.

Chromium

While there is no RDA for chromium, it is considered sufficiently important for our health to warrant an estimated safe and adequate intake range—0.05 to 0.20 mg for adults. Recent discoveries have linked chromium with the hormone insulin, and so, with glucose metabolism. Common food sources of chromium include whole grain cereals, a range of vegetables and fruits, as well as meats, cheese, and peanuts. Less common sources which may find their way into foods as ingredients or nutritional supplements include molasses and brewer's yeast. Refining foods such as sugar and grain products removes their natural chromium. In addition, chromium absorption is very inefficient: no more than 2% of what is taken in. As more and more foods contain refined sugar and grains it is possible that chromium deficiency could emerge as a health problem. In contrast, chromium toxicity range is also a concern. Industrial waste has contaminated some water supplies with chromium. Awareness and pollution management are the answers to this hazard.

Selenium

The nonmetallic trace mineral selenium works throughout the body but is most concentrated in the kidneys, liver and hair. As part of a particular enzyme, selenium is an antioxidant, and it can even replace vitamin E in that function.

Selenium's estimated safe and adequate intake range for adults is 0.05 to 2.0 mg. Reliable sources are wheat and other cereals, animal foods, and some plants. Deficiencies have been documented in China, where ongoing mild deficiencies are associated with heart damage. Several cases of selenium deficiency are blamed for heart failure. In other studies, persons who live in areas where selenium is sparse in the soil have a higher cancer rate. Others report that supervised selenium therapy can retard the growth of cancer. Selenium supplements are not recommended without medical supervision, however.

Too much selenium is evidenced by hair loss, brittle nails, discolored teeth, and tissue swelling. Children can develop gum and dental problems from an excess. Selenium came to the attention of U.S. scientists when cattle in the midwest were getting an excess from plants grown in soil rich in selenium. They developed "blind staggers," in which they would suffer loss of hair, blindness, a staggering paralysis, and eventually death.

Cobalt

The use of cobalt in the body is not clear. Evidently it is not, of itself, essential but it is a constituent of vitamin B_{12} (cobalamin), an essential nutrient available only from animal foods.

Other Trace Minerals

Still more trace minerals are present in the human body, and gradually scientists are identifying them and their activities and attempting to determine whether they are essential.

We would be better off *without* some, for instance, lead. Meanwhile, the investigators work to determine their sources. Does it occur in the body because it is a natural part of what we eat and drink? Or does it crop up in certain products by way of pollution or additives? The presence of certain minerals may be due to the concentration of heavy metal contaminants as they are moved along in the food chain, in water supplies, and in the air. Even essential minerals can be toxic or deadly in large quantities. A day's requirement of potassium consumed in one dose could be poisonous, for example.

Cadmium, titanium, lead, mercury, and even strontium are among the minerals present in the body that may cause damage in minute doses. For example, lead poisoning can result from using water that is channeled through lead pipes. Fish in some polluted waters contain such high levels of mercury that they are unsafe to eat. Such substances can build up to toxic levels in humans.

Remarkably, these same minerals and others, such as gold, silver, boron, tin, and aluminum, may have necessary body functions and may occur naturally in the body in minute amounts. Perhaps even arsenic—a carcinogen and a deadly poison—in minute quantities has an essential role in health. What we know for certain about trace minerals is that there is a great deal more to learn.

SUMMARY

Minerals perform many jobs. Without them life could not go on. The body is known to need over twenty different minerals, but more are probably required. Some are needed in such small amounts that it is difficult to understand what they do. Minerals are important constituents of every body cell and compound—bones, teeth, fluids, muscles, soft tissues and secretions. A second important function is that they act as body regulators; they keep fluids and electrolytes in balance, transfer nutrients in and out of cells, control acid-base balance, and transfer electrical charges between substances for nerve and muscle function. They also catalyze many chemical reactions. Tables 9-11 and 9-12 summarize the sources, need levels, functions, and deficiency symptoms of minerals.

TABLE 9-11
Major Nutritive Minerals

Mineral	Selected Food Sources	Adult RDA Range	Principal Functions	Deficiency Symptoms of Selected Conditions
Calcium	Milk products, fish, including bones, legumes, leafy greens, citrus fruits	800 mg	Builds bone and teeth. Helps transmit nerve impulses. Aids muscles to contract and relax. Assists in acid-base balance. Helps clot blood.	Disturbed bone development, maintenance, and strength: rickets in children, osteoporosis in adults.
Chloride	Table salt, meats, milk, eggs	1700-5100 mg	Hydrochloric acid for stomach digestive juices. Co-regulates osmotic pressure, and fluid and acid-base balance. Activates enzymes in saliva.	Deficiency unusual; fluid and acid-base balance might be disturbed.
Magnesium	Green, leafy vegetables, nuts, soybeans, seeds, whole grains, milk	M 350 mg F 300 mg	Part of energy functions. Helps transmit nerve impulses. Helps muscles relax. Strengthens bones and teeth. Ingredient in laxatives.	Rare, except in alcoholics, then: irregular heartbeat, muscle tremors, weakness, and cramps.
Phosphorus	Meat, poultry, fish, eggs, milk and milk products, legumes, nuts, phosphates in processed foods	800 mg	Calcium's metabolic twin: builds bones and teeth. Transports and breaks down fats. Part of energy and genetic materials. Cell membrane and enzyme constituent.	Shortages uncommon except with prolonged use of antacids.

TABLE 9-11 (continued)
Major Nutritive Minerals

Mineral	Selected Food Sources	Adult RDA Range	Principal Functions	Deficiency Symptoms of Selected Conditions
Potassium	Oranges, dried fruits, bananas, meats, legumes, including peanuts, coffee, tea, cocoa	1875-5625 mg	Co-regulates osmotic pressure and fluid and acid-base balance. Transmits nerve impulses. Involved in protein formation and energy functions. Contributes to muscle tone.	Uneven heart beat, muscle weakness, hardening of cell structure and muscles, kidney and lung failure.
Sodium	Table salt, cured foods (bacon, pickles, olives, sauerkraut) salt or sodium-rich condiments (e.g., catsup, soy sauce), salty chips, nuts, salt-softened water	1100-3300 mg	Co-regulates osmotic pressure and pH and fluid balance. Transmits nerve impulses. Promotes glucose uptake by cells.	Intake is usually too high. Excess is associated with hypertension in susceptible persons.
Sulfur	Protein foods: meat, poultry, fish, milk and cheese, legumes, wheat germ	Deficiency not seen in human beings.	Part of every cell, as constituent of three amino acids. Helps in forming strong links between protein molecules.	Not a problem for humans.

TABLE 9-12
The Trace Minerals

Mineral	Selected Food Sources	Adult RDA Range	Principal Functions Selected	Deficiency Symptoms of Conditions
Chromium	Meat, cheese, eggs, whole grain products, legumes, including peanuts, brewers, yeast, molasses	0.05-0.2 mg	Linked with insulin in glucose metabolism.	Theories point to abnormal sugar metabolism.
Cobalt	Animal foods, especially organ meats	None set (cobalt is a part of vitamin B_{12})	With vitamin B_{12} helps in maturation of red blood cells.	
Copper	Organ meats and other meat, especially oysters, whole grain products, legumes, nuts, grapes (and grape wine)	2.0- 3.0 mg	Hemoglobin formation, Part of enzymes in glucose breakdown. Helps form sheath to protect nerve fibers. Part of muscle and connective tissue.	Rare in humans: In animal development, bone and nervous tissue disorder, loss of elastic quality in tendons and major arteries.
Fluoride	Floridated water, some fish, when bones are included (sardines)	1.5-4.0 mg	Strengthens bones and teeth May de-activate certain enzymes.	Dental decay; perhaps osteoporosis.
Iodine	Iodized salt (fortified) salt-water fish and sea vegetables	150 ug	Vital constituent in thyroxine synthesis to govern BMR. May help utilize carbohydrates.	Goiter; in infants, cretinism.
Iron	Liver, red meat, bivalves, egg yolk, leafy deep green vegetables, dried fruits, legumes, whole and enriched grains, potatoes, molasses	M 10 mg F 18 mg	Part of hemoglobin in red blood cells. As part of hemoglobin and myoglobin, transports oxygen and carbon dioxide.	Anemia pallor, weakness, fatigue.
Selenium	Seafood, meat, whole grains, milk, egg yolks, legumes, garlic	0.05-0.2 mg	Antioxidant Co-worker with vitamin E	Very rare: associated with heart damage; possible link in increasing cancer risk.
Zinc	Liver, meat, poultry, seafood, eggs, milk, legumes, including peanuts	15 mg	Involved with dozens of enzymes. Essential in protein synthesis, including reproduction, the immune system, and wound healing. Facilitates sense of taste.	Reduced appetite and sense of taste, slowed wound healing in children, growth and sexual maturity are compromised.

Chapter Review

1. How many essential minerals can you name? List them and identify as many of the jobs they do in the body as you can. Then check your text to see which ones you missed and which of the very important jobs you omitted.
2. To the list above, add the quantity of each mineral needed daily by an adult. Check again to see whether you are right and add those you missed.
3. To the same list add good sources of the various minerals.
4. What are some of the dangers of consuming these minerals in excess?
5. Explain what electrolytes are. What are several of their special abilities?
6. What is osteoporosis? Explain how calcium and fluorine may play a part in preventing it.
7. How do minerals function in maintaining the body's acid-base balance?
8. What properties of minerals help transmit nerve impulses and make muscles contract and relax?
9. How does iron pick up and transfer oxygen in the body? What role does chlorine play in oxygen transfer?
10. Explain how minerals control fluids in the body. What is aldosterone and what does it do?
11. How do minerals help cells pull in fluids and nutrients and pass out fluids and waste?
12. What physiological functions does water perform in the body? How much should a normal adult have daily? How much of the water the body uses comes from outside sources and how much is a product of metabolism?
13. What are some of the obstacles to getting potable water in certain areas of the U.S.?
14. How does water get polluted? What role does chlorine play in water safety? Are there any dangers in using chlorine to sanitize water?
15. What is hard water? How is it softened using sodium chloride (salt)?

Part 3

The Healthful-Foods Program

Chapter 10

Managing Nutrients in Food Purchasing and Production

- *To provide an understanding of the conditions and forces associated with nutrient damage to ingredients and food products.*
- *To present the measures in a managerial checklist for procuring nutritious food and preserving nutrients until the food is served.*
- *To discuss the nutrient merits of various food processing methods.*
- *To reconcile the kitchen needs of the operation with those for the program.*
- *To indicate proper temperature for storage of perishable food.*
- *To outline general food handling practices that promote preservation of nutrients during storage, preparation, and cookery.*
- *To indicate preferred methods of production for major food categories that are compatible with guest preferences and nutrient preservation.*
- *To review references for avoiding unwanted nutrients and substances and to provide ideas for doing so.*

NUTRITION IN THE KITCHEN

The preceding chapters outline what healthful foods are and what nutrients they provide. This chapter pulls together the nutrient information in a consideration of how to procure and preserve the desired nutrients in menus and how to limit or eliminate substances that should be avoided. Before decisions can be made on which recipes are appropriate for a particular operation (see Chapter 11), it is necessary to have an understanding of ingredient and food product considerations for purchasing, storage, and production that could influence management's decisions on what recipes to include in menus.

In any plan to offer healthful foods to patrons, a fundamental goal should be to procure foods of high nutrient quality and store, handle, prepare and serve them in such a manner as to preserve the healthful qualities of the food. Fortunately, such an emphasis can result in excellent food quality, because techniques used to provide fitness fare and those used to produce fresh, good food parallel one another. Attaining these objectives requires a commitment from management to provide for an excellent staff training program on nutrient management that includes clear, practical instruction and documentation for employees (e.g., notations on recipe cards). This chapter is a companion to Chapter 14, which outlines training needs according to employee roles in the nutrition-oriented foods program.

Management also is responsible for seeing that proper facilities, equipment, and tools are available to achieve program goals. For example, instituting a healthful-foods program may necessitate adjustments in space utilization and storage containers to accommodate more fresh products. It is especially important for nutrient preservation that all food heating, holding, and cooling equipment have good insulation with reliable temperature calibration and control, and that controls receive frequent monitoring. Small-batch preparation equipment and tools should be available, as well as related facilities to allow using cookery methods that will produce both the desired nutrient and recipe results.

Nutrients: Will They Be "Safe at the Plate"?

Just as mishandling a freshly-picked flower can cause it to wilt quickly to a shadow of its former glory, inappropriate food handling can result in loss of nutrients and quality (Fig. 10-1). The energy nutrients—carbohydrate, protein, fats, and oils—are not nearly as delicate as vitamins and minerals, but even they can deteriorate or be lost. Careless *trimming* wastes nutrients, as does *overcooking* or burning. Fats turn *rancid* if not stored properly. Sugars and some starches can *dissolve* in cooking liquid (e.g., broken boiled potatoes). *Dehydration* (e.g., freezer burn) can destroy nutrients. And finally there is plain *spoilage*.

Both water-soluble and fat-soluble vitamins and some minerals are subject to loss when they pass into the water used for soaking or cooking, or into drip loss from thawing or cooking meat. Water-soluble vitamins in particular are unstable in other ways, too; some are heat labile (sensitive to heat) and can be lost in improper cookery or if held too long. Other nutrients oxidize easily (are destroyed by oxygen in the air), or can be destroyed by ultraviolet light or an alkaline environment. Several vitamins and minerals are chemically active and are changed or lost if they are combined with certain food additives or environmental contaminants.

Table 10-1 charts the minerals and vitamins, and their principal sensitivities to *solubility, acidity, alkalinity, heat, light,* and *air* (oxygen). Because we are more likely to think in terms of foodservices *activities* than complicated nutrient reactions, preservation measures are noted at the top of each column. As you study the table, keep in mind that the primary concerns are being aware of the most sensitive nutrients; protecting foods that are particularly good sources of scarce nutrients; and protecting major nutrient *source foods* that are consumed in sufficient quantities to have an impact on nutritional status.

Certain nutrients are quite fragile in the face of the forces of food handling, especially vitamin C and folic acid, followed by thiamine and riboflavin. This knowledge suggests certain procedures needed to protect different types of food during various stages of handling and preparation.

Preparing and cooking foods in large quantities often takes a heavy toll of nutrients, but it is not always possible to modify procedures sufficiently to prevent

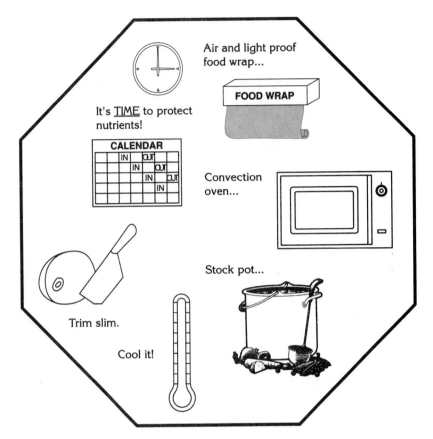

It's <u>TIME</u> to protect nutrients!

Air and light proof food wrap...

FOOD WRAP

CALENDAR

Convection oven...

Trim slim.

Cool it!

Stock pot...

FIGURE 10-1 Stop! Think! How can this food be managed to preserve it's quality and nutrient value?

significant losses. In an ideal situation, paring and slicing of salad vegetables would be done just before they are served to the guest; in the real world of an active foodservice operation, foods frequently must be prepared or cooked well ahead of service time in order to have them ready quickly when people want to eat. The alternative is product shortfall, service delays, bottlenecks, and unhappy patrons. In quantity foodservice work, it is most important wherever possible, to follow a well-planned program designed to minimize losses. Harm to the nutrient integrity of foods best can be avoided by having an awareness of the causes (e.g., excessive heat in preparation) and an understanding of strategies for preventing problems (such as batch cookery). Figure 10-2 illustrates six fundamental emphases for policy and action. Referring to this table, we will supply guidelines for the healthful-foods program, outlining the considerations necessary in a program to secure and preserve nutrients through managing food purchasing, storage, preparation, and cookery or other temperature treatment.

TABLE 10-1
Identifying Sensitivities to Preserve Nutrients

Nutrient	Solubility	Acidity	Alkalinity	Heat	Light	Oxidation	Good to excellent sources of the nutrients that are especially vulnerable.
	Can lose in preparation, cooking liquids, drip.	Acid food or additives.	Baking soda and other base-makers.	Limit heat time; chill at other times.	Avoid sun exposure. Use opaque cover.	Wrap or cover; cook whole or moderately cut.	
Minerals	Water	Some	Some	—	—	—	Any food subjected to leaching possibility
Vitamins							
A	Fat	—	—	—	—	—	Whole or fortified milk, eggs, deep gold fruits and vegetables
D	Fat	—	—	—	—	—	Fortified dairy and margarine products, fish liver oils, yeast
E	Fat	—	Limited	—	Limited	—	Vegetable or cereal oils and fish oils
K	Fat	Yes	Yes	—	Yes	Yes	Eggs, leafy green vegetables
Thiamin	Water	—	Yes	Yes	—	Yes	Meat, milk, legumes, whole or enriched grains
Riboflavin	Water	—	Yes	—	Yes	—	Milk (prime source), meat, eggs, grains
Niacin	Water	—	—	—	—	—	Meat, whole or enriched grains, leafy greens
Vitamin B$_6$	Water	—	Yes	—	Yes	Yes	Bananas, grapes, cabbage, potatoes
Pantothenic acid	Water	Yes	Yes	Dry heat	—	—	Liver, meat, whole grains
Biotin	Water	—	Yes	—	—	Yes	Liver, meat, eggs, milk, whole grains
Folic acid	Water	—	—	Yes	—	Yes	Leafy greens, liver, some other vegetables and fruits
Vitamin B$_{12}$	Water	—	Yes	—	—	—	Animal foods
Vitamin C	Water	—	Yes	Yes	—	Yes	Citrus, fleshy fruits, cabbage family, leafy dark greens, potatoes

Reprinted with permission of Macmillan Publishing Company from Stare, Frederick J., McWilliams, Margaret, Living Nutrition, 4th ed., (New York: Macmillan 1984)

Checklist for Nutrient Preservation

Activity Stage

A. ARE THE NUTRIENTS THERE IN THE FIRST PLACE?

Purchasing
1. Accurately identify and specify in detail the product appropriate for the program.
2. Select unrefined versions of foods when reasonable.
3. Work with vendors who reliably furnish the freshest food and well-preserved products.
4. Audit specifications and product quality on receipt of goods; do not accept products of doubtful freshness.

B. PROTECTING AGAINST TIME, TEMPERATURE, ALKALI, AND OTHER THREATS

Storage
1. Plan deliveries, date products, rotate stock, and otherwise manage inventory to allow the minimum time needed between delivery and consumption.
2. Manage for proper storage conditions, and in particular, for proper storage temperatures. Work with reliable equipment, including accurate thermostats. This applies to products before service and for any required chilling of items remaining following service.
3. Train staff for product sanitation and protection (wrapping, covering); minimizing exposure of products to air, light, pests, and microbial, chemical, and other contaminants.
4. Vitamin C and other alkaline-sensitive nutrients are damaged when baking soda is used in soaking or cooking water to speed cooking or retain green coloring. Using it is a poor practice.

C. KEEPING NUTRIENTS AFTER PURCHASE

Pre-prep
1. Nutrients are lost when food is lost to the knife; refrain from excessive trimming, paring, peeling, and topping.
2. Collect edible trim, cooking, and some canning liquids and damaged but good produce for a stock pot (soup or sauce base) or other use to turn the potential nutrient loss to a gain.

D. PROTECTING AGAINST SOLUBILITY AND LEACHING LOSSES

Leaching occurs when a food is soaked or cooked in water or oil, and the soluble nutrients pass into the liquid.
1. Soak foods as briefly as possible: wash fruits and vegetables before peeling.
2. Do not divide foods into smaller pieces than necessary to minimize the surface area exposed. Store fresh foods whole. When the recipe permits, cook foods in their peels. Cook products whole and divide later.

Cookery
3. Bake (roast), broil, stir-fry, or steam, if possible. Unless the liquid is part of the product (soup, stew) avoid boiling.
4. If the food IS submerged in water, cook in as little liquid as is effective, cook as fast as practical, and utilize any remaining liquid in other foods (see stockpot, C2 above).

E. HEAT HURTS: AVOID UNNECESSARY HEAT IN COOKERY

Pre-prep planning
Especially for vegetables and fruits uncooked
1. Consider, is this a product guests would enjoy?

Cookery
2. Cook fruits and vegetables as briefly as possible while still obtaining the desired recipe result.

Cookery Planning
3. Carefully project quantities to prepare. Holding, re-storing and reheating foods is nutrient-loss double trouble.
4. When larger pieces are cooked, less surface area is vulnerable; however, this should be weighed against the amount that cooking time or temperature may have to be increased.
5. Cook frozen vegetables (and fruits) from the frozen state. Do not thaw or refreeze.
6. Vegetables and fruits should be cooked only until done or slightly undercooked.
7. Cut and cook food as close to serving time as feasible. "Batch cook" vegetables, cooking only the quantity anticipated to be needed in the short term. When food must be held, 20 minutes should be considered a maximum.

F. DRY-UP DRIP LOSS

Drip loss is the "juice" that is squeezed from meat when it is cooked, especially in high heat. All types of nutrients can leach into this "drip," and flavor and yield may be reduced.

Cookery
1. For large roasts, slow-cookery at low temperatures results in less drip than rapid cooking at high temperatures. Manage and use any carving losses.

Pre-prep cookery
2. Thaw frozen meats only as much as necessary prior to cooking.

Cookery
3. UTILIZE pan drippings other than the fat portion in sauces, gravies, etc. (Chill drippings in refrigerator; fat will rise to the top where it is easily removed.)

FIGURE 10-2 Checklist for nutrient preservation.

PURCHASING TO SECURE NUTRIENTS

A healthful-foods program should be supported solidly by a well-designed and conscientiously-executed purchasing program in order to secure appropriate products of high nutrient quality. If the nutrients are lacking in the first place they can not be preserved.

Food Preservation Purchasing Considerations

The highest nutrient and quality yields are available from products that are afforded the best protection from nutrient menaces between the farm and the table. This is as true for animal products as it is for produce; indeed, the optimal nutrient preservation method may vary by product and even by processor or vendor. An important consideration in procurement is to deal with reliable producers, distributors, and other suppliers who are aware of their customers' programs and are knowledgeable and ethical in their provisioning. The route from field to kitchen allows plenty of opportunities for poor nutrient management (Fig. 10-3). The product that comes into a foodservice operation is no better than the practices of those who have handled it up to that point. Getting the right product at the product's peak of quality depends on a good menu plan but must be supported by ingredient knowledge, careful product specifications, and conscientious suppliers.

What form is best to buy—fresh, frozen, canned, dehydrated, or cured? Table 10-2 compares nutrient values of variously processed foods, highlighting vitamin C

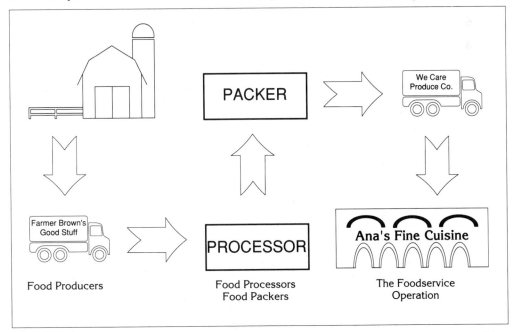

FIGURE 10-3 A reliable system of food suppliers is the best insurance that care is given to retaining nutrients between harvest and delivery to the operation.

TABLE 10-2
Comparison of Nutrients in Fresh and Processed Foods
(Vitamim C and Thiamin)

Item	Fresh	Frozen	Cooked	Canned	Dehydrated
		(mg per 100 grams)			
Vitamin C (Ascorbic Acid)					
Carrots	7	—	6	2	3
Orange juice	50	48*	—	39	43
Spinach**	51	28	27	14	—
Tomatoes**	21	—	24	17	—
Thiamin					
Beef	0.08	—	0.05	—	—
Peas, dry, cooked	0.35	0.32	0.28	0.09	0.15
Ham	0.77	—	0.35	—	0.62***
Potatoes	0.09	0.07	0.09	—	—
Spinach	0.10	0.09	0.07	0.02	—

* After reconstituting at a 3:1 water-to-concentrate ratio
** An acid reaction protects vitamin C, so high-acid products such as tomatoes and orange juice lose less in processing than other items, and can even gain.
*** Commercially cured ham, uncooked.
(Values from USDA Handbook 456) Nutritive Value of American Foods in Common Units, Adams, Katherine F. 1975 Agriculture Research Service of USDA.

and thiamine, two of the most easily lost nutrients. Fresh foods are the best nutrient sources, followed by frozen foods, and matched closely by cooked, and when applicable, dehydrated foods. Canned foods are poorest in these sensitive nutrients. (Highly acidic foods, such as orange juice and tomatoes, offer a protective environment for ascorbic acid, enabling it to endure processing relatively intact.) Because of the perishability of fresh foods and the often considerable delay before they are used, the nutrient value of a frozen product is sometimes superior to that of a fresh one, by the time the food is served. In many areas, fruits and vegetables are frozen within a few hours of harvest, whereas the shipping of fresh vegetables can take days. The nutrient value of quality canned products can be superior to that of out-of-season or mishandled fresh crops in some cases. Preservation may bring with it some nutrient compromises, but these processes enable us to enliven our fitness bill of fare and to serve what we could not otherwise: a lush variety of foods and ingredients; seasonal foods year-round; ready-to-cook foods with less labor; regional foods anywhere; and all at a moderate cost.

To support recipe and menu development, a review of food and ingredient processing and purchasing options should include consideration of alternative products that might fill certain needs (e.g., to store fewer bulky vegetables) or resolve a problem for the operation (e.g., lower labor costs, shorten lead time), without compromising the nutrition and quality goals of the program. Figure 10-4 shows how food ingredient choices can be visualized as following along a *degree-of-processing continuum.* Understanding the nutrient-loss consequences of various food handling techniques is especially important as the industries of foodservices and food processing mature and converge. Judging the most advantageous selection point along the continuum for ingredients (and entire menu items) will be an increasingly critical managerial tactic and will continue to prompt adjustments in back-of-the-house operations.

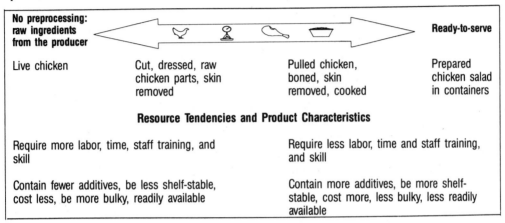

FIGURE 10-4 The Degree-of-Processing Continuum for Foods.

Getting Specific

Fresh Foods. If products are to be served fresh and nutrient quality is to be ensured, no corners can be cut. Fresh fruits and vegetables are at their nutritional peak during their regular growing season. Some authorities contend that field-grown and vine-ripened product has higher levels of vitamin C and other nutrients than that grown in greenhouses. Any food begins to lose quality and nutrients at the moment of harvest, therefore, it is important to work with distributors who handle products appropriately for nutrient retention (see below).

Color in fresh fruits and vegetables is associated with good nutrient value. Bright orange, mature carrots, deep orange sweet potatoes, and gold, blushing apricots contain a greater amount of carotene than pale-colored products. Deep green vegetables contain more iron and vitamins A and C than their washed-out counterparts (e.g., leaf lettuce has more vitamin A than iceberg because its leaf is greener). Excellent vitamin sources—the outer leaves of vegetables, edible vegetable trimmings, and juice from canned vegetables—which are unlikely to be used in other recipes should be added to the stock pot to enrich soups and sauces.

Frozen Foods. The main nutrients lost through freezing are vitamin C and thiamine; both are lost during *blanching*, a quick, partial cooking in boiling water the purpose of which is to shorten later cooking time, to destroy pathogens and to inactivate enzymes that can cause spoilage and alter nutrients. Fresh products suffer similar nutrient losses if they are cooked. In comparison to fresh products, one that is blanched is more stable afterward and resists further losses of vitamin C and other vitamins.

Canned Foods. Some losses of heat-labile vitamins occur during canning, but newer techniques have reduced the losses somewhat. Canning is done in liquid, and if the liquid is discarded, with it goes a portion of the water-soluble vitamins. Canning liquids that are flavorful should be incorporated into other dishes to make optimal use of the nutrients they contain. Unfortunately, some canning brines are too salty to be used in quantity in a healthful-food program. Fruits canned in their own juices avoid the refined sugar in heavy canning syrups. Even with recent improvements, there can be a big difference between the amount of nutrients available in some canned goods in comparison to the amount in carefully processed fresh or frozen versions. Peas, which are otherwise a good thiamine source, lose nearly 75% of it in the canning process. In *Jane Brody's Nutrition Book*, the *New York Times* health columnist, writes, "The losses of B_6 and pantothenic acid can be as high as 91% in canned foods. You can't expect to meet the RDA for these vitamins if you subsist on a menu of refined, processed, and canned foods."

Dehydration. Drying is a good preservation method for some foods. Freeze-dried foods retain more of their nutrients than those dried in the sun or other heat. In sun-drying, a one-third loss of vitamin A or carotene would be normal. In the still costly freeze-drying process, moisture is removed by rapidly freezing the food in a vacuum, then pulling out the moisture as vapor, thus even many of the fragile nutrients remain unharmed.

Other Nutrient Considerations in Purchasing

Dairy Products. Low-fat, skim, and nonfat dry milk products should be fortified with vitamins A and D, which occur naturally in the butterfat but are removed with the cream when milk is skimmed. Margarine also should be fortified with vitamins A and D.

Grain Products. Whole grain cereals and bread products are preferable to refined, milled ones. As the previous chapters point out, whole grains are fine sources of important minerals and both fat-soluble and B vitamins. The greatest concentrations are in the germ and bran (which also contains fiber), the parts that have been removed from refined grain products such as white flour. As mentioned in Chapter 4, the fibers of various grains are now recognized as being genuinely beneficial to health. When whole grains do not suit menu needs, alternatives are enriched, refined grain, or a blend of them and whole grains. Knowledgeable menu planners often offer both whole grain and processed products (e.g., white bread) when both are requested by sufficient numbers of guests.

Federal standards for enrichment have been established for some wheat flours, white bread or rolls, farina, cornmeal and grits, macaroni and noodle products, and rice. Processed grains and products labeled "enriched" do have certain nutrients added after refining, but the fiber is not restored. In comparison to nonenriched refined flour, enriched refined flour contains seven times more thiamine, nearly six times the riboflavin, and about four times as much niacin and iron. Many breakfast cereals are *fortified* (extra added, not just restored) with considerable quantities of nutrients; some packaging promotions even proclaim that their contents provide "100% of the

USRDA" for certain nutrients. Such products must list the quantities of nutrients on their labels.

The last step in securing nutrients to bring into the foodservice is taking delivery from the supplier. Persons with this responsibility should understand the product and quality specifications expected in order to be able to judge the acceptability of the products or product alternates purveyors bring to the delivery dock. Only products that meet or exceed quality standards should be accepted, and they should be moved immediately to the appropriate storage area or to the kitchen for use.

STORAGE CONSIDERATIONS TO PROTECT AND PRESERVE NUTRIENTS

The impact of careful storage and handling on the nutrient value of foods can be great, especially for fresh foods. Under poor conditions significant vitamin losses can occur in just a few hours, and even under refrigeration, regrettable losses can occur in just a day or two if food is mishandled. Considerations for managing nutrient retention center around basic principles of responsible inventory management supported by specific recommendations for foods kept in each of the three major types of foodservice storage facilities: dry, refrigerated, and freezer or low-temperature storage.

Planning should aim to keep the interval between delivery and use as short as possible. In the case of fresh foods, this may necessitate arranging for frequent deliveries. Food must be handled carefully, as bruising can rupture cells, leading to spoilage and to nutrient loss. Products should be dated to ensure proper rotation on a first-in, first-out (FIFO) basis to maintain relative freshness. Items must be wrapped or otherwise covered in the proper manner for that food to confer the appropriate protection from, or (in some cases) exposure to, air, light, or humidity. Products also should be protected from contaminants, including human hands, micro-organisms (bacteria, mold), chemicals, dust, and ashes. A pest control program must be maintained against rodents and insects; they also know the most nourishing and best foods. (For example, some insects eat just the germ portion of grains and legumes.) Cut-up, peeled, and other pre-prepared products in storage, particularly fresh vegetables and fruits, are much more vulnerable to nutrient losses to oxidation, leaching, and light than whole fruits and vegetables, so cutting should be done as close to the time of preparation and service as possible.

The correct temperature, humidity, and air circulation must all be provided to retain the quality and nutrient value of foods in storage. This is a priority. Temperature needs vary for different foods (Figure 10-5 and Table 10-3). As extended storage time compounds the threat of nutrient loss, both tables also provide guidelines on maximum length of time items should be kept in such storage conditions. It must also be kept in mind that, although the product may *appear* well-preserved, the nutrients continue to deteriorate but are invisible. Therefore we repeat; follow-through on having the *minimum* time possible between the delivery of each product and its use.

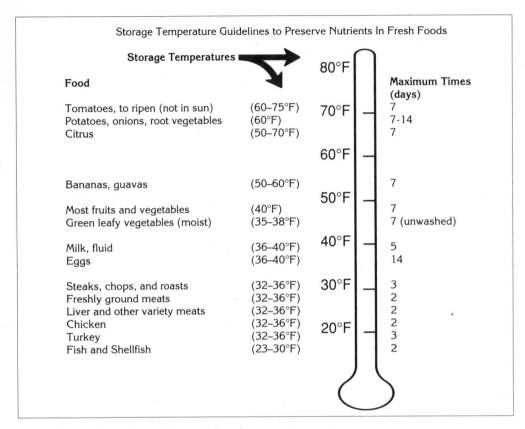

FIGURE 10-5 Storage temperature guidelines for preserving nutrients.

Dry Storage

A cool, dry, well-ventilated area away from ranges, ovens, and broilers is best for maintaining the quality of the canned goods, grains, potatoes, onions, and other staples kept in dry, nonrefrigerated storage. Vitamins are reasonably preserved when dry-storage products are kept around 60°F (15.4°C). Losses of vitamin C and thiamine from good sources of each can result, even in canned goods, when this temperature is exceeded for any significant length of time (Table 10-4). Imagine the losses at common production kitchen temperatures of 85°F and well above. Whether they are stored in dry or chilled areas, products that are sources of riboflavin—dry and fluid milk and its products, eggs, grains, flours, breakfast cereals, breads, and similar goods—deserve special mention. They should be stored in opaque containers that block strong light, which easily destroys the riboflavin.

Refrigerated Storage

At no time is the relationship between food quality and nutrient quality more evident than during handling and storage of refrigerated fresh foods. Steps taken to

TABLE 10-3
**Storage Guidelines to Preserve Nutrients
in Processed Foods**

Food	Maximum Holding Time in Days	Storage Temperature in Degrees F
Dry goods and staples, canned foods, dried milk	180 (unopened) 90 (covered)	60
Processed dairy products, butter, hard and soft cheese	14 180 (wrapped) 7 (covered)	36-40
Other refrigerated processed foods Cooked dishes and leftovers containing eggs, meat, poultry, fish, milk, cream, cream filling	Serve on day prepared	32-36
Other cooked dishes or leftovers Preserved meat, bacon, canned ham, dried beef	2 (covered) 7 (wrapped) 30 (unopened) 30 (wrapped)	32-36
Ice cream and ices	30 (covered)	10
Frozen foods, meats, vegetables, juices, and others	90 (covered)	—20-0

preserve one usually preserve the other as well. For example, the sanitation codes in many areas require that the local health department approve all new refrigeration equipment prior to its use in foodservice operations. Officials want to be certain that it meets standards to attain, maintain, and register the temperatures claimed for it. (A lot of substandard equipment is available.) Happily, for both food safety and nutrition, refrigeration conditions that discourage microbial growth favor nutrient retention. Even in refrigeration, the best conditions for quality and nutrient retention vary for different types of food—meats, dairy foods, fresh produce (see Fig. 10-5).

Fresh fruits and vegetables are living things even though they have been harvested. They "breathe"; they need air and, so, should not be packed too tightly together. Some (leafy greens) need moisture, and most need high humidity to prevent dehydration. Their enzyme systems still function after harvest and can direct continued ripening, spoilage, etc. Their functions can be retarded by chilled storage

TABLE 10-4
Vitamin C and Thiamine Losses During Storage of Canned Foods

Item	Recommended Temperature (°F)	Actual Temperature (°F)	Months Stored	Proportion of Vitamin Lost
Vitamin C	60	65	12	10%
Canned Citrus Products	60	85	12	25%
Thiamine	60	70	3	20%
Canned Meat Products	60	70	6	40%

temperatures, and by providing other favorable environmental conditions (e.g., ventilation).

A loss of natural sweetness can take place in just a few hours if certain produce is held at room temperature. Particular transformations between sugar and starch result in a loss, not of nutrients, but of flavor, when sugar in some produce such as peas and corn is changed into starch by enzymes in the product. Potatoes have different storage needs, and the reverse can happen to them if they are kept too cool: their starch can change to sugar, damaging both cooking quality and flavor.

Most whole fresh fruits hold their nutrients fairly well for several days if properly stored, especially those high in acid (citrus, tomatoes). Tomatoes delivered underripe should be ripened away from the sun at temperatures of 60°F to 75°F. They lose more nutrient value and eating quality if ripened in the sun, in the refrigerator, or above 85°F. Questions often arise about citrus juice. When strained after being squeezed, fresh citrus fruit loses fiber and nutrients: about 1.3 times more vitamin C is available from the equivalent whole fresh fruit. Vitamin C loss is minor during the first several days for refrigerated fruit juice, but even a few hours can result in flavor loss. The United States Department of Agriculture (USDA) states that there is no harm in storing canned juices temporarily in their cans after opening.

Fats and oils can be ruined by oxidation, If oxygen from the air wedges onto the fatty acid chain, it can destroy vitamin A and the eating quality of the lipid. We then say the fat is "rancid" (and useless). Covered refrigerated or frozen storage, with or without the use of antioxidant agents (such as vitamin C and BHT), retard oxidative reactions. Butter, margarine, oils, other fats, and foods that contain them require this care.

Frozen Storage

We may think of "freezing" as 32°F, or 0°C, but in foodservice, the *freezer temperature should be -20 to 0°F*. We want the food to be solidly frozen; that the air temperature registers "freezing" does not produce this. Only when a freezer is designed for such low temperatures can it maintain the products it contains at temperatures below their freezing points. (Home models of refrigerator-mounted freezers may *register* 32°F, but the food in them is likely to be well above the frozen state.) Even in a freezer at 0°F, frozen vegetables such as spinach and broccoli can lose from one third to three fourths of their vitamin C during a year, and losses are greater at higher temperatures. So it is that when the objective is to preserve nutrients, the freezer is still no place for foods to be "parked" for long periods. Foods should be rotated in and out in short order.

The thawing and refreezing of frozen foods damages texture and flavor, destroys nutrients, and can result in additional losses (e.g., when thawing causes excess drip from meats). Flesh products frozen for too long, especially under poor conditions of wrapping and air circulation, can deteriorate in quality and lose nutrients. When freezer burn occurs, there is a marked quality and flavor loss. The outer surface of meat is left dry, pulpy, and light gray in color, and no amount of culinary creativity can bring back the quality of the meat in the burned area. It remains tough, dry, and unappetizing. Oxidation also can destroy flavor and nutrient values in frozen meat, causing some fat, such as that of poultry, to be highly perishable (it can turn rancid). The more saturated fats (beef, lamb) are less susceptible to the oxygen onslaught and can be held the longest.

PRESERVING NUTRIENTS IN PRE-PREPARING FOOD

Care in pre-preparation can go far toward reducing animal and plant product nutrient losses. A first area to address is nutrient losses through food that is discarded because of poor technique in trimming, paring, and other pre-preparation activities employed. Also, usually it is here that foods are sliced, minced, mashed, or otherwise divided, processes that make the nutrients vulnerable to the environment. The smaller the pieces and the more surface area that is exposed, the more nutrient damage is likely to occur. Review Table 10-1 noting especially nutrients likely to suffer when more surface area is exposed. Cooking large pieces of food can require longer exposure to heat; however, net nutrient loss generally increases as surface area and exposure to threats increase.

Nutrient retention during preparation of fruits and vegetables is enhanced by removing them from their optimal storage conditions for as little prep time as possible, soaking a minimal amount of time, washing before peeling, paring, trimming, and peeling minimally, then leaving items whole or in large pieces. The outer leaves of vegetables sometimes are discarded, yet they are likely to contain more vitamin A, iron, and calcium than inner leaves. Vitamins usually are concentrated just under the skin of fruits and vegetables, so if the item must be peeled, as thin a layer as possible should be removed. (Edible skins and peels might be left intact: they can be excellent nutrient sources if guests are interested.)

An acidic additive sometimes is used after washing (lettuce) or paring (potatoes) to retard browning and preserve a fresh look. A mild solution does not seem harmful and can help reduce leach losses. Vitamin C is an antioxidant and, if present in the solution, may increase nutrition.

Rice and other cereal grains should not be washed prior to cooking. In some rice products, the enrichment nutrients are added as a loose, white, powder surrounding the rice; washing simply whisks it away. Legumes usually require thorough washing but should not be cooked with soda to soften them more quickly. Baking soda destroys thiamin and other nutrients.

Pre-preparation losses can be combated with two areas of planning and training: how best to pre-prepare the item and what to do with certain edible imperfect or trim items. An example of both measures would be instruction in exactly how to wash, top, and handle fragile fresh strawberries for minimal product and nutrient loss. A worker might later be assigned to take charge of a stockpot, cut fruit salad, or a similar dish to learn what items should be directed to him or her. For the stockpot, items could include scrubbed vegetable peels, bones and meat scraps, liquid from meats and vegetables, and slightly blemished produce. In this way, the loss is no longer a loss, since the nutrient once again becomes available in soups, sauces and other stockpot derivatives.

PRESERVING NUTRIENTS IN COOKERY

TABLE 10-5
Maximum Cooking Losses* For Vitamins and Minerals

Nutrient	Maximum Cooking Loss! (%)
Vitamin C Folic acid	100
Thiamine	80
Riboflavin Niacin**	75
Biotin	60
Vitamin E	55
Pantothenic acid	50
Pyridoxine Vitamin A Vitamin D	40
Provitamin A (carotene)	30
Vitamin B$_{12}$ (cobalamin)	10
Vitamin K	5
Minerals (in general)	3

 * Maximum cooking losses that would occur under the worst possible conditions short of burning the food beyond recognition.
** Niacin is among the most stable of the vitamins, (see Table 9-1), but since large amounts tend to be lost in leaching under the cooking conditions used in this analysis, niacin cooking losses still can be as high as 75%

(Adapted with permission of Van Nostrand Reinhold from Harris, RS, Karmas, E (eds): Nutritional Evaluation of Food Processing. Westport, CN. AVI, 1975.)

Most foods lose nutrients when we cook them, so why cook? For meat, grains, and many vegetables, cookery increases the ability to chew and digest them, destroys most pathogenic bacteria, and improves the foods' appearance and appeal. Most persons would not accept a regimen of raw meat, raw potatoes, and unbaked bread.

Most nutrient losses in cookery occur in *leaching*, *exposure to heat*, and *drip*. Interfering substances such as intentional and unintentional harmful additives also must be guarded against. A first possibility is to offer guests products like fruits and vegetables in the fresh state, with little or no cooking. Patrons today are requesting more and more of these foods, such as sushi and extensive salad bar selections. The next technique is to minimize the exposed surface area of foods. Foods should be kept covered. When vegetables are cooked whole and in their jackets (if the recipe permits) the nutrient savings can be dramatic. A sweet potato baked whole retains 89% of its vitamin C; one baked as two halves retains only 31%. Reducing exposure to water, heat, etc. also can be achieved through implementing small-batch cookery. For example, rather than cooking vegetables at 9:00 *am* and "holding them" until lunch, smaller quantities should be prepared close to the beginning and throughout the service period. This practice is simply a form of time management. Much of the remaining nutrient protection centers on the selection of appropriate cookery methods and techniques. Building on the precautions above, cooking methods selected should restrict losses from drip and from leaching into cooking liquids, should involve no more heat exposure than necessary, and should involve no avoidable additions of, or contact with, substances harmful to nutrients. Table 10-5 captures a worst-case glimpse of nutrient losses in foods which were subjected to extremely harsh cookery; it is a dramatic testament to the need to use *care*.

Since many nutrients are water soluble, methods that utilize a minimum of water often are a good choice; methods considered to be "dry" (with no lid or wrap, and no added fluids) include baking, roasting, broiling, toasting, and barbecuing. Methods of cookery based on fat, such as deep-frying and pan-frying, etc., also are considered "dry" (no water added) but usually would not be appropriate for preparing fitness fare because they add too much fat and calories. An exception is sauteing or stir-frying in a very small quantity of vegetable oil. Because it is a quick, waterless, and low-fat method, stir-frying cut meat and vegetables in a sparsely oiled and very hot skillet or wok is recommended for preserving nutrients.

Moist methods other than steaming (see below) can be detrimental to nutrient retention but sometimes are the route to the desired menu item; poaching, simmering, boiling, stewing, and braising are examples. Since so many nutrients are subject to leaching and heat damage with moist methods, the following principles should be applied: (1) use minimally cut foods; (2) use the minimal amount of liquid that will assure quick, even cooking without scorching; and (3) keep meats at a maximum of a low simmer, but cook fruits and vegetables as rapidly as possible. This latter can be overdone. Since gently boiling water is as hot as violently boiling water, take care that the water turbulence is used to distribute heat, not to break the food apart. Visible evidence of nutrient (carbohydrate) leaching is the ring of starch one might see at the bottom of a pan of boiled potatoes. Finally, (4) plan to reserve any remaining cooking liquid to be served with the product (as in a stew) or to be utilized elsewhere, as in soups, sauces, and casseroles.

Animal Products

In meat cookery, the objectives are to achieve the taste, color, temperature, tenderness, and healthful qualities desired by the consumer. Meat supplies protein, B vitamins, iron, and other minerals; nutritionists often use thiamine as an indicator of nutrient retention in meat products. We have discussed ways to minimize surface exposure and to preserve nutrients by preventing them from leaching into foods. Meat brings an additional challenge: to minimize drip loss. When protein is exposed to heat and coagulates, the cells may squeeze out moisture, or "drip." This water and fat

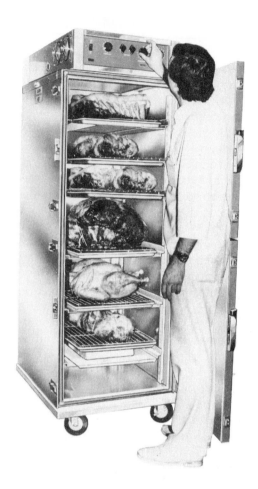

FIGURE 10-6 A slow Roast'n'Hold Convection oven, the Crown-X Mobile Roast-N-Hold oven. *(Courtesy CRES-COR/CROWN X, Crescent Metal Prod., Inc.)*

"juice" can travel through the meat tissue and dissolve or carry with it protein and both water-soluble and fat-soluble nutrients, eventually "dripping" onto the bottom of the pan or into the coals. Drip loss is to be avoided because of its multiple loss disadvantages: loss of nutrients, of meat moistness, tenderness, and flavor components and of product yield or weight.

For large roasts, slow roasting (at temperatures at or below 300°F) is a good technique to minimize drip (Fig. 10-6). For steaks and chops, the high-but-short-term heat of broiling is effective. On a related healthful-food issue, fat in meats cooked at high temperatures may contain substances suspected of being carcinogens; for this reason, some people do not want their broiled meats cooked at too high a heat. (The suspected substances are in the smoke produced when the drip hits the coals or heating element.) Broilers are available in which the heating element is situated beside the meat, allowing the drip to fall harmlessly into a tray below.

Extended simmering (braising, stewing) methods often are an effective way to tenderize tougher cuts of meat: the moist-cookery guidelines above apply to them. About 10% of even the sturdy protein in meat, poultry, and fish can be lost in these methods. Some meat proteins are soluble only in cold water, and these proteins and other nutrients leached into the cold water often rise to the surface, to be removed later as "scum." Starting stew meat in hot water is recommended because in this way, most of these proteins are more likely to coagulate in the meat.

Frozen meats drip less if the product is cooked in the frozen or partially thawed state than if it is thawed totally. Freezing can rupture cell walls in meat. If the meat is thawed, the liquid from these cells drains out readily; studies have shown that significant quantities of B vitamins can be lost in the drip of thawed meats. If cooking from the frozen state is too difficult, as with a thick roast, it is best to partially thaw to an almost pliable state before cooking. (Cooking time and temperature adjustments usually are small.) There are times when frozen products must be thawed, as when ground beef must be reworked into meatballs or otherwise manipulated before cooking. Strategies here include thawing no longer than necessary and making use of the resulting drip loss.

Carving leads to drip loss as well. A turkey or other large roast should be allowed to "rest" for 15 to 20 minutes after cooking and before slicing, to let the juices set; this reduces the losses when carving begins. To the extent possible, what drippings remain should be made relatively fat-free and used for sauces or low-fat gravy. This is easy to do, by chilling the drippings and then removing the fat after it rises to the top and firms.

Milk

Pasteurization affects few of the nutrients milk is prized for, but prolonged high heat can be detrimental and can precipitate the protein (cause it to separate and sink) in milk. Acid can do this also, so caution is required in combining them smoothly, as in making cream of tomato soup.

Plant Products

Fruits and vegetables are relied on for vitamins A and C, while grains are major B vitamin sources, and all supply minerals. For greatest nutrient retention, the cooking method selected for a given vegetable should be the one that produces the desired outcome with the shortest period of heat exposure. For both fresh and frozen green vegetables, steam cookery is the method of choice for nutrition (and color) because it provides a rapid, penetrating heat treatment without submerging the food in water. Since steam is hotter than boiling water, it cooks in less time, though there is the issue of possible harm to heat-labile nutrients from the steam; but avoiding nutrient leaching losses by steaming offsets this. Using vitamin C as a yardstick of vegetable cookery recommendations, in general, pressure steam cooking preserves more than 70%, steam cookery retains 66%, boiling averages about 45%, and boiling in far more water than is needed multiplies the loss. A wide range of approaches to steam cookery are available, from a simple lidded pan with a rack used atop the range to the microwave oven. Even spinach and other foods that tend to pack together easily can be steamed in today's convection type (forced-air) oven steamers using perforated pans (Fig. 10-7). Often these steamers require no added water, utilizing only the moisture on and in the food itself.

Did you realize that canned vegetables have been fully cooked before you open the can? Accordingly, to preserve nutrients, they should undergo as little further heat treatment as possible. A quick steaming to heat them is the best method. Alternatively, their liquid can be drained and heated, then the vegetables may be returned to the liquid briefly for heating. However, in some instances such as in foodservices for the military, it is required that canned foods be heated above 210°F for at least twenty minutes to destroy any

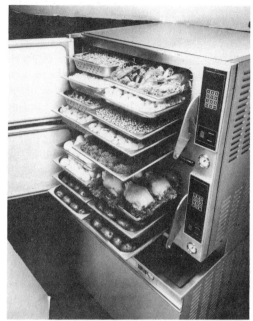

FIGURE 10-7 Convection steamer. *(Courtesy Cleveland/ALCO, Division of ALCO Foodservice Company)*

botulism microbes which could cause illness. For most, however, the need for this caution can be avoided by using reliable food brands, trusted vendors, and sensible storage procedures.

Adding baking soda to cooking water to speed the cooking time of legumes or to protect the color of green vegetables is very poor practice. Especially when heated, this alkaline water is damaging to the alkaline-sensitive nutrients; that is, vitamin C and most of the B vitamins. Vegetables also may develop a slimy, soft texture and lose flavor. The degree of alkalinity of most hard water is so mild that it does not seem to have the same effects.

Except for starchy ones (potatoes, corn), *cooked vegetables should be slightly undercooked.* Most health-conscious guests prefer them to be served this way, and undercooking is insurance against a common foodservice problem, namely that vegetables reach (and often pass) the fully cooked stage while being held for service.

Grains

The B vitamins and minerals we count on from grains are vulnerable to leaching, oxidation, and heat; plus riboflavin is sensitive to light. Most nutrients in rice, bulgur, or rolled oats are retained well if the grains are cooked in a covered pan, along with just the right amount of water or other liquid that the particular grain will absorb during the cooking period. For example, the measure for regular rice is about two parts water to one part grain. With proper measuring the necessity of pouring off nutrients in excess liquid can be avoided. (Enriched rice is not washed before cooking.) Surface area exposure counts in baked grain products as well. Baking cornbread in one large metal pan exposes less area than baking muffins or cornsticks.

The materials used for utensils and cookware that come into contact with food can affect the nutrient value. Good choices are stainless steel, aluminum, glass, and good enamel ware. Copper pots should be lined, as copper destroys vitamins C and E and folic acid, and causes other problems. Some vitamin C also can be destroyed by brass and even iron cookware. (Ironically, vitamin C helps the body utilize iron.) Iron skillets can add usable iron to foods cooked in them.

Allied industries are supporting the delivery of healthful foods and changing the way some foods cook by developing deterioration-resistant product packaging and improving microwave and other cookery and reconstitution packaging and equipment. Boil-in-bag items and microwave pouches bring to the kitchen prepared foods, often sealed and chilled immediately after their initial preparation, and which can remain sealed until the moment of service. They may be individual portions or tray packs, and they may require cooking or simply tempering. With proper storage and use such products have excellent prospects for retaining nutrients and are a sign of additional innovative products to come.

POLICING NUTRIENTS IN PURCHASING AND COOKERY

Of course, purchasing and producing recipes also is an opportunity to avoid certain nutrients. Chapter 4 pointed out the various guises of simple sugar and typical product sources to avoid. Chapter 6 discussed ways to avoid too much fat and choices for balancing meals with more polyunsaturated fat and less cholesterol. Chapter 9 set forth the sodium content of common foods. Finally, an awareness of issues and alternatives, coupled with attention to ingredient labels, may be necessary to side-step the use of particular ingredients and chemical additives in foods that guests may wish to avoid. For example, chemical preservation and processing practices such as those sometimes used in curing meats or even in decaffeinating coffee can be offensive to committed nutrition-oriented guests, so the menu planner and purchasing persons must work around such issues. The following discussion presents ingredient and cookery ideas gleaned from chefs and others who have had success with healthful foods programs.

Fat Control Tactics

When possible, use low-calorie substitutes for ingredients that are high in fat, cholesterol, and calories. Read labels for terms that reveal the presence of saturated fats or cholesterol: egg, egg-yolk solids, whole-milk solids, palm, palm kernel, or coconut oils, imitation or milk chocolate, shortening, hydrogenated or hardened oils, lard, butter, suet, and animal byproducts. Substitute more acceptable products for foods with these ingredients. Use lean meat cuts, trim well before cooking, and remove fat separated out during cooking. Use cooking methods in which fat need not be added, such as broiling or roasting meats and steaming green vegetables.

Specific Tactics. For creamy salad dressings, cut back on the oil or other fat by half or more, using low-fat, plain yogurt in its place. Use low-fat cottage cheese blended with yogurt instead of cream cheese or heavy cream. Adding cornstarch helps prevent curdling when this combination is used in cooking. In place of mayonnaise or sour cream, combine two thirds low-fat cottage cheese with one third plain, low-fat yogurt in a food processor or blender. Use vegetable purees to thicken lean, cooked sauces. Mashed or pureed potato makes a good thickener. The smooth, creamy texture of custards and flans can be achieved with evaporated skim milk instead of whole milk or cream. Consider substituting egg whites for a portion of the whole eggs in custards or flans. Substitute sherbet, ice milk, nonfat frozen yogurt, or tofu desserts for ice cream. For coffee use low-fat milk instead of nondairy creamers, which generally are high in coconut oil, which contains saturated fats.

Substitute low-fat cheeses such as part-skim mozzarella and ricotta for full-cream varieties. Avoid cheeses that contain more than 3 grams of fat per ounce. Some products are promoted as substitutes for cheese; read the labels to see whether they contain saturated fat.

Avoid products that come pre-breaded because the coating often is loaded with fat. Instead, coat food with whole wheat bread crumbs after dipping it in skim milk mixed with an egg white.

Experiment with baked products to minimize added fat. Often one third to one half of the fat in muffin and other bakery products can be eliminated. If commercial mixes are used, purchase those to which the oil is not yet added. When making up the product, use a polyunsaturated oil and, for example, if the recipe calls for one cup of oil, use two thirds cup oil and one third cup water. (Test the quality of the resulting product, noting on the recipe whether the same, more, or less oil should be used next time.)

Saute food in a nonstick pan, using a small amount of stock in place of butter and other fats or, if necessary, a thin coat of oil applied to the pan with a pastry brush or wax paper. Because cold oil is absorbed more readily than hot oil, always heat oil thoroughly before sauteing food. Avoid adding oil to grill marinades; instead, brush food lightly with oil before grilling. The use of teflon-coated pans or using vegetable coating sprays can reduce the amount of fat on food.

FLAVOR FAVORS

In general, season with herbs, spices, and other flavors instead of butter, margarine, or cream or cheese sauces. To sweeten dishes without table sugar, syrup or honey, use concentrated fruit juices, such as frozen apple or orange juice. Choose olive oil instead of the less flavorful vegetable oils when the flavor should shine through. Alternatives to salt include acidic ingredients such as lemon and vinegar; hot seasonings such as ginger, Szechuan peppercorns and hot chilies; strong flavorings such as garlic and onions (especially browned onions); and strong herbs and spices. Wine infuses cooked dishes with flavor, and the alcohol calories evaporate in cooking. (Be certain of the acceptability of the use of alcohol to the guests.)

Reducing Sodium in Foods

Substitute herbs and spices for salt and salt-based seasonings such as garlic salt, seasoned salt, salty condiments (mustard, soy sauce) and monosodium glutamate. Avoid high-sodium processed foods by reading labels. Avoid regular canned vegetables and fish. Avoid excessive baking powder and soda (*sodium bicarbonate*). Use low-sodium or unsalted ingredients during cooking.

SUMMARY

Managers of nutrition-oriented foods programs should ensure that, along with being appealing, quality foods, that program menu selections actually contain the expected and implied nutrient characteristics. Even when a product of high nutrient value is purchased, a significant loss of nutrients can be inflicted on foods due to inappropriate handling, cookery, and holding procedures. While some compromises may be called for in order to meet the volume demands in quantity foodservice, guidelines can be established to assist personnel in seeing that appropriate products are procured and that their nutrient qualities are retained in storage, preparation, production, and service. It is management's responsibility to support the service of nutritious food with training, facilities, equipment, tools, and a spirit of commitment.

Energy nutrients can be lost or rendered unappealing through excess trimming, by dissolving into liquids that subsequently are discarded, from drip-loss of meats, and through damage to the edible quality (overcooking, dehydration, spoilage, fat rancidity). Minerals, though not destroyed, are subject to being discarded and can be changed chemically in combination with certain substances (e.g., pollutants). Vitamins are the most delicate nutrients. Precautions should be in place to guard against needless losses, taking into account the vulnerability of certain vitamins to solubility, acid, alkali, heat, light, and oxidation.

To obtain products of high nutrient quality, foods that are reasonably unrefined should be purchased from vendors who reliably furnish products that have the best nutrient promise (e.g., deep orange cantaloupe) and have been handled appropriately since harvest. Only products that meet program standards should be accepted.

Among common food preservation methods, freezing usually retains the highest proportion of nutrients; canning is much less effective. Each item should be stored as briefly as possible in appropriate conditions of temperature, humidity, ventilation, and packaging for optimal nutrient preservation.

Exposure and losses are avoided in preparation and production by minimizing soaking, cooking, and holding time, cutting vegetables no smaller than required (leaving unpeeled, when possible), cooking frozen foods without thawing, and using appropriate cooking methods (e.g., steaming vegetables instead of boiling). Nutrients in meat drip, other liquids and trim should be preserved in stocks for other recipes. Batch cooking minimizes holding cooked foods too long.

Chapter Review

1. What is meant by the phrase "preserve the healthful qualities of the food"?
2. As manager or owner of a foodservice how would you go about setting up a program to ensure that nutrients were retained in the foods served?
3. What support must management provide to ensure foods have and retain a maximum quantity of nutrients?
4. Name a food that is a major source of each of the three energy nutrients. What kitchen procedures can result in the loss or ruin of energy nutrients? What do employees need to know and do to avoid such problems?
5. What kitchen procedures can result in the loss or destruction of vitamins? Minerals? What do employees need to know and do to avoid such problems?
6. If you wanted to purchase fresh foods with good nutrient values, what would you consider regarding the journey of that food between harvest and the foodservice site? About the vendors?
7. Describe the relative nutrient quality of fresh, frozen, and canned foods in general. Under what circumstances might preserved foods be more nutritious than those termed fresh?
8. Using broccoli as an example, describe the different forms it might take along the "degree of processing continuum" for foods. What considerations for facilities, labor, time and nutrients might apply when deciding what form to buy and serve?
9. Name several examples of color as an indicator of nutrient quality of foods.
10. What is blanching? Why are frozen foods blanched? How does it affect vitamin content?
11. What nonvitamin substance does whole grain bread have that refined, enriched bread lacks?
12. What might the nutrient consequences be in storing foods: (a) for too long, (b) in too warm an environment, and (c) unprotected from pests and contaminants?
13. Describe the recommended storage temperature and duration for fresh fish and for frozen vegetables.
14. What is freezer burn and what does it do to meat? Explain how an unappealing item represents lost nutrients.
15. Describe the main nutrient preservation points in pre-preparing and cooking fresh vegetables.
16. What is drip loss in meat? What damage to quality can drip loss produce? Name guidelines to avoid drip losses.
17. How does steaming compare with boiling in nutrient retention? Why?
18. Explain two separate views on heating canned vegetables? To avoid added exposure to heat, how might they be prepared?
19. What does heat and an alkaline medium do to vitamins C and B_1? What happens to green vegetables when baking soda is put into the cooking water? To legumes?
20. To what stage of doneness should nonstarchy vegetables be cooked?

21. Describe the relationship between nutrient preservation and the amount of surface area of foods exposed to heat, water, etc. What implications does this have for storing, preparing, and production steps?
22. How can new product packaging contribute to the effort to preserve nutrients?
23. What are some culinary tips for avoiding unwanted ingredients while offering tempting sauces and flavors?

Chapter 11
Marketing the Healthful-Foods Program

Chapter Goals

- *To indicate the scope and variety of components that comprise a nutrition-oriented foods program*
- *To provide typical objectives for implementing such a program.*
- *To present a guide for planning a program.*
- *To integrate management and marketing considerations into a program that meets both the desires of guests and the objectives of the business.*
- *To discuss the importance of knowing the market, while providing program-relevant information on how and what to know.*
- *To profile potential market segments that may seek special menus.*
- *To explore a foodservice industry view of patron interest in special menus according to the operations' main consumer markets.*

For many establishments, providing healthful foods is part of a carefully thought out strategy that is necessary for being competitive. The National Restaurant Association (NRA) estimates that more than 45 billion meals are eaten in restaurants, schools, and work places every year; this means that, on average, each person in the U.S. eats over 190 meals out each year. Nearly half of all foodservice guests are interested in nutrition-oriented fare—potentially billions of meals annually. With an eye to the *overall* opportunity, nearly 200 restaurants open every *week* in the U.S., but according to *Standard and Poors'* business reference, nearly 7000 foodservice operations failed during 1986 alone. Only operators who understand and responsively cater to their markets will thrive, or even survive, in such a competitive environment today. Is a healthful-foods program part of the answer?

THE NUTRITION-ORIENTED FOODS PROGRAM—WHAT AND WHY?

There are as many ways to have a healthful-foods program as there are operations. In general in these chapters we are referring to programs with one or more of the emphases and subofferings noted in Table 11-1. Chef Jeremiah Tower provides an example of the *menu item emphasis* with program fare that is low in fat, low in

218

TABLE 11-1
What's in a Nutrition-Oriented
Foods Program?

Emphasis on Menu Items May Include:

Low in calories, often called "light" (see also, low fat)

Low in fat; may include less saturated fat and less cholesterol

Often this means smaller portions or dual portion-size choices, an emphasis on fish and poultry products, and de-emphasis on fatty sauces

Plentiful fresh fruits, vegetables, and whole grain products

Emphasis on quality and freshness of major ingredients

Noted items may be low in sodium, additive-free, all natural, locally grown, meatless, cooked simply, etc.

A willingness to accommodate at least a moderate degree of product substitution and special preparation requests

More involved programs:

May feature highly creative preparation and unusual but healthful ingredients and combinations

A greater preparedness to accommodate individual dietary needs and to honor more complex special requests

Program Emphasis on Information May Include:

The following two items often are used with the menu item emphasis:

Products: designation of menu selections that meet certain criteria, e.g. low in fat and calories

Overall menu: provide information on substances to seek or avoid, e.g., menu items with less than 500 mg sodium

Those below are more typical of fast food operations:

Overall menu: focus on nutrition advantages of existing menu items as one element in promoting good health

Overall menu: highlight how certain nutrient needs are met by selected menu items or combinations of them

---

calories, and high on appeal. His trademark is a dedication to the use of fresh, locally grown ingredients, simple cookery, and creative use of fresh herbs instead of sodium and fatty sauces. For his work with several West Coast restaurants he is credited with being a pioneer in The New American Cuisine, regional and light. On the other hand, by featuring placemats depicting the way its fast food hamburger menu fits into the Basic Four Food Groups Plan, McDonald's cleverly uses the *information emphasis* to draw attention of consumers away from any nutrition drawbacks of the menu and to highlight the benefits of their menu, without resorting to "shaping up" any specific items.

Why have a healthful-foods menu? From a business viewpoint there are a number of reasons to include healthful foods (Table 11-2). When selected reasons are adopted as program objectives, they become the yardstick of success. One or

TABLE 11-2
Is a Healthful-Foods Program Needed?

According to the needs of the company, will the program support the foodservice operation in meeting one or more of these objectives? Being or becoming:

1. More competitive in the market place?
   - Preserve or expand market share.
   - Enhance menu breadth; (overcome veto factor).*
   - Exploit market opportunity.
   - Be able to service possible health-related foodservice contract needs or requirements.

2. More responsive to guests?
   - Answer guest product requests.
   - Cater to guest service requests.
   - Lend positive "We care" image.

3. More profitable?
   - Increase net profit.
   - Increase total sales, average check, average cover.
   - Offset costs.
   - Increase customer counts: more new customers, more frequent repeat customer visits.

* The "veto factor" refers here to a group member who rules out selecting a restaurant for the whole group because it fails to offer menu choices he or she perceives as healthful.

more of the interwoven objectives—being more competitive, more responsive to guests, or more profitable—could spur the concept along. For example, a spokesperson for the Four Seasons hotel chain stated that they wanted to respond to the requests of their health-conscious guests (traveling executives) by providing food moderate in fat and calories. Their measure of resounding success is that nearly 40% of dining room luncheon orders now derive from the low-calorie selections! Nonbusiness reasons, such as personal convictions, were an impetus behind many of the early programs, but conviction *alone* may not pave the way for success. Commercial foodservices can afford to market healthful foods as a part of their offerings only if it pays; they must operate for profit. An editorial in the *NRA News* stressed this, saying, "Make it profitable and we'll use it. We are not in the education business. We're not in the business of telling people what to eat. We are in the business of providing people with a choice of the food they want, and we will adjust our offerings to meet their needs and desires."

Some foodservices have been incorporating health considerations into their foods for a long time. Hospitals, nursing homes, schools, and other operations in institutional settings made health a sales factor in days when there was little nutrition awareness. Many foodservices today are finding it advantageous to promote some foods as healthful to please present and potential patrons (Table 11-3).

Healthful-foods programs are not for everyone. If the operation's customers have little or no interest in a healthful-foods program or if they find that the program

TABLE 11-3
Representative Major Hotel Chains That Offer Nutrition Programs

Best Western International
Days Inn
Fairmont Hotel Company
Four Seasons Hotels, Ltd.
Hilton Corporation
Holiday Corporation
Hyatt Hotels Corporation
Le Meridien Hotels
Loews Hotels
Marriot Corporation
Radisson Hotels
Ramada Inns
Sheraton Hotels
Stouffer Hotels
Thunderbird/Red Lion Inns
Westin Hotels

is inappropriate or confusing, then providing it is unlikely to pay off. In addition, as noted in the following chapters, implementing a program can involve added resource costs, from recipe development to employee training.

Thorough and realistic planning supported by accurate market information can constitute a solid foundation upon which to build a successful healthful-foods program. Without such preparation, or with shoddy planning, the program is likely to be weakened by poor decisions, be shaken by unanticipated problems, and perhaps defeated by the resulting chaos and unpredictability in operations and guest response. Astute foodservice competitors *first* do their homework on the likelihood of meeting goals, and only when that picture looks good is a decision made to undertake a healthful-foods program.

BRINGING THE NUTRITION-ORIENTED FOODS PROGRAM TO LIFE

There is much more to a successful-healthful foods program than deciding to do it and immediately offering new items to guests. A market study should be made, and thought must be given to recipes and a menu plan, preparations for marketing, and staff training. Finally, the items are offered and the market study cycle resumes.

The complexity and time involved in planning and implementing a healthful-foods program depend largely on the scope of the program. Is it for one unit or for an entire chain? Will new cooking or serving equipment be required? Will there be many program items for each meal, or will a few light selections be added at breakfast only?

It is of course necessary to be knowledgeable about nutrition and food as they apply to a healthful-foods program, but it is equally necessary to know how to apply such knowledge in a foodservice operation. Essentially, the managerial demands of a healthful-foods program are very similar to those of any other new or separately identified menu (or menu portion). The important difference is the knowledgeability about foods and nutrition needed to plan and carry out a consistent, appropriate, and responsive healthful-foods program with style and skill.

As for any successful menu program, a well thought-out checklist is in order to organize a thorough consideration of the recommended steps and options. Figure 11-1 is an example of a Program Evaluation Review Technique (PERT) chart representing a possible type of "to do" list for implementing a healthful-foods program. Whatever type of checklist is used, the method should prompt the planner (as PERT does) to consider and to forecast the answers to questions such as these regarding the program:

1. What events must occur? (A market study? A new recipe?)
2. In what sequence must these events occur?
3. What activities must be done to make events happen?
4. What are the interrelationships or interdependencies (e.g., can item 2 be begun before item 1 is completed?)
5. How long will it take to complete the activities?

The foodservice plan may seem complete and foolproof, but it is always good to consider different possible conditions or circumstances and to be prepared to respond to them. Contingency, or back-up, plans should be outlined. In the language of planning, constructing alternative plans to meet a variety of possible outcomes is called *premising* or testing for "what if?" For example, if a vendor is unable to provide particular ingredients in fresh form year-round on acceptable terms, some options are indicating "available in season" on the menu, identifying an acceptable substitute, finding an alternate source, or eliminating the menu item. Plans should be kept flexible so they can be modified as necessary. Plans are made to arrive at goals and objectives, but sometimes even well-planned routes are subject to roadblocks, detours, and other hazards.

In this chapter we will explore events 1 to 6 of Fig. 11-1, defining a healthful-foods program and identifying potential guests for clues as to who and how many are interested in patronizing such programs. The go/no-go program decision is the bottom line. Chapter 12 addresses the menu itself and the activities requiring attention for events 7 to 14. Considerations and decisions involved in selecting appropriate menu items and identifying and developing healthful recipes are the focuses. Attention turns in Chapter 13 to marketing, or selling, the planned menu items. Activities to be completed (or considered) for this effort include plans for menu promotions and for getting feedback. Decisions also must be made about responding to guests' special requests. Formulating descriptions and information for menu copy, handouts for guests, and staff training materials may require special nutrition expertise.

Chapter 14 presents considerations for training programs to support the healthful-foods menu. Knowledge and skills needed to support foodservice employees so that they can carry out their responsibilities effectively within the program are outlined. Whether it is the host person who cheerfully introduces the "Light Touches" menu items in one of the lavish Neiman Marcus department store dining rooms or the chef for a local coffee shop's fitness fare, foodservice employee training is critical to the success of the program.

Checklist for Implementing a
Nutrition-Oriented Foods Program

An example of a simple PERT chart, designed to capture a
sequence of inter-related events within a time-frame.

GUIDE: Circles represent the numbered events listed below: event sequences are shown by numbers inside circles. Arrows between circles represent activities to complete in accomplishing an event. Numbers above arrows represent the estimated days required to finish those activities. The critical path is the longest route (in days) from start to end.

EVENTS:

1. The idea is born: "Should we have a program?"
2. Gather facts, investigate demands, competition, opportunities, etc.
3. Obtain adequate information about foods and nutrition to understand patron and food handling needs. (Some operators may possess this information.)
4. Identify target markets: establish ways (feedback) to understand, influence, and satisfy them and to learn of evolving wants and needs.
5. Set program and menu objectives (e.g., Be more competitive).
6. Decision to go ahead (e.g., after feasibility study shows that an envisioned program or change "fits" and should meet objectives).

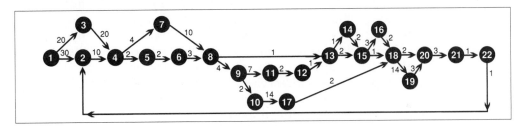

7. List menu ideas consistent with available resources (see Nos. 2, 3, 4, above).
8. Select possible healthful food products and recipes. Adapt or change existing recipes and or develop new ones.
9. Adjust ingredients, check suitability, market costs and access, etc.
10. Announce program and general features and rationale *to staff.* (For optimal staff morale and enthusiasm, be certain this comes before event No. 11).
11. Test recipes for healthful qualities and overall acceptability.
12. Re-assess program based on "fit" and cost versus objectives (see No. 5).
13. Decide which menu items are to be used.
14. Plan selected recipes into program's menu. (For *this* example, it is assumed that the menu necessitates no new equipment or tools.)
15. Plan the terms and scope for menu item descriptions to be made available on employee fact sheets, menu and other promotions.
16. Ready marketing mix elements for new items and/or services. Notify press.
17. Determine program training needs; train trainers.
18. Place orders for needed printed materials (e.g., menus or clip-ones, packaging, fact sheets, flyers, and media advertisement copy).
19. Begin staff training.
20. Review entire program to see that all elements are in place.
21. Program roll-out! With or without fanfare, announce and offer new menu items.
22. Loop to No. 2, fine tuning for a successful, guest-pleasing program.

FIGURE 11-1 Checklist of implementing a nutrition-oriented foods program.

The Guest In The Driver's Seat

The "this-is-what-we-have-and-you-better-like-it days are over," says Steve LaHaie, General Manager of a Chicago restaurant featuring fresh seafood in combination with a healthful-foods program. In a nutshell, this is known as "the marketing concept." If a decision-maker fails to understand and provide what patrons want, would-be patrons will exercise their plentiful options and satisfy their wants elsewhere. No single operation, operator, or program is "the only game in town." Patrons are shoppers; many like to graze, sampling here and there. Competition for dollars, appetites, and eating occasions comes in many forms. To compete successfully, the marketing concept says that one should not push products at patrons; rather, patrons should be attracted to (pulled, not pushed) a product because it offers what they, the guests, want.

One of the challenges in setting up a program of healthful-food choices is that patrons have so many ideas of their own as to what "nutrition" is and how foods affect health. To some, healthfulness means getting plenty of certain foods. To others it means eating foods that are no fun. To still others it means calorie control. One must ask, "If we offer healthful foods, will patrons recognize it? Will they agree with our ideas?" Some will; some will not; and some will be indifferent. This is natural. While it is true that the business of marketing is the business of pleasing, it is also true that there is a great deal of misinformation about concerning what is and what is not good to eat, and in setting up their programs, foodservices should be aware of this and should avoid going too far. Trying to cater to those who want very unusual foods or eccentric diets is not good business. Interest is often short lived. Usually such requests come from only small, sometimes outspoken groups, and in obtaining information on how the market is segmented, this group should also be identified for what it is. Over time, dozens of these ideas may be tried by operators who failed to identify and serve the right markets; eventually they may find that there are as many different ideas on how to eat to stay well or thin as there are patrons. After a period of trying to meet fickle demands, an operator may throw up his or her hands and say, "No more healthful menus here!" Aristotle's famous rule of "nothing in extremes" applies to foodservice operations as well as other areas of life. A solid segment of patrons with reasonable healthful-food desires can be alienated by the practice of going to extremes to satisfy small inappropriate market sub-groups.

Who Will Buy?

Through ongoing formal and informal market research, information should be collected and interpreted to assist in shaping a healthful foods program. The need never ends to study the competition, trends, and especially, the customers in order to attempt to understand their general and specific wants; attitudes (e.g., "health is important to me."); actions (what patrons actually buy, as opposed to what they say they want); and their wish-lists (e.g., low-fat strawberry shortcake). It is important also to know their potential buying power and how they are best reached and attracted (e.g., whether they read a local newspaper). A *customer market* can be defined as a number of individuals, groups of individuals, business enterprises, or other organizations that (1) have wants and needs, or believe they do, (2) have resources (money in most cases), and (3) will buy or exchange their resources for a given product or can be influenced to do so.

According to this definition, the potential market for foodservice customers includes just about everyone. To attempt to match the needs and wants of the mass market with the objectives of any particular foodservice, significant subgroups of the market must be identified by characteristics they share, for example, the frequency with which they eat out and customary spending level; these are termed *market segments*. The diverse tastes and needs of consumers together create a multiplicity of different segments. Many segments include among their needs and wants healthful foods. Foodservice marketers must tailor not only their menus but their marketing programs to relate to what they learn about who potential patrons are and what they are seeking. Only then can they hope to begin to influence a buying decision. It is impossible to sell everything to everybody. A specific product or products should be offered for sale to meet the wants of a specific kind of patron. The marketing program should make potential patrons aware that their wants can be satisfied by certain foods within the operation's overall setting.

But not all patrons have an interest in healthful foods, (Fig. 11-2). Recognizing who the market is *not* is an important part of knowing the market. It can be a waste of effort to attempt to please those who are inconsistent or indifferent in their response to healthful-foods programs. Importantly, it is up to the operator to match product and market. Healthful foods could be a completely inappropriate merchandising tool for some clientele: a market segment that consists principally of persons who engage in heavy physical labor has no reason to respond to a menu that offers only portions of a size appropriate for the weight conscious.

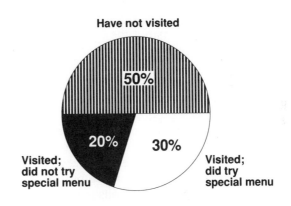

U.S. Adult Population

FIGURE 11-2 Restaurants offering special menu items. *(Reprinted from "Consumer Nutrition Concerns and Restaurant Choices," published by the National Restaurant Association, 1986)*

GETTING TO KNOW THE MARKET

A secret intelligence mission may sound more glamorous in an adventure movie, but an intelligence system should be very much a part of any foodservice operation. This refers to the ongoing system of information gathering needed to assist in investigating, developing, and maintaining a successful operation. Information supports making informed decisions and taking appropriate action when necessary. A well-tuned intelligence system is paramount to a program for healthful foods because of the constantly shifting demands of customers and the dynamic, competitive environment, and because the business of managing foodservices from a nutrition standpoint is in its infancy. It requires close attention, but offers valuable rewards.

Among other techniques, information can be collected through personal discussions with guests, interactions with staff, formal or informal surveys (including comment cards), through dining visits to the competition, by regularly reviewing pertinent publications relating to foodservices, nutrition, and health, and by attending foodservices shows. No matter how sophisticated or simple this intelligence system is, its purpose is to keep decision makers abreast of actions, forces, and feedback that could affect the business and could suggest opportunities or needed changes.

Intelligence information to review may provide an update on activities *internal to the foodservice*, such as monitoring patron response to waitstaff knowledgeability about healthful menu offerings or about production personnel morale and attitudes. It is important also to look beyond the front door. It may seem relatively easy to respond to patrons' comments but the intelligence system that stops there has no input from people who do not participate or visit but who might be persuaded to do so if their desires were known. Intelligence also should bring in information from sources external to the operation. Figure 11-3 presents some of the major external forces that are always present but frequently overlooked in the long-term scheme of managing a healthful-foods program.

Learning about the marketplace is a complex but worthwhile undertaking. Good research means asking questions to learn about consumers, the market forces, competition, etc. The better the research, the more useful will be the results. Who and what to ask? How should questions be phrased? And finally, the responses and other feedback must be interpreted realistically and applied sensibly. This is a good time to invest in the services of a business research specialist or even a promising graduate student at a nearby hospitality or business school.

Markets and Target Markets

Knowing that people are interested in healthful foods is not enough information around which to design a sales program. The market has to be described and segmented into groups that can be targeted, attracted, and won over. Once a profile has been drawn, a reasonable estimate of the numbers of potential patrons in different segments can be made using both published information and that derived from guest and waitstaff comments, surveys, and other input. Knowing these segments and their size is fundamental to decisions on the scope and emphasis of the program, (e.g., fresh foods, weight control, low salt, etc.). Before money and effort are expended on programs, it is only good business to establish that enough people are sufficiently interested and willing to pay for them to make the investment worthwhile.

Like a cake, the market can be sliced, or segmented, in innumerable ways. Many surveys on patron actions have been conducted. Though no single survey can ascertain how strongly patrons feel a need for more emphasis on healthful foods, reviewing several surveys can be revealing. Fortunately, we can look to certain indicators, or clues, such as demographic descriptors, and from them, draw inferences as to whether different segments exist and their size and strength. Demographics are fundamental in understanding guests. Such information is available in public census records such as those categories in Figure 11-4. In the paragraphs that follow, note how specific combinations of patron demographic characteristics suggest the most likely candidates for healthful-foods programs. As an example, consider the

Forces:	Competitive	Economic
Social		Labor
Technological		International
Political/Legal		Medical

Forces Outside the Company	"Intelligence Information Examples Pertinent to Managers of Healthful Foodservice Programs
Social:	Demographics: A growing proportion of the population is composed of nutrition-conscious seniors.
Competitive:	Direct: Customers often choose one restaurant over another because it offers a salad bar.
	Indirect: Will customers use their limited time and money to dine out, or to enjoy their own healthful foods preparation at home with a video?
Economic:	Local: Regular patrons from a nearby plant may soon lose their jobs and their usual income.
Technological:	Succulent beef with 30% less saturated fat than usual herds provide is now a reality.
Labor:	How can we attract and retain good employees? In some areas, the most pressing issue for day-to-day operations has been recruiting able people.
Political/Legal:	When and if so, in what form will menu labeling become law? How can we now honor the "intent" of the law?
International:	Providing new markets, new products, and able competition, this sphere is a growing force in the environment of healthful menus.
Medical:	A medical report reveals new evidence that a diet with ample fiber can be beneficial.

FIGURE 11-3 Examples of external "forces" on healthful-food service programs.

over-50 market. A recent *Wall Street Journal* article reports that between 1978 and 1988, the amount of dining out by senior citizens increased by 21%, though it increased only 6% in the population overall. This trend is significant, because seniors frequently prefer modest portions and low-fat foods and, surprisingly, they now constitute one third of restaurant breakfast and dinner patrons. The magnitude of this opportunity comes to light when it is noted that, as of 1988, the following major corporations were in various stages of entering the continuing-care market, preparing to pamper aging baby boomers: Holiday Corporation, Marriott Corporation, Hyatt Hotels, and TW Services, (parent of Denny's and Canteen Corporation).

Age
Sex
Education
Family size
Income range
Marital status
Employment type
Ethnic heritage
Family income level
Rural urban residence
Region of the country
Family members working
Stage in the family life cycle

FIGURE 11-4 Demographic and common descriptive information often usable in customer market segmentation.

Consumer Interest in Nutrition

In their study of patron attitudes, the NRA revealed their findings that *more than half of the population says that they would be "likely to try nutritious and unprocessed foods at restaurants if given a chance."* The NRA has studied restaurant patrons in general over many years and, in the late 1980s, stated "Consumer interest in health and nutrition is a trend that has had, and will continue to have, a significant impact on the foodservices industry.... Consumers' interest in nutrition when eating away from home is undiminished."

The findings in these and in the studies below point to other nutrition-related foodservices opportunities and to distinctions among Americans surveyed. Some recurrent themes are apparent in the findings discussed in this and future chapters. In general, consumers appear to be split between seeking novelty or creativity, and seeking mother-love foods, the old favorites such as bakery sweets. Also, it appears that the nutrition-related concerns of a broad spectrum of guests have placed them on dietary alert to:

1. *Include* certain foods or substances perceived as healthful.
2. *Restrict* certain nutrients or substances perceived as unhealthful and foods containing high levels of them.
3. Seek *alternate preparation* methods, (in line with the above)
4. Have *access to information* about the health-related qualities of menu choices to support making informed decisions on items 1 to 3.

A look at a small handful of studies can shed light on such consumer interest. Table 11-4 presents the results of a 1987 study that reveals the high interest in the idea that foodservice operators should offer guests low-sodium, low-fat, and low-calorie foods. From one half to two thirds of restaurant patrons say they consciously choose to avoid such items as fat and to include plenty of fiber in their diets (Table 11-5). In 1984, Lipske studied the public's interest in nutritious foods (Table 11-6).

TABLE 11-4
Patrons' Interest in Being Offered
Healthful Foods

	Yes (%)
Low-sodium food	63.5
Low-fat/low-cholesterol food	61.7
Low calorie food	58.0

Pratscher M, Lydecker T, Weinstein J, and Bertagnoli L: "Tastes of America: How America Loves to Eat Out," Restaurants and Institutions, vol. 97, pp 30-84, 1987.

The study cautioned that what was reported was *attitudes* and that patrons might behave quite differently when the time came to order from a menu.

THE NRA'S FOUR SEGMENTS: OPPORTUNITIES ABOUND

Traditional Customers. The NRA in the mid-1980s identified four distinct customer market segments based on attitudes of foodservice patrons toward healthful foods (Figure 11-5 and Table 11-7). The largest group is *traditional consumers*, who constitute 37% of the population, but consume 43% of all meals served; in other words, they eat out more than the average person. The group, which also accounts for nearly half (46%) of reported visits to fast food outlets, is dominated by single, young men who earn less than $40,000 a year. They show little or no interest in selecting foods for their healthful qualities. They want primarily flavor. They evidently come to eat traditional meat-and-potatoes meals without regard for health concerns. Some may be dieting but decide to forget the diet because they are going out. Such a youthful group would normally have few health problems and little concern about future health. Targeting such a group for a healthful-foods program would be unlikely to lead to success.

Many establishments, including fast food chains, have found that offering alternatives of one or more healthful menu choices counteracts the *veto factor* (i.e.,

TABLE 11-5
Nutrition-Minded Food Choices

Percentages of Americans Who Consciously Include or Restrict Selected Foods, Nutrients, or Substances When Making Food Choices

	Include (%)		Restrict (%)
Foods high in calcium	68	High-fat foods	68
Foods high in fiber	67	Salt	68
Foods high in starch,		Sugar	68
(e.g., rice, pasta, bread)	67	High-cholesterol foods	65
		Additives (artificial	
		flavors and colors)	50

Reprinted from Consumer Nutrition Concerns and Restaurant Choices, published by the National Restaurant Association, 1986.

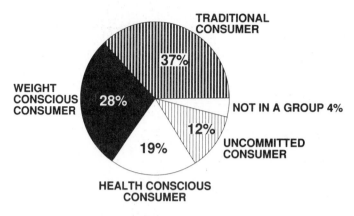

U.S. Adult Population

FIGURE 11-5 Restaurant market segmentation according to interest in nutrition. *(Reprinted from "Consumer Nutrition Concerns and Restaurant Choices," published by the National Restaurant Association, 1986)*

when one member of a group sways the others from going to an operation because he or she is particular about diet). Wendy's, Burger King, and Carl's Jr. introduced salad bars as such a measure. On the higher end of the price scale, planners point out that diners in their gourmet rooms and bistros have diverse clients and guests to please. They take away the veto obstacle by an artful blending of items for the health conscious consumer. Compare Figures 11-2 and 11-6 for evidence that 49% of the NRA's traditional consumers do patronize operations that have special menu items. Realizing that traditionals are not very interested in special menus, some of those visits may have occurred because a well-rounded menu offered something appealing to each type of consumer in their group, so it was unnecessary for the veto factor to come into play.

Weight-Conscious. *Weight-conscious consumers*—28% of the population who eat 25% of restaurant meals—want food that is low in calories. While they eat out less often, they spend more, accounting for 31% of all visits to fine dining establishments. The group is made up largely of middle-aged, career homemakers, married women living in urban areas with household incomes of more than $40,000.

TABLE 11-6
Special Food Interest of Restaurant Patrons

Preference	(%)
Those wanting diet foods	26
Those wanting natural foods	23
Those wanting "meat and potato" type foods	20
Those wanting "kid foods"	16
Those wanting sophisticated foods	10

Lipske S.N: "The Eating Out Public's Interest in Nutrition," Position Paper and Research Summary, GDR-CREST, NRA, 1984.

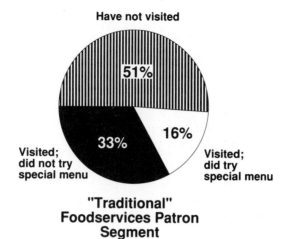

Have not visited

51%

Visited; did not try special menu 33%

16% **Visited; did try special menu**

"Traditional" Foodservices Patron Segment

FIGURE 11-6 Restaurants offering special menu items do attract the "NRA Traditional" (meat-and-potatoes) consumer, perhaps because the menu helps to overcome the "veto factor." *(Reprinted from "Consumer Concerns and Restaurant Choices," published by the National Restaurant Association, 1986)*

Health-Conscious. The third NRA group makes up 19% of the population and consumes 17% of all restaurant meals. Like weight-conscious diners, these people demonstrate a willingness to spend more for what they want and account for 26% of all fine dining visits. The demographics of this group are 55 to 64 years old, female, married, child-free, exercise regularly, and well-educated. They probably represent the group most likely to respond in numbers to a healthful-foods program, but they may want "the works": low calories, fiber, whole grains, low-fat. They are likely to be loyal if the program is well-conceived and consistent.

Though there is certainly ample cross-over between these two groups, NRA's weight-conscious and health-conscious consumers in general differ both in the food choices of interest to them and in their eating attitudes. Many (not all) weight-conscious consumers may have little regard for nutrient density, additives, and sodium. Total calories often are the sole focus. The health-conscious person, on the other

TABLE 11-7
NRA Study Segments Consumer Attitudes

Consumer Attitude Segment	% of Adult Population	Reported Eating Out Occasion			
		Total (%)	Fast Food (%)	Moderately Priced (%)	Fine Dining (%)
Traditional	37	43	46	39	32
Weight Conscious	28	25	23	26	31
Health Conscious	19	17	16	16	26
Uncommitted	12	12	12	14	8
Not in Group	4	3	3	5	3

Reprinted from Consumer Nutrition Concerns and Restaurant Choices, published by the National Restaurant Association, 1986.

hand, may have a litany of criteria for menu selections (low fat, low cholesterol, no additives) and might expect a modest calorie count to be part of the package. Figure 11-7 contrasts the responses from members of each group to typical menu items they might be likely to try if they were available at restaurants. Notice that the top choices of the weight conscious-consumers include items likely to contain additives or "artificial" ingredients that save calories. The health-conscious consumers ranked such "real," whole foods as fish, whole grains, and vegetables atop their list.

In attitudes, NRA's weight-conscious consumers report that they believe calorie control is an essential part of their weight program, but they sometimes feel they are giving up a lot of pleasure when they order low-calorie items. Although they may occasionally order very high-calorie foods, in general, they make a point of ordering nutritious foods when they eat out. They prefer broiled foods and consider fried foods "bad for you." Significantly for alert restaurateurs, they report that they "would eat out more often if it wasn't so fattening."

In contrast to other patrons, health-conscious diners do not feel that flavor is the most important thing about food, but neither do they think that foods that are good for them do not taste good. They know about nutrition, know what they want, and are conscientious about sticking to their dietary objectives. Rather than feeling

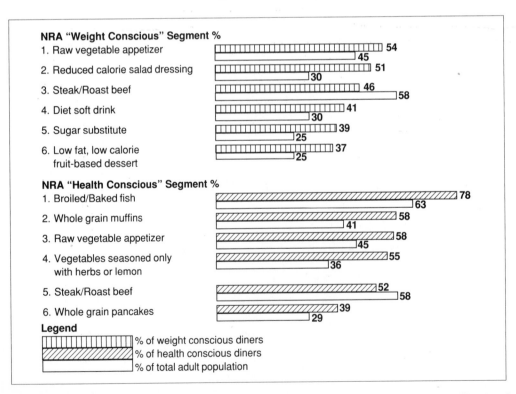

FIGURE 11-7 Menu items patrons are most likely to try if they are availale at restaurants. *(Reprinted from "Consumer Nutrition Concerns and Restaurant Choices," published by the National Restaurant Association, 1986)*

as if selecting healthful foods is self-deprivation, they regard it as another facet of a lifestyle along with exercise and other health concerns.

Uncommitted Consumers. The fourth NRA group accounts for 12% of the population and 12% of all meals eaten out. (Four percent of the population [3% of meals eaten out] did not belong to any of the identified groups.) Typically the uncommitted are persons in transition from one set of values or circumstances to another, 35 to 64 years old, who live in the suburbs, have no children, and earn more than $40,000 per household. Members typically patronize fast-food and mid-scale restaurants. Few have strong opinions about diet, but many are somewhat conscious of the need to restrict fat, calories, cholesterol, and perhaps sugar. Their motivation to exercise *some* dietary restraint probably is not entirely their own but is based on the urging of a physician or family member, often a loved one concerned with the person's weight gain or the risk of heart disease.

Beyond the NRA Segments

Other indicators of opportunities for offering healthful foods abound. It is estimated that between one third and one half of all U.S. adults are on some kind of diet. Most of these "dieters", an estimated 65 million, do so to control weight, but there is also a significant group who have cardiovascular problems or at least are concerned about them. Half of all deaths from disease stem from disorders of the heart and blood vessels. Moderation of intake of foods thought to be associated with high blood pressure, stroke, and heart attack is an important consideration in food selection for a significant number of diners and may be medically prescribed.

A substantial market, nearly 10 million people, suffer from diabetes, and many of them must control their diet very strictly. Most of them have a type of diabetes that can be managed by good diet without drugs. A menu that meets their needs offers a selection of foods that provide adequate nutrients and are low or moderate in calories. Some restriction of refined carbohydrate is often necessary, but diabetics who handle insulin treatment well can usually eat a normal amount of carbohydrate without any problems. Choices appropriate for a diabetic can also serve as balanced, nutritious choices for the general public, and vice versa.

Many people must, or should, follow diets of various kinds, particularly the 10% who are over 65. Those with gout, kidney, or gastrointestinal problems and persons with needs associated with pregnancy, among others, are potential patrons for healthful food selections. Five percent of Americans are estimated to have food intolerances: allergies represent about 1% of them. These persons look for appropriate food items and for clear ingredient information to guide their selections.

Restaurants in and near hotels can look to the more than 2 million persons who stay in hotels each night as a potential market for a nutrition-oriented program. For them, eating away from home is a must. Among other interested segments, many of these are fitness-conscious business persons who are pleased to find special menus designed to help them stay in shape while they are on the road.

Finally, many men and women, especially those between 30 and 50 years old, are fitness-conscious. Many are relatively affluent and are prepared to pay for products and services that promote their well-being. Typically, they take nutrition seriously and certainly might be attracted to an appealing and appropriate menu of healthful foods.

AN INDUSTRY PERSPECTIVE: WHO SERVES NUTRITION-MINDED GUESTS?

With an idea in mind of the wants and characteristics of potential program patrons, clues for program planning can be derived from a broad look at the foodservice industry. Consider the profile of persons most likely to visit foodservice operations of the main types as presented in Table 11-8. A survey by Sherwood (Fig. 11-8) helped capture patron attitudes on the availability of nutritious foods at *operations* targeted to different consumers (or their varying moods). An operation's concept or theme offers clues to probable patron interest in nutrition.

The existing or planned menu concept also can provide insight into the probable "fit" of a healthful-foods element and to patron interest. If patrons come to a restaurant for heavy barbecued ribs or for rich, traditional French cuisine, such a program may be inappropriate. But not necessarily. *Friendly's Family Restaurants*, famous for their ice cream (which still makes up 40% of sales), continue to expand their popular "light" menu.

The Feasibility Study

Any start-up or major change in the way a business is operated should be preceded by at least an informal feasibility study, which enables the operator to avoid many pitfalls, develop stronger and surer plans, and perhaps determine that a wiser decision, under the circumstances, is no-go rather than go. The NRA has recommended five steps for making a feasibility study, a highly simplified view of which is given in flow chart form in Figure 11-9. The explanations of the five steps follow.

Step 1. Collect information about the market area. Learn about the population to be served. Collect demographic and attitudinal information, such as the age and income level of the potential group. Are they fitness-conscious? Do they eat out often? Where? Who decides? Are they concerned with healthful foods when they eat out? Which foods or what kinds of foods? Why? Planners also need to investigate such variables as traffic volume and patterns, customer sources (e.g., nearby shops or office complexes), and city/county/state zoning and other regulations and plans that could impact the area in the foreseeable future. If the budget allows, a more sophisticated marketing survey might be launched to learn about the consumer area in greater detail.

Step 2. Investigate other competition, including operations that may also be promoting healthful foods. *Competition* is "anything else that people who might otherwise come to one's operation can and do choose to do with their money, time, appetites, and occasions." Competition has varied faces, such as operations in a similar price range, those with similar menus, and those that are equally convenient. Competition for a particular meal, time of day, or occasion is another way to zoom in on the picture. Where do people go for breakfast? Where would they go after the gym?

Such questions cannot be answered by driving down the street and counting the number of fast food stands. Some of the questions can be answered only by using intelligence data to learn the attitudes and actions behind patronage patterns and competitive strategies.

Step 3. Assemble and interpret the information collected about the market, the area, and the competitive environment. This step requires objectivity and realism. Who are your patrons? Will they pay for healthful foods? Sketch out a menu and service plan, and establish basic goals. For example: What proportion of income is expected to come from this market? What level of orders is expected per meal period?

Step 4. Next, extend the menu and service concept in the light of what has been learned from steps 1,2, and 3 about the needs and preferences of the population in the market area. Begin to formulate strategies and programs to be used to attract this market. At this point, write out detailed (but still tentative) decisions on what will

TABLE 11-8
Tendency of Major Foodservice Markets to
Incorporate a Healthful Foods Program

Major Food Service Markets and Typical Sub-Markets	Tendency to Incorporate Nutrition in the Menu		
	High	Moderate	Low
Public Settings			
Free-standing eating establishments			
Fine dining		+	
Family dining		+	
Fast food			+
Cafeterias		+	
Social caterers		+	
Hotels/motels	+ *		
Transportation (air/rail)	+ *		
Leisure			
Concessions (arenas, theatres)			+
Clubs		+	
Retail			
Department stores	+ *		
Convenience stores			+
Less Public and Institutional Settings			
Plants and business offices	+ †		
Schools	+ *		
Health care			
Hospitals	+		
Senior centers	+		
Detention	+		
Military	+		

* Particularly in "first-class settings
† Particularly when linked with a wellness program

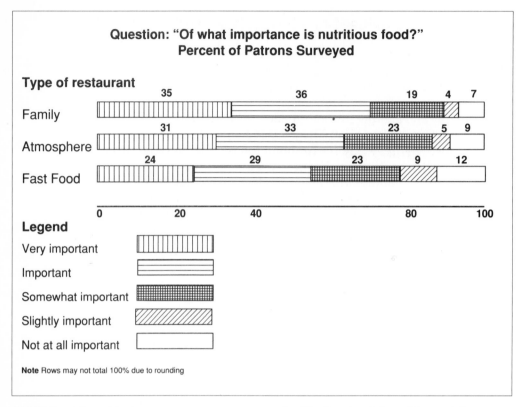

Question: "Of what importance is nutritious food?"
Percent of Patrons Surveyed

Type of restaurant

Family: 35 | 36 | 19 | 4 | 7

Atmosphere: 31 | 33 | 23 | 5 | 9

Fast Food: 24 | 29 | 23 | 9 | 12

Scale: 0, 20, 40, 80, 100

Legend

Very important
Important
Somewhat important
Slightly important
Not at all important

Note Rows may not total 100% due to rounding

FIGURE 11-8 *"Of what importance is nutritious food?" (Reprinted from "National Restaurant Association's Current Issues Report, Nutrition and Foodservices and Food Product Information".)*

be offered, prices, the service style, decor, entertainment, staffing level, hours of operation, etc. Step 5 depends on carrying out this step comprehensively and accurately.

Step 5. Question: Is the addition of the envisioned healthful-foods program a sound venture for implementation? Step 5 is intended to lead to an answer or decision: go, no-go, or modify the plan and reevaluate. The decision should take shape from summarizing and analyzing information from Step 4. Computerized spreadsheet software can speed calculations of the quantitative impact of the new menu (e.g., expected volume per weekday lunch, perhaps broken down by number of guests, costs, sales, program menu item type, and ingredient requirements). Either manually or with the help of a computer, project ahead, using both pessimistic and realistic forecasts of patronage, costs, and other parameters. Explore contingencies: "What if we were to add a third chicken item to the menu? How might this change the estimates on costs and sales?" Try different forecasts to see whether particular changes in the plans might achieve better results.

If new healthful foods will comprise a substantial portion of the total menu, it is advisable to prepare from forecasts such financial statement tests as a profit-and-loss statement, an income statement, a cash budget, and a balance sheet. A sources-

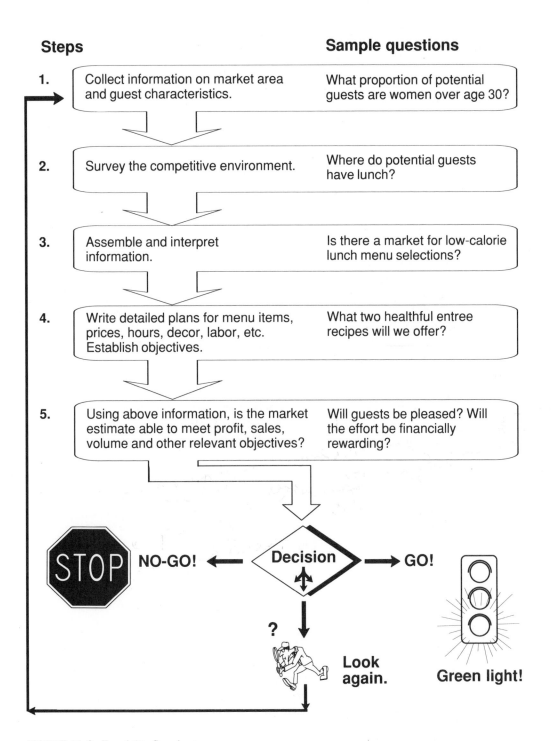

FIGURE 11-9   Feasibility flowchart.

and-uses-of-funds statement could provide a view of financing and potential profitability of the program. The venture must also satisfy company objectives such as profitability, cash flow, sales volume, growth, and goodwill. Other preliminary considerations pertain to company resources. Will such a program bring sufficient benefits (e.g., sales, repeat business) to justify any required investment for inventory, facilities, equipment, and preparation and service training?

It is possible that the information in the financial statements will show that the business cannot support a health-related foodservice program. Other obstacles may also surface, such as production bottlenecks or an incompatibility between the menu and the operations' image. If this is the case, it is best to re-evaluate the information in Step 3 to see whether there is another practical way to serve the market that was neglected or put aside earlier. If so, repeat Steps 4 and 5 for that approach. If the planned outcome seems neither attractive nor practical, it is best either to begin the process again using the insight gained or simply to drop the idea for the present time.

As protracted and time-consuming as this process may seem, and it is indeed, it offers many benefits. The most important might be avoiding an unsuccessful program and developing a potential winner. A second benefit is that, rather than having many untested concepts floating vaguely in the mind, the process of writing out a plan, as in Step 4, requires a degree of commitment to important decisions, and can point to contradictions that would go unnoticed were the plan not put on paper (e.g., the intended hours of operation for the "*A.M. Naturelle*" breakfast program might conflict with the expected staffing schedule). For a new operation, a third benefit is that a lending institution, such as a bank or the Small Business Administration, requires business plans similar to that outlined here. The lender needs to know that management has researched the situation, that a clearly detailed projection of the business has been completed, and that financial statements based on the plan of operation point to the ability to repay borrowed funds.

It's Feasible

When the feasibility study points toward a "go" situation, the time has arrived to finalize the healthful-foods menu. The next chapter provides guidance for menu planning and recipe development for guests interested in dining out with an eye to nutrition.

SUMMARY

Nutrition-oriented foodservice programs usually emphasize menu items that have qualities perceived as health related (e.g., fresh, low-fat) and/or nutrition information. Because of the widespread interest in health and the popularity of eating out, a nutrition program may be part of the foodservice operator's answer to meeting such objectives as being more competitive. Plans, based on a thorough understanding of the market, guests, and operations, should constitute the first step in establishing a new or revised healthful foods program. A checklist should be prepared to guide the activities necessary for taking the program from idea to service success.

The collective opinion of consumers drives the market today. Thus, the market concept refers to the need for foodservice decision-makers to satisfy patron demands based on factual information on their present and potential desires for a dining experience.

A marketing intelligence and feedback system is vital to study the market, its needs, and, eventually, the program's performance. Marketing program changes might be prompted by information from internal and external sources.

The total market includes subgroups of persons with similar attitudes on eating, including those for whom the healthful foods program specifically is structured and those for whom it has no appeal. The NRA has identified four segments based on dining-out food choice attitudes. Thirty-seven percent are considered traditional and prefer fast food, meat-and-potatoes menus. Another 12% are uncommitted; their attitudes are changing. The two groups seeking healthful-foods choices are the weight-conscious (28%) and the health-conscious consumers (19%), although the menu demands of the two groups differ. A healthful-foods program can overcome a patron veto factor by broadening the appeal of a menu across segments. Many other indicators also point to an ongoing, undiminishing but shifting interest in healthful foods, including the large number of persons on various medically imposed diets.

A feasibility study is an evaluation tool for making decisions on whether or not to go ahead with the plan. Five steps in the feasibility study are (1) collect information about the market area and population; (2) investigate the competition; (3) assemble and interpret information from 1 and 2 and establish operational objectives; (4) plan in detail the menu and service concept, including expected costs and sales levels; (5) evaluate whether objectives are met and whether the target market is large enough to provide a worthwhile business base. Finally, make the decision to go/no-go, or to look again.

Chapter Review

1. What types of nutrition-related emphases on menu items might be included in a foodservice nutrition program?
2. How could a nutrition-oriented foods program support the objective of remaining competitive? Responsive to guests?
3. What is the purpose of planning? Why should planning come first in starting a new operation or business?
4. A planning timetable provides guidelines for accomplishments and coordination of times and events, as well as a measure of due dates and deadlines. As an exercise, write the numbers 5, 4, 3, 2, 1, 0 across the top of a page. The 5 represents your decision to investigate establishing a healthful-foods program, and the 0 represents the day the program is introduced. The numbers 4, 3, 2, and 1 represent the months preceding opening. Under each month list the major categories of planning activities that might need attention that month. Remember, some items must come in a particular sequence (e.g., planning what to

communicate to the waitstaff about the new menu must come after planning the menu).

5. What is premising? Why is premising an important part of planning?
6. Should the types of plans discussed in this chapter be flexible or should they be rigid and followed absolutely as written? Explain your answer.
7. What is "the marketing concept"? Explain a consumer-driven market. Should *each* individual consumer be in the driver's seat, in terms of dictating menu and service demands? Why or why not?
8. Why is it important to get to know the wants and needs of guests and potential guests?
9. Describe some of the different ways members of the general public are likely to interpret the concept of healthful food choices.
10. Define a customer market. What is a market segment? A target market segment? Is the target market segment part of the customer market?
11. What are three qualities a customer market must have?
12. Why is marketing to a target market segment a good answer to the challenge of responding to the many possible opinions on what is healthful eating?
13. What is the purpose of an intelligence system? Give an example of an internal force relevant to healthful foods. An external force.
14. Name several guest demographic characteristics that seem to be associated with wanting healthful foods.
15. According to Table 11-5, what substances did half or more of survey respondents say they restrict?
16. Describe the relative size and characteristics of each of the four NRA consumer segments.
17. Discuss the types of differences one might expect in menu selections preferred by the *NRA's* health-conscious and weight-conscious consumers.
18. What is the veto factor and how can a nutrition program help avoid this problem?
19. Name several indicators (other than the NRA survey) of the probable demand for nutrition programs.
20. In matching a foodservice concept with guests' nutrition interests, name several types of foodservices for which a nutrition program may be less in demand. More in demand.
21. What are the five steps of a feasibility study? What should one know after Step 3? In which step should a decision be made as to which specific healthful menu items are to go on the menu and on the volume expected to sell? When should one look at the bottom line to see whether the program is feasible?
22. What are the reasons for conducting a feasibility study *before* beginning a foodservices program of healthful foods?

Chapter 12
Bringing the Menu to Life

Chapter Goals

- *To stimulate interest in and understanding of planning menus that suit the desires of nutrition-oriented guests.*
- *To indicate objectives and limits in recipe and menu decisions.*
- *To provide examples of nutrition-oriented recipes and menu programs suitable for various types of foodservices.*
- *To outline the objectives and considerations of major foodservice diet programs that are in use regionally and nationwide.*
- *To provide examples and potential sources of healthful recipes.*
- *To examine nutritional considerations in healthful recipe development.*
- *To list and illustrate approaches to nutrient analysis of recipes.*
- *To discuss the purpose and aspects of recipe testing and evaluation.*
- *To discuss the opportunity in viewing menu item accompaniments and special requests as part of menu planning.*
- *To explore distinctions between menu and meal development.*

THE MENU OPPORTUNITY

The decision to "go" with a nutrition-oriented foods program calls for a menu worthy of success. As the PERT chart in the previous chapter lists (Fig. 11-1) recipes must be collected, selected, developed, and tested, then artfully incorporated into the overall program of the operation. An operator does not just decide to serve healthful food and begin serving immediately. Menuing healthful foods can be profitable. It is not a good will effort, but it certainly can enhance the public image of an operation. When healthful eating is among the desires of one or more targeted market segments, operators are wise to build healthful foods into their foodservices. Marketing at least several lighter, more nutritious menu selections can broaden the customer base without driving away those who come for the operation's usual offerings. Well-executed meals and snacks that conform to healthful standards also are attractive to patrons other than those who consciously seek healthful foods. An exotic fresh fruit juice "mocktail" could appeal to a broad market, including youngsters. In some patrons' minds, there is a stigma to healthful foods that evidently stems from the old idea that diet is denial. It should be an aim of the operation to prove this false, through the appeal and quality of program selections. Over days, months, and years, such menu choices tend also to be ordered by many of the

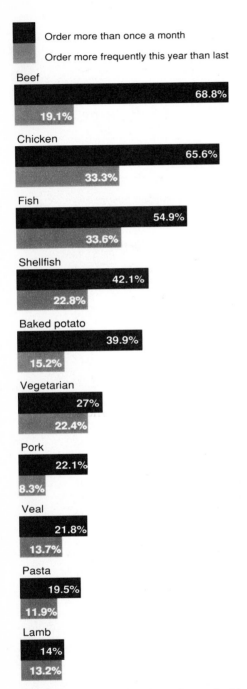

Order more than once a month

Order more frequently this year than last

Beef
68.8%
19.1%

Chicken
65.6%
33.3%

Fish
54.9%
33.6%

Shellfish
42.1%
22.8%

Baked potato
39.9%
15.2%

Vegetarian
27%
22.4%

Pork
22.1%
8.3%

Veal
21.8%
13.7%

Pasta
19.5%
11.9%

Lamb
14%
13.2%

FIGURE 12-1 Changing menu choices: In this cross-sectional survey of restaurant patrons, it is easy to spot the popularity of chicken, fish and vegetarian entrees. (*Pratscher M, Lydecker T, Weinstein J, Bertagnoli L: "Tastes of America: How America Loves to Eat Out" Restaurants and Institutions, Vol 97, p 49, 1987*)

uncommitted and by those who vacillate between selecting and neglecting nutrition-oriented menu options.

Figure 12-1 shows how patron orders have changed in just one year. They are ordering more items considered to be low in fat, such as fish and chicken. Between 1983 and 1986, the NRA found that four out of 10 consumers said they had changed their restaurant eating patterns because of health and nutrition concerns, and six out of 10 said they had changed their eating patterns at home for the same reasons. The study further showed that breakfast sandwich orders more than doubled from 1982 to 1985; in the same period, broiled or baked fish orders jumped 51%, salad entrees 38%, and rice dishes 37%. During this time, steak sandwich orders declined 33%, seafood dropped 17%, (perhaps because it was fried) and steak platters fell off 15%. Also consistent with this trend toward more healthful foods, 26% of all consumers said they ordered more vegetables. Table 12-1 offers a look at changes in recipes and menus that a handful of fast food chicken chains have undertaken recently in the scramble to broaden their market by attracting nutrition-oriented guests.

Which Came First, the Menu or the Recipe?

This question is as vexing as the chicken-egg puzzle. Once menu ideas are in place, recipes

TABLE 12-1
A Sampling of Recent Nutrition-Oriented Recipe and
Menu Changes by Chicken Chains

Chick-Fil-A	Changed to peanut oil for chicken cookery.
Church's	Classic "broiled chicken" with one-third the calories and one-half the fat of the fried product.
El Pollo Asado	Spanish for char-broiled chicken, this marinated flame-broiled dinner claims to be "changing America's taste in chicken."
El Pollo Loco	The American Heart Association has approved their non-fried chicken.
Kentucky Fried Chicken	Oven-roasted chicken, a chicken quarter marinated and sprinkled with a specialty seasoning mix.
Lee's	Puts out roast chicken.
Mrs. Winner's	Thinner dinner salads and sandwiches and a boneless, skinless chicken breast.
Pioneer Take-out Corp.	Lighter products in testing: signs in all units to tell guests that pure vegetable shortening is used.
Popeye's	Barbequed chicken sandwich, with sides of red beans and rice or "dirty rice."

can be sought. Similarly, when an understanding of guests' wants is in focus, then promising recipes can be tailored for the menu and resource and foodservice nutrition management needs can be spelled out. To seize the program opportunity in putting together menus and recipes, it should be all the more apparent that a seat-of-the-pants technique is unlikely to succeed. Program objectives and information about changing desires of markets should be kept in mind throughout the recipe and menu planning processes, and for the life of the operation. The new healthful menu must not be just a cosmetic—like painting over blistered boards—it must have a solid concept and a well-prepared foundation of recipes.

MENU MANAGEMENT FOR NUTRITION PROGRAMS

The menu is the major control instrument in managing a foodservice. It establishes what is to be served; what is to be done; food, labor and other costs; service; facility, equipment, and tools; purchasing, and a host of other factors. Once written, it establishes the operational program for the facility. In writing a menu that incorporates a healthful-foods program, one must be sure the new or revised items blend with the others and that they are properly presented and marketed. Descriptive material must be prepared with care so that it sells and is accurate.

GENERAL MENU CONSIDERATIONS

Many factors must be included as general considerations in establishing menu offerings. The degree of responsibility an operation has to provide healthful foods was discussed in Chapter 1. This depends largely on the type and needs of patrons, the type of operation, and on its goals. Will *all* patrons want healthful foods? Normally, a foodservice does best to offer some healthful foods and some foods that might not be so designated (see Chap. 11). One must also remember factors such as what kind of image the operation wants to project, how to achieve profit objectives, how to win patron satisfaction and good will, and how to appeal to relevant demographic patron characteristics such as religion, ethnic background, financial status, and age.

Some admonitions bear repeating: Don't overdo the healthful aspects of foods: not all patrons like or want it. Remember that, though patrons claim to want healthful foods, quality and flavor may come *first*. Give patrons alternatives, in terms of the number of menu items offered and their variety.

Why Resources Are Part of the Menu Plan

Capital and Budgets. In most cases, available money governs what can and cannot be done. For example, if investment capital for a larger oven to make yeast breads in-house is unavailable, this menu option is out. Other cost considerations are discussed later.

Facility. Available resources or those that need to be obtained must be considered; one of the most important questions is whether the facility has the proper space, equipment, and tools to accomplish the goals. If an existing facility has one small broiler and the decision is to add a number of broiled entrees, perhaps another must be obtained, in which case money and space will have to be found for it. Can a new high-speed broiler replace the old one? Can oven-baked items be offered instead of broiled ones? Is sufficient storage space available for the kinds of foods that will be required? Storage space may be adequate when many items are stored dry, but if the program is to offer many new fresh or frozen foods, what then? New fitness fare items also may suggest the need for special serviceware (casseroles, goblets, etc.) to display each item to best advantage.

It may be possible to retire some equipment. If only a few items are now to be grilled, the grill might be removed. Grilling could be replaced by sauteing on the range top, and a high-speed pressure cooker could be installed that would be more suitable for vegetable steaming. It is advisable to review food holding needs because it is often here that nutrients are lost. Preparing food, then giving immediate service is desirable, if not always practical. If such a facility review is done with an eye to coordination and detail, there should be few hitches in this area when the program starts.

It is also important in considering facilities to see that menu offerings are planned so that no piece or group of equipment is overloaded while others stand unused. This can defeat a program. Those who plan the menu selections should know expected recipe volume, needs, production times, and how long it will take to process foods through various pieces of equipment. When planning new facilities or remodeling, planners often set up detailed flow charts showing how foods can be processed through equipment. This helps assure that the equipment as established will be sufficient to handle the need.

Worker Skills and Labor Costs. Menu decisions in any operation should be made with close attention to the number of hands on deck. Staffing can be thought of as coverage of specific tasks, including the number scheduled per time period in which the particular task needs to be done. Persons with the proper knowledge and skill must be the ones available. This often is an important limiting factor. Preparation times of menu items must also be reasonable. If patrons have only 45 minutes for lunch, foods must be produced and served quickly. The volume of food that must be processed in the kitchen requires consideration so that workers can turn the dishes out. Waitstaff number and skill must be coordinated with menu demands. Too elaborate a service can overload waitstaff and impede proper dining area responsiveness and turnover.

The cost of labor is an important consideration. If they require too much staff or time, certain menu items may not be feasible to offer. Putting highly skilled workers on vegetable cleaning duty is very uneconomical. Fresh foods generally take more preparation time, and this has to be considered.

Of course, those *supervising* the accomplishment of these tasks should be *knowledgeable enough about nutrition* and its applications to see that the program is designed and implemented properly. Without such knowledge and adroit application, the program is almost sure to fail. The program must be built solidly on sound and correct preparation.

GENERAL MENU DECISIONS ABOUT THE SCOPE AND SHAPE OF THE MENU AND PROGRAM

Usual Meal Periods and Patron Sources

Reports from operations that are offering healthful foods with success and consensus in the Gallup Reports both indicate that healthful foods are most in demand during the morning and noon dining hours: 50% of customers in one study ordered healthful foods at noon but only 35% at night. Travelers and business persons are the groups who most often select such foods.

Menu Extent

Experts recommend that the program start out simply, with a small number of menu selections expanding as acceptance grows. A period of familiarization may be needed by employees and patrons, so it is wise to undertake an easily manageable list. For the most part, operations that devote all or a major portion of their menu to health-conscious diners have met with disappointing sales. The menu must maintain a balance to suit the desires of different kinds of patrons, so a blend of dishes is usually most successful. Freshness, cleanliness, and quality are always imperative.

Claire Regan of the NRA suggests that a typical, full menu operation might have a total of two to three salads and appetizers in the healthful-foods class, two to four entrees, and about two desserts. Of course, low-fat salad dressings and low-calorie sweeteners should also be offered to complement healthful-foods, and are not part of this count. Regan notes that appetizers and salads are often regarded as healthful by interested patrons but that the opposite is true of desserts. The healthful desserts offered might be fresh fruits, low-calorie frozen desserts, light, delicate mousses and the like. She cautions that even health-conscious consumers often want traditional desserts, making a trade-off of prudent, low-fat, low-calorie selections early in the meal for an old-fashioned, rich dessert.

Menu Plan Format

There are many variations. Menus can be *a la carte* (priced individually), or *table d'hote*, (offered together as a meal). Some operations' menus seldom change; this is considered a fixed menu. Some places have a fixed menu and another that changes more often—sometimes by the meal or daily. Items usually are presented on a menu in the order eaten, so appetizers might come first, followed by soups, salads, entrees, vegetables, breads, then beverages and desserts.

SPECIFIC NEEDS: PLANNING NOTES BY FOODSERVICE TYPE

Few markets are rigidly uniform; instead they are composed of several diverse groups, some of whom care not at all about healthful choices. Anyone planning a menu, therefore, must look toward satisfying not one but several markets.

Dr. Beth Carlson* reported a study to isolate patron's desires for healthful-foods in 33 various operations—hotels, restaurants, fast food operations, and other typical restaurants. She found pronounced differences in patrons' desires. Anyone contemplating a healthful-foods program should study the market to learn the specific desires of potential patrons. That done, planning can be tailored to satisfy these specific desires.

In Chapter 11, we looked briefly at the types of foodservice operations most likely to have success with a nutrition-oriented foodservice program. The profile below offers insight into Menu Planning considerations for various types of foodservice operations.

Hotel Restaurants

Nearly 2 million people stay in hotels nightly, as mentioned previously. Restaurants in and near hotels hosting business persons have made the most progress in catering to the growing number of health-conscious travelers by developing healthful-foods programs. They are finding that the programs pay—not only in customer satisfaction but on the bottom line. Many such operators who have tried nutrition programs rate them among their most successful promotions. Healthful-food items are offered in appetizers, soups, salads, entrees, and desserts. Most operators have created new items rather than altering their regular recipes. Business travelers are the best patrons, and they often take advantage of the hotel's entire fitness package, including the health spa. Conventioneers, tourist groups, and persons who are upper middle-class and above also tend to like the programs. Some hotel foodservices provide separate menus of healthful fare, but most include the items alongside regular ones, either identifying them with copy or symbols or putting

*Carlson, Beth L, "Meeting Consumer Needs—The Basis for Successful Marketing of Nutrition in Foodservice," *International Journal of Hospitality Management*, 1986, Vol. 5, #4, pp. 163-169.

them in a special section. The selections are varied enough so that patrons seeking healthful items can find items that suit their nutrition-oriented wants.

Ethnic Restaurants

The food staples of many ethnic recipes have a built-in advantage as they provide plenty of complex carbohydrates and little animal fat (Table 12-2). Some cuisines, such as classic French food have a reputation for richness, but the Newport Beach, California Le Meridien Hotel (see Fig. 12-2) has demonstrated that where there is demand, there is a way to appeal to nutrition-oriented guests in French.

Les Appetizers
Terrine de Crabe a la Mousse de Champignons   6.50
Terrine of Alaskan Crab Legs with Seasoned Mousse of Fresh Mushrooms/90 calories

Gaspacho Glace, Royale D'Herbes   4.50
Gaspacho with Royale of Fresh Herbs/40 calories

Confit de Legummes en Salade   6.00
Assorted Salad Greens with Cooked Vegetables and Fresh Herbs/70 calories

Coque de Melon aux Pamplemousse et Menthe   5.00
Marinated Melon and Grapefruit with Fresh Mint/70 calories

Salade d'Asperges Vertes a Huile de Noix   7.00
Fesh Green Asparagus Salad, Walnut Oil Vinaigrette/92 calories

Les Entrees Froides
Salade Supreme de Volaille au Citron Vert, Vinaigrette de Soja et Sesame   12.25
Supreme of chicken Salad with Sesame and Soya Sauce/225 calories

Saumon Froid, Salade de Concombres, Huile d'Olive Vierge   13.50
Cold Peached Salmon with Cuccumber Salad and Virgin Olive Oil/205 calories

Salade de Homard aux Artichauts sur Lit de Poireaux a l'Huile de Basilic   14.50
Lobster Salad with Artichokes on a Bed of Leeks and Basil Oil/126 calories

Ramequin de Gambas au Beurre Citronne   13.50
Ramekin of Shrimp with a Lemon Butter/110 calories

Les Entrees Chaudes
Escalope de Saumon a la Creme de Basilic   15.00
Scallopine of Salmon with a Basil Cream Sauce/360 calories

Loup de Mer Roti aux Fines Herbes, Petits Farcis Californiens   14.50
Fresh Seabass Roasted with Herb Crust and Stuffed California Baby Vegetables/392 calories

Paupiette de Volaille aux Cepes et Epinards, Crepes d'Aubergines   13.50
Boneless Breast of Chicken filled with Cepe Mushrooms and Spinach served with Eggplant Crepes/490 calories

Filet Mignon Grille a la Moutarde et Poivre Vert   15.00
Broiled Filet Mignon with Green Pepercorn flavored Mustard/379 calories

Cote de Veau a la Creame d'Estragon, Pates Fraiches   16.00
Broiled Veal Chop, Tarragon Sauce and Fresh Pasta/295 calories

Les Desserts
Souffle au Chocolat Amer/*Choice of Pastries/300 calories*   4.50
Souffle au Chocolat Amer*Frozen Bittersweet Chocolate Souffle/275 calories*   4.50
Bavarois aux Poires, Sauce Chocolat*Light Pear Flavored Pastry with Chocolate Sauce/195 calories*   4.50
Panache de Sorbet et Fruits Frais/*Assortment of Sorbets and Fresh Fruit/166 calories*   4.50
Baies Rouges/*Fresh Red Berries/112 calories*   7.00

Les Boissons
Selection de Thes, Infusions/*Selection of Traditional or Herbal Teas*   2.00
Cafe/Coffee   2.00   Expresso   2.25   Double Expresso   2.95   Cappucino   2.95

FIGURE 12-2 The menu at the Bistrot Terrasse, of Le Meridien Newport Beach highlights healthful foods. *(Courtesy Le Meridien Newport Beach)*

Fine Restaurants

White-tablecloth, or expense-account, restaurants also find a market for healthful foods, but it is smaller, perhaps because even people who follow a healthful-food regimen compromise on it when they visit such operations. The market is

TABLE 12-2
Highlighting Healthful Foods on Ethnic Menus

Highlight These	Avoid Including These
Chinese	
Steamed dishes	Fried foods (fried rice, egg rolls)
Lightly stir-fried items	Soy sauce
Brown rice	MSG
	Sweet and sour dishes
French	
"Light," or classic, stew	Au gratin dishes
Chicken, veal	Rich saues, (bearnaise,
Lean beef	bechamel, hollandaise)
Seafood	
Italian	
Tomato, marinara, and	Heavy sauce and cheese recipes
red clam sauces	Butter, cream, heavy cheese,
Pasta primavera & vegetables	meat, fried eggplant
Japanese	
Sushi	Rich condiment sauces
Sashimi	
Pickled vegetables	
Tofu dishes	
Mexican	
Lean meat tostadas	Tortilla chips, nachos
Mexican salads	Fried foods (including refried beans)
Seviche (marinated fish)	Heavy cheese, sour cream
	Guacomole
New American (Regional)	
Fresh fruit and vegetable salads	Deep-fried fish and chicken
Broiled fish	French fries
Tex Mex (fajitas, meat/	Deep dish pie
vegetable items)	Pizza with deli meats and
Low-fat pea/bean-based	extra cheese
stews, soups	
Pizza with vegetables	

predominantly middle-aged professional males who are affluent, well-educated, and somewhat prominent. They shy away from so-called diet foods. What they want is high quality dishes, and healthfulness is just one part of the considerations. They want food that is delicious; its RDA score is secondary. A few offerings presented with the regular ones but identified as healthful in a subtle way is all that is needed. Prices can be on a par with those of regular items. The market is a challenge to menu planners because these patrons may want something somewhat different, very appealing, and of excellent quality. The program sells better at lunch than at dinner; at dinner guests seem to be more relaxed and less concerned with health.

Family Restaurants

Family restaurants have a broad market, a small segment of which is interested in healthful fare, so menus must be more varied and flexible. Some attention must be given to offerings for teenagers and children, who often are not concerned about healthful food even if their parents are. (Parents may even tolerate some rebellion to avoid a confrontation.) It is still good business to include some healthful food items, but they should not be over-emphasized. If the items are available, the interested patron will note it and often will take advantage of them. Merely listing these offerings can enhance the image of the operation, even if most patrons do not select them.

Fast Food Operations

Fast food operations have received some bad press when it comes to nutrition. They have been criticized for serving foods too high in sodium and fat and too poor in vitamins and minerals for the calories involved. Operators of such establishments have to work out healthful food programs within the limits of established menus, which has been difficult, but some very successful steps have been taken: side and entree salads and salad bars have been added, vegetables such as tomatoes and lettuce have been added to hamburgers, and buffets offering foods other than the standard fried chicken or hamburgers have been introduced. Some have lowered fat content by changing their method of cooking from frying to broiling (e.g., charbroiled hamburgers). Switching from animal fat to vegetable oils for much of the frying has allowed some firms to substantially reduce the saturated fat and cholesterol absorbed by foods. Some fish houses have been able to modify recipes and cooking procedures to "lighten up" dishes without too much menu variation. Most find that their patrons are more interested in freshness and consistent quality than in healthful foods beyond the measures noted.

Many fast food operations have gone out of their way to offer information about the nutrient value of their foods, though few patrons ask for it. The operators do find that the availability of the materials helps improve their image, helps them compete, and reduces criticism.

Some fast food operations have not been enamored with their experience with healthful-food offerings, because they can be more costly to produce and the extra cost may not readily be passed on to patrons. Often they have had to add more perishable foods, such as fresh fruits and vegetables, which require more careful and skillful storage and preparation techniques.

Business and Industry Feeding

Planners in business and industry foodservice settings frequently find that establishing a healthful-foods program is desirable. Often it ties in with the company's employee wellness or health program. It sells less well in foodservices for blue-collar workers than for white-collar workers. White-collar groups in all settings are apt to give some patronage. In most cases, emphasis is placed on the overall program rather than on specific menu items, and some programs have gone so far as to meet special dietary needs of employee sub groups. Sometimes staff physicians or dietitians may request that the foodservice provide for special dietary needs of individuals. Management of many businesses realize how important good nutrition is to health and productivity, and they want their foodservice operations to do all they can to serve healthful foods. They often try to have a general information program on health, exercise, nutrition, and other wellness issues aimed at educating employees and bringing together a united effort to promote health and fitness. Some use low-key promotion, but others have health fairs, use the company newsletter, set up weight-reduction clubs, make loudspeaker announcements, use clip-ons or table tents in the employee dining areas, or otherwise try to get across the message that proper eating promotes health and fitness.

A sparkling example is The Litehouse, which serves healthful items as a special part of the employee cafeteria of New York Chemical Bank's restaurant services operations. With six cafeterias, they serve herbal teas, salads, yogurt, and among many other items, fresh fish, which is displayed on ice and prepared as customers watch.

RECIPES AND MENUS: SPECIAL PROGRAMS FOR FOODSERVICES

The nutrition-oriented efforts of various operations such as those discussed above often reflect the traditional approach of developing several recipes and menus to suit a special diet plan. In the past, public foodservice diet "specials" nearly always were weight-wise selections. In the health-conscious climate of today's marketplace, restaurateurs see opportunity in branching out to include selections for those on restricted (e.g., low-fat, low-sodium) diets and for those who eat to promote and maintain their health and fitness.

Some restaurateurs are developing their own cuisine and diet standards. While many are excellent, not all are based on facts. "Nonnutrition" selections—those that are *mis*represented as having one or more healthful qualities—have been with us a long time. Some restaurants still offer the high-fat, supposedly "low-calorie" beef and cottage cheese plate. On the "Light Delights" section of a metropolitan coffee shop recently was pictured their fat-laden special; a bacon, peanut butter, granola, and honey sandwich on a (white) English muffin; such a nonlight selection portrayed as light could lead the knowledgeable patron to doubt any other claims on the menu. Assuming the basic ideas for the types of menu items to offer have been formulated, it takes skill to put together the right ingredients and recipes. Many operators seek help from experts. A network of affiliations has grown of this outreach which includes health organizations, diet programs, consultants, and medical centers that are resources for both formal and informal nutrition program assistance for operators. By their nature, these programs are both informational and product-based. Most are designed to let consumers know about the program and to represent program health goals in a positive and persuasive light. At the same time, they help operators manage the planning, procuring, producing, and serving of items to meet these health goals.

The American Heart Association's (AHA) Creative Cuisine program has been in effect since 1975. Creative Cuisine and sanctioned local chapter variations probably have had more impact on more operations than any other nutrition-related program in the country. It has expanded to a program of guidance for restaurant recipe and menu planners, and is an attempt to work with and through operators to serve the needs of a populace seeking food choices that are low calorie, low fat, and low cholesterol. (Sodium reduction also is encouraged by AHA). A look at the objectives, guidelines and marketing of the Creative Cuisine program offers an overview of the considerations involved in nutrition-oriented recipe and menu planning, no matter what the nutrition emphasis. While the basic national Creative Cuisine program is described below, chapters have flexibility to make certain variations to meet local needs. Many have adopted other names for their program version, including Heart's Content, Eat Well, Good for You, and Hearty Heart.

For its part, the AHA program seeks out restaurants, corporations, and large hotel chains (e.g., Marriott) that are willing to offer a certain number of dishes that meet AHA diet guidelines. Such items generally are flagged on the menu and noted as being approved by the AHA. They might be designated with the AHA's heart logo *or* in one of a variety of menu treatments AHA provides. The AHA stresses that basic menus need *not* be changed necessarily, but rather that certain existing items are emphasized.

What the restaurant gains is new or broader exposure to a health-oriented clientele. It enjoys instant credibility and the public relations benefit of the AHA alliance. It also benefits from the ready-made support provided: such a program can be relatively easy to adopt and promote. In fact, the AHA describes the program as a total program, one that takes aim at everyone involved, from chef to patrons. The AHA furnishes program guides, managers' guides, chef's preparation lists, waitstaff tip sheets, patron's brochures, table tents, self-adhesive logos, window cards, some initial publicity, and even recipes, on request.

At the center of the Creative Cuisine program are ingredient, recipe, and menu guidelines. For example, participating restaurants must agree to offer at least four qualifying entrees. Qualifying entrees may include no more than 6-ounce portions of cooked meat, fish, or poultry, with a maximum fat content of 15%. The item must be trimmed of fat or skin and baked, broiled, boiled, steamed, rotisseried, or sauteed with *approved* fats and oils. (The AHA provides lists for approved polyunsaturated, cholesterol-free fats and oils.) Dairy products used must be low-fat (2%) or nonfat milk, low-fat (under 10%) cheeses, and nondairy creamers must be made from approved oils.

Other criteria are set out for salads and their dressings and for vegetables, breads, desserts, and spreads. Often the stumbling block of program acceptance by operators has been the restrictions on saturated fats. Reducing entree portion sizes can be an effective strategy for reducing fat. Also, some regional chapters are more flexible in the types of fats and oils allowed for use in AHA selections, sometimes even supplying brand name and supplier information for reference.

SELECTING AND DEVELOPING HEALTHFUL RECIPES

Collecting potential nutrition-oriented recipes and ideas for the program menu can begin early during the planning period. Keeping in mind the operation's objectives, resources, and present menu, the opportunities lie in providing quality, healthful versions of foods guests are looking for. As always, identifying good recipe prospects can be guided by knowing guests' preferences. Table 12-3 shows the relative popularity of specific menu item possibilities. Although these rankings are based on claims rather than actual behavior, the high ranking of many wholesome, healthful foods can be used as an indicator of patron responses to such menu choices. Preparation preferences for four categories of entrees are ranked in Table 12-4. Methods requiring no additional oil or fat rank at or near the top for each type. These are patron choices the recipe decision-maker should keep in mind.

Sources of new recipes include magazines, newspapers, and other general publications as well as government agencies and health-related facilities. For example, the source of the enticing recipe in Figure 12-3, from world-famous Caesar's Palace, was a community International Nutrition Event, a free, public health promotion that was cosponsored by the Cooperative Extension Service and a major area hospital. Large food companies such as Heinz, General Foods, General Mills, Standard Brands,

TABLE 12-3
Ranked Popularity of Foods Patrons Might Try in a Restaurant*

Rank	Item	Percent Very Likely to Try
1	Fresh fruit	78
2	Lean meats	64
3	Broiled/baked fish or seafood	63
4	Whole wheat breads, rolls, crackers	60
5	Steak or roast beef	58
6	Poultry without skin	47
7	Raw vegetable appetizer	45
8	Whole grain muffins	41
9	Vegetables seasoned with herbs or lemon juice only	36
10	Food cooked without salt	36
11	Regular soft drink	35
12	Fried fish or seafood	34
13	Low-fat cottage cheese	33
14	Cereal with low-fat or skim milk	33
15	Fried chicken	32
16	Reduced-calorie salad dressing	30
17	Diet soft drink	30
18	Caffeine-free soft drink	30
19	Whole grain pancakes or waffles	29
20	Caffeine-free coffee	28
21	Premium ice cream	28
22	Low-fat, low-calorie, fruit-based desserts	25
23	Sugar substitutes	25
24	Bagels or bread with low-fat cream cheese	24
25	Rich, gooey or chocolate dessert	22
26	Fruit ice or sorbet	22
27	Calorie-controlled entree	20
28	Low-cholesterol egg substitute	9

* Survey question was: "How likely would you be to try particular items if offered in restaurants?"
(Reprinted from Consumer Nutrition Concerns and Restaurant Choices, published by the National Restaurant Association, 1986)

TABLE 12-4
Patrons Preferred Cooking Methods for Various Entree Categories

Poultry	%	Meat	%	Fish	%	Shellfish	%
Baked/ roasted	52.4	Broiled	54.3	Deep-fried	42.7	Deep-fried	47.2
		Grilled	52.9	Broiled	38.5	Broiled	18.2
Deep-fried	35.7	Baked/ roasted	39.0	Baked/ roasted	22.3	Stir-fried	13.2
Broiled	27.3					Sauteed	12.6
Grilled	21.2	Stir-fried	18.2	Sauteed	17.3	Poached	5.8
Stir-fried	17.7	Mesquite-grilled	15.9	Grilled	16.5	Baked/ roasted	5.3
Sauteed	12.0			Poached	9.5		
Mesquite-grilled	7.5	Sauteed	12.6	Blackened	8.5	Grilled	5.3
		Deep-fried	7.9	Mesquite-grilled	4.6	Mesquite-grilled	2.1
Poached	2.8	Blackened	4.7				
Blackened	2.0			Stir-fried	4.1	Blackened	1.5

Patrons place broiled and baked selections high on their list of each main entree type.
(Pratscher M, Lydecker T, Weinstein J, Bertagnoli L: "Tastes of America: How America Loves to Eat Out" Restaurants and Institutions, Vol 97, p 48, 1987)

Uncle Ben's, and Kellogg's have departments that test foods and publish recipes. Product councils are delighted to share recipes—from the Cling Peach Advisory to the United Dairy Industry Association. A number of nonprofit health organizations also offer assistance.

Recipe Development

It is especially desirable to maintain and use standardized recipes in nutrition-oriented programs because the foods produced from them must contain precise *amounts of nutrients* and be consistent in quality, quantity, and cost. A standardized recipe is one that is written in clear culinary terms so that other users can duplicate the intended product outcome. Ingredient descriptions, recipe quantities, procedures, and serving standards should be spelled out unambiguously. If the recipe is not in *written* form, or if the recipe is not followed, the item is bound to be made differently each time, depending upon who is making it (even, sometimes on his or her mood). With such mismanagement, offerings vary, and patrons expecting something they once had that pleased them may get something very much different the next time. It is also poor management practice to allow one employee to have the recipe in his or her head and not written. There is the potential for power games, and if the employee is absent or quits, the recipe is lost.

Choosing which recipes to offer as part of the program is a challenging task. At least three routes are open for recipe composition, but it can be unwise to assume that guests see them as equivalent (e.g., those who dislike the idea of "substitute" foods). Which direction or directions will the program's recipes take? The options are: (1) to use foods that are *naturally* low in calories, such as fresh fruits and

CHICKEN SCALLOPINI WITH SWEET PEPPERS
MICHAEL TY
FOOD DIRECTOR
CEASARS PALACE

YIELD:	4 SERVINGS
1 lb	Chicken Scallopini (Chicken breast cut in thin cutlets and pounded)
¼ cup	All purpose flour
¼ tsp.	Salt
¼ tsp.	Dried whole basil
1/8 tsp.	White pepper
2 teas.	Vegetable oil
¼ cup	Dry White Vermouth
1 ea.	Small red bell pepper
1 ea.	Small yellow bell pepper
1 ea.	Small green bell pepper
2 teas.	Minced shallots
2 teas.	Margarine

Cut all three sweet peppers into julienne stiprs.

In hot boiling water, blanch sweet peppers in water for 30 seconds. Remove and chill immediately.

Combine flour, salt, basil and pepper in a small bowl and mix well. Lightly dust chicken scallopini.

In large skillet heat margarine and lightly saute minced shallots and sweet pepper. Stir frequently until crisp and tender. Remove from skillet and set aside.

Add oil to skillet and heat until it smokes lightly. Saute chicken scallopini on each side (lightly browned.)

Add vermouth and peppers and cook for 10 seconds

Serve over steamed rice. One-half cup per serving.

NUTRIENT INFORMATION PER SERVING

Calories	359
Protein	44%
Carbohydrate	34%
Fat	22%
Sodium	234 milligrams
Cholesterol	77 milligrams

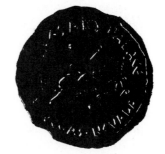

FIGURE 12-3 *(Courtesy Caesers Palace, Las Vegas, NV.)*

vegetables prepared in low-fat recipes; (2) to serve "regular foods" in ways that are relatively low in calories, such as a *modest portion* of roast pork, or a salad with dressing *on the side*; and (3) to *substitute* foods, such as low-calorie salad dressing, or "nearly forbidden" desserts made with non-nutritive sweetener, whipping agents, and products imitating the mouthfeel of fats.

Entirely new items can be offered, or it may be that some of the items already offered fall into the healthful-foods category and need only be identified on the menu. Recipes in the restaurant's collection should be reviewed to see whether and how they might be adapted to suit program needs. Recipes might need adjustment to cut back on salt, fats, or rich sauces. Portion sizes may be reduced, but care must be taken to maintain the patron's satisfaction and value perception: sometimes a smaller portion is offered at a lower price. Vegetables and other salads are likely targets for simple menu modification as they may require little more than making available low-fat, low-sodium dressing choices. A seafood house has a great opportunity for offering healthful foods, since many people perceive fish as healthful, by simply offering fish dishes baked, broiled, steamed, boiled, poached, microwaved, or grilled with little fat, instead of fried. A steak house might offer beef items that are trimmed of all visible fat as well as some skinless poultry choices and especially fish and seafood. Recipes for soups might be adjusted to include less salt and fat. Convenience entrees that conform to dietary demands are also available.

Often a recipe must be modified to meet the nutrition standards of the program. An example recipe for baked veal breast with herb dressing and sour cream sauce calls for bacon to be fried, with the bacon fat used to saute the vegetables and herbs; it specifies sour cream and eggs for the dressing, and sour cream is also an ingredient in the sauce. Substituting vegetable oil for the bacon reduces the salt, saturated fat, and cholesterol, adds some unsaturated fat and adds no cholesterol. Using egg whites, white sauce or an egg substitute would reduce fat and cholesterol in the dressing, as would replacing sour cream with yogurt. The recipe calls for 1/2 pounds of dry bread crumbs which can be replaced with 4 pounds of cooked brown rice (less sodium, more fiber). While the basic recipe is little changed, the product now is reasonably low in calories and is low in saturated fat, oils, sodium, and cholesterol. It could be called baked veal breast with brown rice herb dressing and yogurt sauce. The revised recipe is in Table 12-5, and the breakdown included therein shows the difference in selected nutrients for the "before" and "after" versions.

Recipe Nutrient Analysis

If a healthful-fare program is instituted, it likely will be necessary to calculate nutrients for the total recipe and per portion before making any claims for the nutrient qualities of the food. It is wise to be sure that such statements are based on facts. One avenue is to use a pre-evaluated recipe. The ratatouille recipe in Figure 12-4 and hundreds of others come complete with nutrient information and are widely available in cookbook form.

If the recipe must be analyzed, good information often can be obtained from the labels of packaged ingredients. Food processors and industry groups representing different food products make available leaflets and other materials noting nutrient values for common recipes and portions using their products and generally provide them free upon request. If such information is not available, tables of nutrient values can be consulted and the nutrient yields of the recipe can be calculated. An example is offered in Table 12-6. The *USDA's Home and Garden Bulletin No. 72* (see appendix), or the *USDA Handbook No. 8*, among others, give reliable information of this kind.

Although the calculations using tables of food values are not difficult, they can be quite time consuming, and many questions of interpretation can arise. A recom-

TABLE 12-5
Selected Nutrient Values for 50-Portions Veal, Dressing, and Sauce*

Ingredient	Calories	Fat (grams)	Carbohydrate (grams)	Protein (grams)	Cholesterol (mg)	Sodium (mg)
Dressing						
Oil, vegetable, 6 ounces	1504	170				
Onion, chopped, 1 1/2 lb	261	1	54	9		40
Mushrooms, sliced 1 1/2 lb	206	2	29	18		49
Parsley, minced, 12 ounces	8			2		48
Celery, chopped, 12 ounces	44		10	1		210
Dill, fresh, chopped, 6 ounces	18					
Tarragon, dried, 1 tsp	4		(not significant)			
Ground veal, lean, 3 lb	1813	81		271	1230	675
Brown rice, 1 lb†	1633	9	351	34		119
Egg substitute, 3 cups	480		82	36		1548
Yogurt, plain, low-fat, 3 1/2 cups	395	14	42	27	26	560
Pepper, black, 2 tsp			(not significant)			
Totals for dressing	6366	277	568	398	1256	3249
Per 5 ounce portion	127	5	11	8	25	65
Veal and Sauce						
Veal breast, 19 lb	11481	513		1716	7790	4275
Veal stock, 3 qt‡			(not significant)			
Cornstarch, 3 ounces	308		75			
Yogurt, 3 cups	340	12	36	23	22	480
Totals for veal and sauce	12129	525	11	1739	7812	4755
Per 4 ounce cooked veal and 2 ounce sauce	243	10	2	35	156	95
Totals for recipe	18496	802	679	2137	9068	8004
Per portion	370	16	14	43	181	160
Savings Realized by Revising the Recipe						
Savings per recipe	2614	247	78	78	4852	14167
Savings per portion	52	5	2	2	97	283

*Most values from USDA Handbook No. 8; others from Barbara Kraus' *Sodium Guide* (1983) and *Calories and Carbohydrates,* 5th ed., both published by Signet, New York City; some values were verified by reference to values in Hamilton, Whitney and Sizer, *Nutrition: Concepts and Controversies,* 3rd ed., St. Paul, MN. West Publishing Co., 1985.
†Dry weight before cooking
‡From bones from breast

mended alternative is to let a computer handle most of the work. No-frills dietary analysis software for popular personal computers is available at a modest price, but more powerful programs can be costly. Figure 12-5 shows an example of one of the many nutrient analysis formats available using capable software.

Alternatively, for the smaller operation, it costs relatively little to deliver recipes to experienced consultants who already have these computing systems and perform recipe analyses for others. In general, their prices are reasonable and are based on the number of recipes analyzed and the complexity of each. A reputable firm can provide rapid turnaround and reliable analysis of any usual nutrient. Most also can

RATATOUILLE
B. Kuntz, La Costa Spa & Resort, Carlsbad, Calif.

Ingredients	5 portions	24 portions	Method	Nutrient Analysis	
Whole tomatoes, cut into bite-size pieces	1 16-oz. can	5 16-oz. cans	Combine in heavy saucepan; toss. Heat to boiling; reduce heat; simmer until fork-tender.	Calories	41 kcal
Zucchini, cut lengthwise in quarters, seeded, core removed; cut into bite-size pieces	1 cup	4¾ cups		Protein	1.9 gm
				Fat	0.4 gm
				Carbohydrate	8.8 gm
				Fiber	1.3 gm
Eggplant, pared, cut into 1-in. cubes	1 cup	4¾ cups		Cholesterol	0 mg
Small bell pepper, sliced	½	2		Iron	1.1 mg
Small red onion, pared, thinly sliced	½	2		Sodium	121 mg
				Calcium	59 mg
Oregano	1½ tsp.	2½ Tbsp.		Vitamin A	1021 IU
Parsley, chopped	1½ tsp.	2½ Tbsp.		Thiamine	0.12 mg
Garlic clove, pared, crushed	1	5		Riboflavin	0.05 mg
Black pepper	pinch	as needed		Vitamin C	29 mg
				Potassium	391 mg
Salt substitute	as desired	as desired	Taste and adjust seasonings. Better when held and reheated. Serving size: ⅔ cup.	Niacin	1.1 mg
Artificial sweetener	as desired	as desired		Phosphorus	45 mg

SPECIAL DIETARY SYMBOLS
As you use the cookbook, look for the following symbols
as special dietary indicators:

 indicates two grams or more of dietary fiber per serving and is a good recipe to include in a dietary plan for increased fiber.

indicates less than 60 milligrams of cholesterol per serving and a recipe which could be included in a dietary plan for lowered cholesterol intake.

 indicates less than ten grams of fat per serving and a recipe which could be considered in a dietary plan for lowered fat intake.

indicates a sodium content falling under 140 milligrams per serving.

FIGURE 12-4 The ratatouille recipe from La Costa Spa. *(Reprinted with permission from Dietitians' Food Favorites. The American Dietetic Association Foundation, 1985.)*

calculate the number and types of dietary exchanges per menu item or per meal, for those interested in providing this information. Once a menu has been computer analyzed, menu modifications can be recalculated with speed and ease. Firms offer software or services to measure both small and large portion sizes; nutrient counts can be requested for just a specific portion of a single ingredient or food; for the totals of ingredients in a recipe; for a collection of recipes (or a meal); or for a larger collection of menus which could represent an analysis of the menu plan for a full day. The latter is especially appropriate in a health care setting.

While management would have all the nutritional information from these analyses, patrons usually will not be interested in detailed nutrient information. Some might be interested in the final, per portion, figures for certain nutrients. Alternative

TABLE 12-6
Calculation of Selected Nutrients Using Nutrient Value Tables for Foods.
50-Portion Recipe for Apple Snow Pudding with Low-Calorie Vanilla Sauce

Ingredient	Amount	Calories	Selected Nutrients			
			Carbohydrate (grams)	Sodium (mg)	Fat (grams)	Cholesterol (mg)
Snow Pudding						
Applesauce, unsweetened	16 lb	1488	400	80	6	0
Nutmeg	1 tsp	11	1	trace	0	0
Vanilla extract	1 1/2 ounce	97	0	42	0	0
Egg whites	1 1/4 lb	291	5	960	0	0
Sugar, granulated	2 1/4 lb	3928	1015	40	0	
Gelatine, dry	3 ounce	270	0	40	0	0
Total		6085	1421	1162	6	0
Low-calorie Vanilla Sauce						
Milk, low-fat	6 lb	978	138	1524	3	trace
Non-nutritive sweetener	1 ounce	18	4	50	0	0
Vanilla extract	1 ounce	65	0	28		
Cornstarch	4 ounce	410	98	4	trace	0
Total		1471	240	1606	3	0
Total for two items		7556	1661	2768	9	0
Nutrients per serving*		151	33	55	.2	0

Calorie, carbohydrate, fat and cholesterol values from USDA Handbook No. 8 and sodium values from 1983 Sodium Guide to Brand Names and Basic Foods, (Kraus, Barbara) New American Library, New York, 1983.
* 1/2 cup pudding and 1/4 cup sauce

ways to provide this information to guests are provided in the following chapter. It is often good to let patrons know that information is available in brochures or other formats (even though few are likely to ask for it) as it is a public relations enhancement. Management should keep the additional information in the files, to be able to back up claims or inferences if necessary. At the bottom line, the advice is to put forward a healthful-foods program with style and with restraint, make no claims that cannot be supported, and not overdo it.

Nutrition information can be placed on the back of standardized recipe cards, or a separate file may be maintained for this information. In some cases, the file of regular recipes and of healthful food program recipes may be kept separate. It is usual to see different food groups differentiated by different colored cards (meats often are on pink cards, salads on green ones), but because so many items may fit into two or more categories, this kind of classification may not work best for the operation.

It is desirable to put on recipe cards some charge to employees to follow directions carefully and observe good methods for preserving nutrients (e.g., caution against oversoaking or overcooking vegetables or against using too much fat might be noted on recipes). Some indication that a recipe has specific healthful values such as being low in sodium or in fat can be given to inform workers of the reasons the

Sample Computerized Printout: Recipe Analysis

The "2001" Cafe / Recipe: SALAD, Fresh vegetable / Eight Ingredients / Portion Cost $x.xx

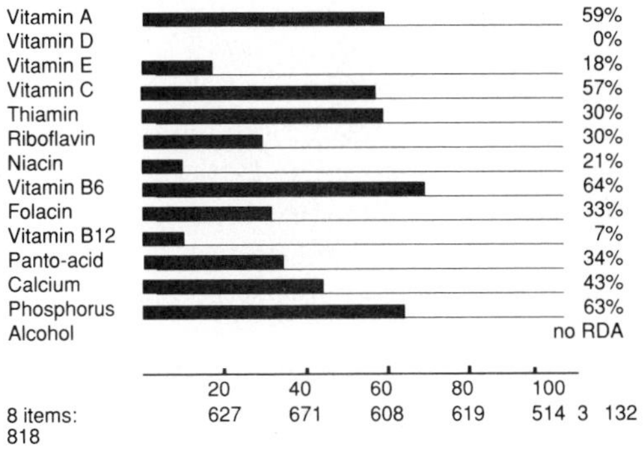

Nutrient	Bar	%
Vitamin A		59%
Vitamin D		0%
Vitamin E		18%
Vitamin C		57%
Thiamin		30%
Riboflavin		30%
Niacin		21%
Vitamin B6		64%
Folacin		33%
Vitamin B12		7%
Panto-acid		34%
Calcium		43%
Phosphorus		63%
Alcohol		no RDA

```
         20    40    60    80    100
8 items: 627   671   608   619   514  3  132
818
```

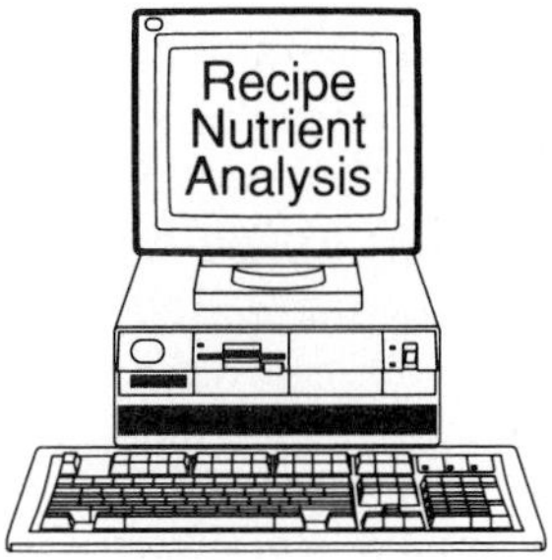

Item	Food Name	Portion	Serving	Amount
627	Lettuce-iceberg-raw	1/4 head	100%	135.0 gm
671	Tomato-raw	1 tomato	100%	135.0 gm
608	Celery-pascal type-raw	1 stalk	100%	40.0 gm
619	Cucumber slices-no peel	6-9 slices	100%	28.0 gm
514	Beans-cnd-red kidney-s/l	1 cup	100%	255.0 gm
30	Cheese-cheddar-cut pieces	1 oz	100%	28.0 gm
132	Salad dressing-blue ch.	1 tbsp	100%	15.0 gm
818	Pepper-black	1 teaspoon	25%	.5 gm

Nutrient Values (%RDA)

KCalories	476 kc	(23%)	Riboflavin	.36 mg	(30%)
Protein	25.7 gm	(58%)	Niacin	2.78 mg	(21%)
Carbohydrate	54.3 gm	(-%)	Vitamin B6	1.28 mg	(64%)
Fat	18.5 gm	(-%)	Folacin	136 UG	(33%)
Fiber	4.06 gm	(-%)	Vitamin B12	.23 UG	(7%)
Cholesterol	39 mg	(-%)	Panto-acid	1.92 mg	(34%)
Saturated FA	7.78 gm	(-%)	Calcium	346 mg	(43%)
Oleic FA	3.8 gm	(-%)	Phosphorus	509 mg	(63%)
Linoleic FA	4 gm	(-%)	Thryptophan	249 mg	(152%)
Sodium	423 mg	(19%)	Threonine	987 mg	(226%)
Potassium	1364 mg	(36%)	Isoleucine	1396 mg	(213%)
Magnesium	43.5 mg	(14%)	Leucine	2069 mg	(237%)
Iron	6.56 mg	(36%)	Lysine	1815 mg	(277%)
Zinc	1.38 mg	(9%)	Methionine	359 mg	(105%)
Vitamin A	2368 IU	(59%)	Cystine	217 mg	(105%)
Vitamin D	0 IU	(0%)	Phenyl-anine	1275 mg	(257%)
Vitamin E	1.51 mg	(18%)	Tyrosine	961 mg	(257%)
Vitamin C	34.5 mg	(57%)	Valine	1473 mg	(193%)
Thiamin	.3 mg	(30%)	Histidine	706 mg	(-%)
			Alcohol	0 gm	(-%)

Percentages by calorie (4:4:9:7)
Prot: 21% Carb: 45% Fat: 34% Alco: 0%

FIGURE 12-5 Computerized nutrient analysis for recipes assists in totalling many common nutrients or just a few. Exchanges (and costs) also can be calculated. *(Nutritionist diet analysis printout from N-Squared Computing, Silverton, OR.)*

recipe calls for specific ingredients or substitutions, or requires specific procedures or cooking methods.

Recipe Testing and Evaluation

Efforts in recipe development and product testing cover a broad spectrum. For example, an independent operator may test and develop any one recipe for only a short time. At Hilton Hotels, Inc., menu writers work closely with suppliers and nutritionists, taking months to fine-tune recipes for use across the country. General Mills Restaurant Group (including Red Lobster) is supported by extensive test kitchen facilities and a professional nutrition advisor. Even in fast foods, not everything is fast. The salad product line introduced by McDonald's in 1987—1988 was an investment based on *10 years* of recipe testing and development.*

Any recipe that is new or has to be changed should be tested in small quantity before being used in regular production. Each recipe should be production tested, performance tested, and taste tested. *Production testing* evaluates their practicality and the way they use available resources—their ease, speed, conflicts, etc. *Performance testing* is important for healthful-food items, because freshness is so essential to nutrient preservation, to the appearance of the dish, and to its eating quality. The products of recipes that stand up best to the rigors of handling, production, and service are favored. Do the aesthetic and healthful qualities survive handling, quantity preparation, holding, etc?

Taste testing never should be overlooked. When guests are involved with taste tests during recipe development, their input can guide recipe developers in creating products that have greater appeal for the intended audience. Tasters can help establish what *they* consider to be a generous or poor salad portion, for example, or what they consider to be too salty or too bland.

Figure 12-6 offers an informal evaluation sheet that guests might use to judge recipes. The form includes many of the most typical criteria for evaluation (e.g., flavor, texture), but these may need adjustment for different products and purposes. Discussions with "judges" can help discover what recipe qualities they feel are important to criticize that may have been overlooked, (such as the texture of take-out food when it arrives at its destination).

Overall testing for nutrition-oriented recipes should be *two*-pronged. Imagine that you are visiting a restaurant and are asked if you would participate in judging the products of three different recipes for marinated roast chicken which are being tested as a potential light menu item. In this case, you are involved in the first type of testing, which is to determine what is considered more and less desirable for each area (flavor, freshness, etc.). In this phase, the question is what do guests think of the product *according to the way they like their food*. In the second type of taste-testing, imagine that you are the supervisor who is now evaluating the selected chicken recipe according to what the taste should be each time the standardized recipe is used. In this case, you are expected to judge the taste *based on standards established from the first phase*, according to whether the employees produced the desired outcome. Personal preferences should rarely enter in at this phase. Of course,

---

*For more information on recipe testing, see Kotschevar: *Quantity Food Production, Standards. Techniques and Principles, Ed. 4.*, Van Nostrand and Reinhold, 1988.

Recipe Evaluation Form

Recipe reference # _____   Date _____

Tested by (optional) _____   Menu price_____

Name of recipe: **Vegetarian Hearty Vegetable Soup with Sourdough Bread**

Would you <u>ordinarily</u> be inclined to order such a menu item? Yes_____No_____

Please circle the figure which best corresponds to your opinion. We invite your comments throughout.

	Love it	Like it	It's O.K.	Not Quite	Awful
Flavor					
Freshness					
Temperature					
Seems low in calories					
Texture (vegetables)					
Portion size:					
Main dish_____					
Luncheon_____					
Value					
Overall quality					

Would you buy this?   _____

Why, Why not?   _____

Comments: _____

_____

_____

Thank you for your help in our continuing effort to serve you better.

_____
The Management

FIGURE 12-6 Recipe evaluation form.

recipe standards always should be flexible and open to adjustment if future testing indicates shifting guest preferences.

Menu Development

An operation's decision makers usually will compile a list of acceptable menu items and select from it the menu items actually to be offered. The number in each food category, such as appetizers, salads, entrees, desserts, should be modest at first, as described in General Menu Decisions, above. In most establishments, the nutrition-oriented items are just one part of the total menu, so it is important that the selections fit in with the composition, style, price range, and sophistication of other items.

Different operators use different objectives to help them determine which recipes to select for the menu. For example, in addition to meeting nutrition guidelines, Stouffers' is most likely to give the nod to recipes for their "Look of Lean" program with: a "quality" look, regional product availability, and excellent eye appeal. Hilton's "Fitness First" recipes must be: appealing to guests, easy to pre-prepare, and simple to produce. Others look for such criteria as increasing the number of menu options using available inventory and adding to their flexibility in meeting various consumer nutritional demands.

After deciding which items will be offered on the menu, an operator must decide how to present the items. Although menu layout and design is beyond the scope of this book, considerations specific to nutrition-oriented menu items are described in Chapter 13. (For a thorough treatment of menu planning and printing consideration, see L. Kotschevar: *Management by Menu, ed. 2.* New York, N.Y., John Wiley & Sons, 1986.)

An important aspect of menu planning is the accompaniments. What is appropriate, expected, or desirable with this menu as a whole? Would guests prefer potatoes or rice? Bread, crackers, or rolls? A spread, butter, or margarine? Condiments? Figure 12-7 ranks preferences of guests for typical choices.

Another question is when to "enlighten" or surprise consumers. While creativity can be commendable, tradition and a respect for the familiar also are important in menu development. For example, there are those who say it is monotonous constantly to serve cranberry sauce with roast turkey; they might offer chutney instead. Our sug-

Taking Sides

Which side dish do Americans like best to accompany an entree? The people's choice would make their moms proud: vegetables. And they made no bones about liking their potatoes baked.

Vegetables	79.1%
Baked potato	79.0
Fruit	47.5
Rice	42.2
French fries	39.2
Pasta	24.3
Potatoes (prepared other ways)	21.0
Stuffing	17.0

FIGURE 12-7 Survey results like these suggest plenty of opportunity for nutrition-oriented menus. (Pratscher M, Lydecker T, Wienstein J, Bertagnoli L: *Tastes of America: How America Loves to Eat Out. Restaurants and Institutions*, vol 97, p 48, 1987)

gestion is to serve cranberry sauce, maybe cranberry-orange relish sometimes, but unless you are very sure of your guests' preferences, offer the chutney *only* if the guest has the option to choose the cranberry as an alternative. Otherwise even so small a deviation could leave the guest with a bad feeling about the entire meal.

The Menu Plan and Special Requests

Anticipating the common special preparation or service requests patrons will make regarding their food can be a wise investment of time as it allows management to plan how to respond. Such decisions also may need to be reflected in printed menu materials and in staff training, which are discussed in subsequent chapters. Realistically, a foodservice has only certain resources available to fill guests' requests, and the services offered must fall within a reasonable range of required activity, "fuss," time, expertise, and labor and product cost. It is not the responsibility of all foodservices to go to extreme lengths to cater to patrons' requests in the name of health simply because the operation offers nutrition-oriented items. One also should ask whether the resulting item or service will be at least as desirable as the original in terms of visual attractiveness, flavor quality, access, and timing. Many patrons still are attracted primarily by flavor and visual appeal and frequently by convenience; even though they ask for modifications, they do not want to be disappointed. After considering these parameters, one should decide which types of requests can or cannot be accommodated by the operation and determine policies and procedures for saying "yes" or "I'm sorry."

A survey of foodservice operators by the Gallup organization and the NRA revealed agreeable responses to questions about accommodating special cookery and service requests (Table 12-7). The survey data is based on the nearly 75% of operators who responded that, "on request," they would alter the way food is prepared or served. The results of the same study show typical product substitutions along with the responses of operators in providing them (Table 12-8). The attentive manager should consider making a regular menu item out of a method or substitute that is requested constantly, as has occurred generally with low-calorie soft drinks and decaffeinated coffee.

Meal Development. The nutrition demands in planning a menu for a meal are quite different from those for planning a menu from which a guest can select this or that item. Even in *a la carte* settings, in which menu items are priced individually, combinations, such as a sandwich with a salad, often are available. This can take some of the choice away from guests and place it with the menu planner. For nutrition-oriented menu items, be alert that the overall package of the menu selection reflects the message of healthful food. This means that each component (salad, roll, entree, condiments) as well as the meal collectively should be evaluated for appeal and for nutrients and substances that guests may wish to have or to avoid. Since a principal objective of a fitness-fare program is to meet the healthful-foods demands of interested consumers, a criterion of the meal is that it incorporate, with accuracy and style, the desired qualities (e.g., fresh, additive-free, low in calories, low in sodium, low in fat and saturated fat, low in cholesterol). Association with a program

TABLE 12-7
Patrons' Preferences for Special Requests

| | Type of Restaurant | | | | |
Types of Changes	All Restaurants %	Fast Food %	Family Style %	Fine Dining %	All Others %
Serve sauce on the side	96	90	95	100	97
Serve salad dressing on the side	93	78	93	100	95
Cook without salt	90	88	87	97	92
Prepare foods in vegetable oil or margarine	83	71	84	90	81
Broil or bake food rather than fry it	80	48	85	96	78
Skin chicken before preparing	61	36	64	87	47

(Reprinted from Gallup/NRA Operator Survey, published by the National Restaurant Association, June, 1986.)
Percentages are based on the 73% of respondents who said they would modify preparation services.

name such as Fitness Fare or Heart's Desire suggests that the meal as a whole conforms to an expressed or implied healthful purpose. Patrons are likely to expect not only that wholesome ingredients are included but that in general the meal is designed to provide an appropriate type and amount of nourishing food, (although not necessarily exclusively healthful foods). This is a most important consideration because on it rides the total image of the program to patrons.

In addition to healthful qualities, the *variety and appeal* of the meal is the responsibility of the planner who selects the various items in it. It must be remembered that people eat with their eyes, and the visual impression of a well-planned and well-presented meal that expresses quality as well as healthfulness can be a big patron pleaser. Meals should have appealing contrasts in colors, flavors, textures, and shapes. Contrasts in temperature are also desirable as are different methods of cookery for different items. The plate topography, or "landscape," should be interesting: a slice of turkey beside a slice of bread looks flat and monotonous. Stacking, rolling, garnishing, or otherwise enhancing the presentation can make the meal more appealing. Arrangement on the plate should be done carefully and its techniques and importance should be communicated to employees. Each meal served should present an appetizing picture for the pleasure of the diner.

Menus in Less Public Places

The menus for captive diners, who get all or most of their food from the foodservice, should be planned to meet the specific dietary needs of the patrons, so most items offered probably will qualify as healthful food. For example, elementary and secondary school menus must meet basic USDA requirements for growing, active youngsters. Dormitory and other feeding operations serving older students may need menus that offer plenty of healthful, fresh, and natural food. Jails and other

TABLE 12-8
Percent of Operators Who Offer Selected
Substitutions on Request

Make Available on Request	Type of Restaurant		
	All Operators %	Fast Food %	Non-Fast Food %
Diet beverages	95	92	96
Sugar substitutes	92	85	94
Caffeine-free coffee	84	61	90
Margarine	66	40	72
Whole-grain bread/rolls/ crackers	62	38	68
Fresh fruit for dessert	59	32	66
Reduced-calorie salad dressing	37	32	39
Low-fat or skim milk	33	21	36
Salt substitutes	33	24	35
Bran cereals	31	17	35

(Reprinted from Gallup/NRA Operator Survey, published by the National
Restaurant Association, June 1986)

detention facilities also come under government regulation in menu nutrition requirements. Selected special menus are discussed more fully in Chapter 15.

It must be remembered that all food is healthful when consumed in balance and
moderation.

Table 12-9 provides a menu checklist for planners. It includes typical nutrition-
oriented considerations as well as more general ideas that appear to offer excellent
opportunities for healthful-foods menu planners.

SUMMARY

Selecting items to feature on the menu must be done with patrons' needs in
mind. The menu is the major control center in managing foodservices. Food and
labor costs, facility and equipment needs, training requirements, purchasing,
preparation, and even service activities all arise from the recipes and menu. Sales of
healthful foods appear to be highest at the morning and midday meals. Most programs
begin with only a few selections and allow the list to grow.

Planning considerations will vary with the type of foodservice operation involved. Hotel restaurants have found solid success in marketing to business travelers
and upper middleclass conventioneers and tourists. A smaller but important market
for the upscale restaurant is expense-account executives and their guests. Family

TABLE 12-9
Checklist: Opportunities for Menu Planners in a Healthful Foods Program

Does it include...
☐ Low-calorie foods?
☐ Low-fat, low-cholesterol foods?
☐ Low-sodium foods?
☐ Fiber rich foods?
☐ Additive-free items?
☐ Ethnic or regional recipes?
☐ Fresh and seasonal features?
☐ Nutritious mini meals or appetizers for grazers?
☐ No items misrepresented as low-calorie, etc,?

For overall menu...
☐ Does the customer think the food is worth a return visit?
☐ Does the menu fit with the operation and its objectives?
☐ Does it offer variety in flavors, color, texture, cookery, etc.?

When appropriate, are some nutrient-oriented menu items...
☐ "Packageable" and promoted for take-out?
☐ Reliably available for delivery?
☐ Included if they are awkward to make at home?
☐ Included on a "kids menu"?

and ethnic restaurants find healthful foods please a worthwhile segment, but these foods may be blended carefully into a menu of mostly traditional items. In spite of their limited menus, fast food operators have found profit in healthful items, such as salad bars, and in less obvious product changes, such as reducing fat in burger cookery by broiling instead of frying.

The AHA's Creative Cuisine program is a prominent diet program designed to assist foodservice operators in recipe and menu planning. Program participants comply with such agreements as meat portion maximums and use of approved types of fats and oils. In return, the restaurant receives the notoriety of AHA affiliation for healthful menu items and can obtain a wide variety of printed information and promotional materials through the AHA.

Healthful recipes are widely available. Existing recipes can be adapted or modified, or new ones can be developed to accommodate such demands as low-calorie, low-fat, low-cholesterol, low-sodium, high-fiber, or meatless selections. All recipes should be standardized and tested in production, performance, flavor, and overall quality. Recipes to be used in connection with nutrient claims (e.g., "under 400 calories") should be analyzed for nutrient content, either manually or by computer. The results should be retained by management; details rarely are appropriate for menu depiction. Recipes selected to be used on the menu must fit with the existing menu and the operation's image and must meet other criteria, such as level of production complexity.

Guests *will* make special requests, so part of planning is to anticipate these requests, to the extent possible, and to decide whether to respond to them and, if so, how. For such requests as menu substitutions, management must balance probable patron satisfaction with the use of resources involved in the change. Recipe accompaniments and plating are an important part of the healthful-menu package.

Meal development involves pulling together food and recipes for a complete meal that is healthful as well as attractive, appealing, and nutritionally complete. In less-public settings, such as institutional operations, there may be a greater commitment to healthful foods to meet the needs of patrons who have fewer foodservice options.

Chapter Review

1. Discuss the possible menu opportunity in planning into the menu at least several selections with healthful characteristics. Tie in Figure 12-1 with your response.
2. Why is the menu considered to be the major control instrument in managing a foodservice?
3. List main foodservice resource categories that must be taken into account in planning recipes and menus.
4. During what meal period(s) do healthful foods seem to sell best?
5. Why do you think it is recommended that the program menu begin small?
6. Restaurants in moderate- and high-priced hotels excel in their ongoing, successful programs for healthful foods. Considering their clientele and facilities, describe the guest market they are reaching. Describe the types of menu decisions that support their success.
7. If the majority of the patrons at a family restaurant in fact are not interested in ordering healthful foods, why might the program still be worthwhile? Besides income, what other benefits can be gained by offering healthful items?
8. How have some fast food operations changed their original menu plans to accommodate the demand for healthful foods?
9. Describe entree, ingredient, and recipe guidelines to which participants in the AHA foodservice diet program must adhere. What does the operator receive in return?
10. Name at least five separate categories of recipe sources for beginning recipe development.
11. In modifying or developing a recipe for a healthful foods program, what nutrient culprits would changes in ingredients probably be designed to reduce? What guest concern should be kept in mind if portion sizes are reduced?
12. What specific changes might you suggest for the following menu selections to make them more healthful? What diet needs might your changes accommodate?
    - Pan Fried Brook Trout.........$8.95

- Chicken Carmel.................$8.95 (boneless chicken breast stuffed with shrimp in a rich cream sauce and topped with crumbled bacon)
- Grilled Half-Pound Burger, Francaise....$7.45 (ground from the choicest beef and served under a blanket of cheese sauce with mushrooms and onions)

Note: All entrees are served with cole slaw in a creamy dressing and your choice of ranch-style beans, hash browns, French fried potatoes, or buttered rice.

13. Name as many sources and methods as you can for obtaining nutrient value information about food products. What should be done with recipe nutrient analysis results?
14. What types of considerations should recipe testing cover?
15. Why is it a good idea to involve guests in taste testing recipes?
16. Give examples of objectives operators may have for choosing which recipes to use.
17. Discuss the foodservice operator's considerations in deciding whether or not to honor a special request, such as broiling an item that is offered fried?
18. From Table 12-7, what types of changes were made most frequently to accommodate guests?
19. What meal development considerations are of extra importance in the program when a collection of recipes is marketed as a meal.
20. In less public operations, such as schools and senior care centers, how might the nutrition emphasis in menu planning be different from that in more public operations? Why?

Chapter 13
Nutrition-Oriented Programs: Telling and Selling

Chapter Goals

- To emphasize the opportunity and need for providing guests with meaningful, accurate information about the healthful-foods program and menu items.
- To provide guidelines for phrasing and formatting menu information.
- To present the concept of thinking through guests' potential nutrition information needs.
- To describe the marketing mix elements and to show how managing them properly can shape guests' views of the program.
- To encourage program managers to apply "selling" tactics.
- To outline steps in the "roll-out" of the program.
- To discuss the need for and provision of a system for program feedback, evaluation, and adaptation.

TELLING ABOUT THE HEALTHFUL FOODS PROGRAM

Even the most creative, appealing, and nutritious menu means little if patrons don't know about it. Sometimes patrons cannot obtain nutrition information about menu items or they somehow develop a bad feeling about them and decide not to try the items or even to avoid the operation. In 1987 a National Restaurant Association (NRA) spokesperson reported that only 25% of restaurateurs were promoting the health and nutrition benefits of their menu items. Others offer a few healthful menu items or preparation alterations, but few have yet taken advantage of the business potential and enhanced image of a well-targeted menu coupled with focused selling or marketing efforts. Thus, the next planning step is to "get the word out;" it should take place after preliminary planning has produced recipes and menus for the operations' nutrition-oriented foods program. It is then time to finalize plans for: menu item communications, the program "marketing mix," and for a final sweep including the program review, its "roll-out," or introduction, and the continuing effort to keep in touch with the marketplace and the program's performance. Program objectives are most likely to be realized when managers provide unpretentious, clear, and consumer-relevant information in "telling" intended audiences about the program.

MENU ITEM COMMUNICATION

The availability of delicious, wholesome, menu items specially prepared for nutrition-conscious patrons is doubtless the most important message to communicate about a healthful-foods menu. But when the time comes to select specific menu items, consumers look for certain information to make distinctions on healthful characteristics and to suit tastes, judge value, etc. Food service operators are responding to guest information demands through such means as; (1) training waitstaff in responding to guests' health-related questions, (2) providing a level of printed menu item information on the menu itself and, (3) providing supplementary printed information, available in a display or on request.

MENUS: MARRIED OR SEPARATE?

Operations that offer healthful fare as part of the available menu items, must decide early whether or not to intermingle this list with that of regular dishes into one menu. For most operations, the better course is to marry the two: listing healthful menu choices on the same menu with regular items can enhance the perception that the two menus blend together smoothly. In addition, regular menu items also qualify often as healthful selections, so it makes good sense to present them together. Using a *separate* "health menu" may be perceived as an odd separation of choices, perhaps implying that the regular menu items are unhealthy or that the healthful-food offerings are a management afterthought. Two separate menus also complicates the work of distributing and collecting menus, and either one may be overlooked in the bustle by staff or patrons. Guests also tend to dislike having to juggle two menus at the table.

GUIDELINES FOR OPERATIONS

Patrons who want healthful foods want assurances that they are getting just that. Sometimes they need further information or special accommodation; perhaps they wish to know whether the sauce is low in sodium or whether the flounder might be broiled rather than baked in cream sauce. The excellent practical and public relations value of good, factual menu information should not be overlooked for these patrons. Knowledgeable patrons can be put off by nutrition information that is inappropriate, inaccurate, or exaggerated. Descriptive copy should not contain propaganda, puffery, or empty promises, but written descriptions and other information about the program's menu selections can be presented in a way that tells patrons that the operation values the opportunity to meet their desires for healthful foods. The best approach is moderation. Keeping in mind the facts, which, when presented honestly and simply, both entice patrons and help them make informed decisions, the following eight guidelines may be applied to writing menu copy.

The right message, the right way, the right "fit." Relevant questions are: Is this the message we want to send? Does the form of the message detract—is it too clinical or technical? Does it clutter the menu and obscure the healthful-foods message?

Does it harmonize with our image? Does it foster a positive perception of operation and healthful-foods menu alike?

Be certain that information is accurate. This means that recipes must be standardized and followed and that any published nutrient values (e.g., calorie counts) must be accurate and must be updated if ingredients or portions change. It also means that production and service staff should be familiar enough with foods to answer reasonable questions that are not explained on the menu, without misrepresenting them by making incorrect assumptions or guesses.

Use terms correctly. The Food and Drug Administration (FDA) has defined certain terms used to describe values in packaged foods sold at retail. If these terms are used on the menu, it is sound practice to use them in the same way consumers experience them on product labels. Table 13-1 lists some of the more prevalent terms and provides the FDA's legal interpretation of each for packaged goods. If the salad dressing pictured in Figure 13-1 were offered, what terms might be used to describe it meaningfully and accurately to nutrition-minded guests?

Be specific. Instead of merely "chicken," the menu copy might read "matchsticks of skinless chicken breast with broccoli florets and fresh mushrooms, lightly stir-fried in pure vegetable oil." Instead of "our chef's secret sauce," a meaningful description is appropriate, such as "our low-fat tomato-basil sauce with

TABLE 13-1
Menu Terms the FDA Way

Dietetic or diet:
>   Foods claiming to be "dietetic" or "diet" must be low- or reduced-calorie foods, as outlined below. They must be intended for special dietary purposes such as a low-fat diet and not for weight control alone.

Light or lite:
>   The FDA says these terms describe a low- or reduced-calorie food and acknowledges that they can refer to properties other than calories. The term "light" (or "lite") is a buzzword used variously to describe a number of factors in foods such as calories (lite beer, or "Lite and Lean" cuisine), sodium (light ham), and sugar content ("packed in light syrup").

Low-calorie:
>   The FDA says such a food must contain not more than 40 calories per serving or no more than 0.4 calories per gram (11 calories per ounce).

Reduced-calorie:
>   Such a food must be at least a third lower in calories than its regular (non reduced) counterpart.

Significant source:
>   We might say that liver is a significant source of vitamin A and iron, meaning that a serving provides 10% or more of the U.S. RDA of that nutrient.

Sodium-free:
>   Not more than five milligrams of sodium per portion.

Reduced-sodium:
>   Sodium is reduced 75% below the normal sodium content.

Unsalted:
>   No salt has been added in processing (as in unsalted crackers).

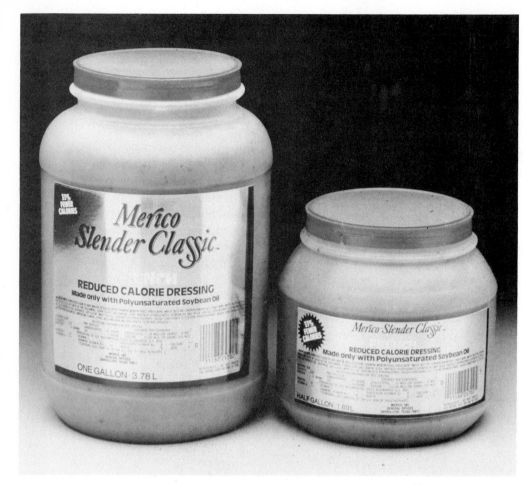

FIGURE 13-1 Terms such as "reduced-calorie" have a legal meaning for packaged goods. When writing menus, use each term's correct interpretation. *(Photo courtesy Merico, Inc.)*

coriander." "With all the trimmings" is not nearly as meaningful as "served with yogurt dip, sliced tomatoes, and chunks of fresh pineapple."

KIS: Keep it simple. Is there too much information? Is it confusing to patrons (see Table 13-2)? Patrons may be uncomfortable, or even misled, when they must make too many interpretations. It is far too easy for misinterpretations, confusion, and hard feelings to result. It is advisable to keep information meaningful and specific but to be cautious and to KIS.

Stay flexible. Avoid being tied too tightly to the descriptive menu copy. If a minor recipe change is made, it shouldn't require a menu reprint. Good planning can afford flexibility. It is usually best to avoid being too specific; for example, nutrient quantities, if provided at all, should be approximate rather than specific.

Do not make health claims. It is unlawful to make insupportable claims (and "supportable" refers to scientific proof, not tabloid headlines). Alternatively, it is

TABLE 13-2
**Familiarity of Patrons With Nutritional and Ingredient
Terms and Their Meaning ***

Term	Very Familiar	Not Familiar
Vitamins	79	1
Caffeine	78	1
Starch	66	1
Vegetable shortening	65	2
Animal fat	60	2
Meat protein	58	3
Carbohydrate	55	3
Fiber	54	3
Minerals	53	3
Enriched flour	53	2
Empty calories	36	25
Vegetable protein	35	10
Soy protein	25	17
Nitrates/nitrites	23	16
Amino acids	22	20
Whey	21	19
Trace materials	19	30
Complex carbohydrates	18	24
Nutrient density	7	44

*The total sample base is 3366 persons. It excludes those who gave no answer and those who claim "some familiarity" with the term.
(Reprinted from the National Restaurant Association's Current Issues Report, Nutrition and Foodservice and Food Product Information. September, 1986, and; "Food, Nutrition and Dieting," Universal Foods and the Wheat Industry Council, 1983.)

proper to state that items are low in salt, if that is true. It is better yet to state that they are low in sodium. FDA Consumer Protection regulations for labels state that "food shall be misbranded if its labeling represents, suggests, or implies, that the food, because of the presence or absence of certain dietary properties, is adequate or effective prevention, cure, mitigation, or treatment of any disease or symptom."

Do not give dietary advice such as "We suggest our fruit plate for those who want to lose weight". Provide facts only.

Four Information Headings for Healthful Menu Items

Guests concerned about health-related qualities look for menu item information that helps them make informed decisions about foods from a dietary viewpoint. Four information areas to consider for particular concerns of nutrition-minded guests are general information, nutrition information, dietary practices and food sensitivities, and substitutions and special requests. Table 13-3 summarizes the types of ingredient, food processing, and food production topics that may be appropriate to include on menus for these guests.

General Information. In general the issues of greatest concern to consumers are whether the food is fresh, frozen, or canned; the portion size; and what main ingredients it contains. Nutrition-minded guests search the menu further for facts that are relevant to their health objectives. For example, usually they insist on fresh foods and want assurance that the chicken and asparagus are fresh (or even locally grown). A statement of portion size may be used to assess calories as much as to make a value or appetite decision. Examples of the way portion size can be indicated unobtrusively include weight (5 ounces of peeled shrimp), volume, or size of serviceware, by count (large steamed artichoke); diameter (pizza), and a simple notation of small, medium, large, or "macho." Diet-conscious diners and grazers also look for such information about appetizer, snack, and side dish items in their quest for satisfying food in clearly understood portions. Information providers should place themselves in the position of the health-conscious guest and provide *useful ingredient information*. Guests might reasonably expect to look to the description of menu items for clues about fiber, calories, fat, and sodium. Such menu information is not yet required by federal law, although some states have taken action to force food service operators to offer consumers information. Perhaps as a warning to the remainder of the industry to respond voluntarily to consumer requests for ingredient information, New York's Attorney General came to an agreement with McDonald's as early as 1986 that outlets would provide ingredient information in all New York units. In fact, a nationwide study in 1987 revealed that over three fourths of consumers were in favor of ingredient listing by fast food chains, arguing that these are packaged foods

TABLE 13-3
Topics of Consideration for Meaningful Communications about Healthful Menu Items

General Information needed to support informed menu choices.

The "real" name of the item (e.g., "fresh halibut fillets," not "deep-sea delight")

The size of the portion

The quality or grade, if applicable

Whether and how preserved (fresh, canned, frozen, cured, etc.)

Relevant processing, preparation, or service notes (e.g., breaded, reformulated, skimmed, trimmed, butter-basted, flambeed with alcohol)

The principal ingredient, including those in any sauce (Restriction of certain ingredients is a therapeutic necessity to many potential guests.)

The cooking method

Any "unexpected" qualities, such as very spicy seasonings

Available dietary accommodations (e.g. menu item substitutions, low-fat cookery)

Information for More Formalized Presentation of Healthful Menu Items

Diet-related "classification" (.eg., low-fat, low-calorie, low-sodium, etc.) Many include nutrient value ranges.

Food preferences indication (e.g., items without meat or that are natural, organic)

Types of fat used in cooking and available for guest use

and, so, should be regulated like those in supermarkets (see Fig. 13-2). (Voluntarily doing this is the responsive path to follow, and may help forestall over-regulation.)

Nutrition Information. The *calorie* quantity, range, or category (low, light) of menu items is the nutrition information most requested by restaurant patrons. The *amount and type of fat (polyunsaturated? vegetable?)* and the range of sodium content are concerns of many other health-conscious guests. Note how these can be revealed through providing information in the categories in Table 13-3. Print formats for communicating this information to guests include listing specific nutrient values on the menu; supplying supplementary information on request; grouping menu items under health-related headings; designating items by using symbols and footnotes; and using footnotes alone. Opinions vary on whether or not to provide specific nutrient values (numbers) on menus. The menu in Figure 13-3 lists approximate quantities of calories, fat, sodium, and other nutrients, with enticing descriptions of healthful fare. A study on supermarket product buying lends support to this strategy. A 1986 report by the Food Marketing Institute cautioned that 35% of respondents "frequently *avoid* purchasing products *without* nutrition information."

Thus far, however, most operators have concluded that food-service guests do not want to know too much about what they are ordering, nor do they want too much gratuitous "technical" information at the point of sale. Although patrons concerned about their diets

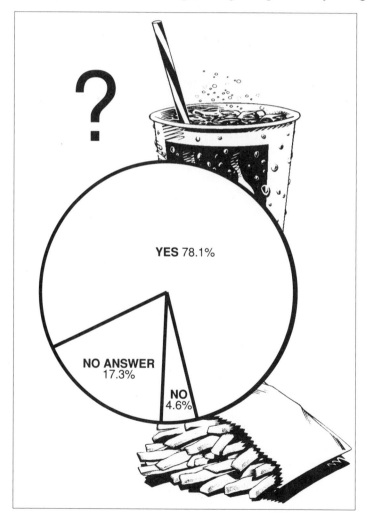

FIGURE 13-2 Should fast-food restaurants list ingredients in foods? *(Praetsher M, Lydecker T, Weinstein J, Bertagnoli L: Tastes of America: How America Loves to Eat Out. Restaurants and Institutions, vol 97, p 82, 1987)*

YES 78.1%

NO ANSWER 17.3%

NO 4.6%

usually have a good grasp of nutrition as it concerns them, it is easy to overestimate their familiarity with terms, as illustrated in Table 13-2.

Only 4% of restaurateurs reported listing calories, according to a 1987 FDA survey. A mere 2% revealed the fat, sodium, or cholesterol content on the menu; however, an additional 1% said this information was available on request (Fig. 13-4). Today it is common for fast food operators to make such information available.

If quantities are stated on the menu, it is recommended and more accurate to state them as a range, since it is unlikely that a recipe would actually produce precisely the same number of calories or other nutrients twice. One might say, "Fresh-Starters with 300 to 400 calories" or "De-Light-Ful Luncheons under 500 calories."

When menu items for the healthful-foods program are presented on the same menu with regular fare but specific nutrient quantities are not stated, another way must be provided to indicate which they are and what are their healthful qualities. Often the items are simply listed under a heading in one portion of the menu:

Perfect Balance ®

For that special balance between taste, nutrition and low calories, Hyatt Hotels is proud to present.

Bird of Paradise

Chilled breast of poached chicken, garnished with kiwi fruits, alfalfa sprouts, sliced tomato and cucumber with a lime yogurt dressing
$8.25

APPROXIMATELY

Calories	507
Protein (grams)	79
Fat (grams)	11
Carbohydrates (grams)	19
Cholesterol (mg)	191
Sodium (grams)	.2

Fresh Artichoke with Chicken Salinas

Chilled artichoke filled with marinated salad of white meat chicken, crisp vegetables, and lemon-herb dressing
$7.95

APPROXIMATELY

Calories	340
Protein (grams)	51
Fat (grams)	7
Carbohydrates (grams)	21
Cholesterol (mg)	125
Sodium (grams)	.2

Vegetable Crepes

Thin crepes made with low cholesterol egg beaters filled with tomatoes, zucchini, peppers and served with fresh vegetables and seasonal fruit
$6.75

APPROXIMATELY

Calories	646
Protein (grams)	19
Fat (grams)	49
Carbohydrates (grams)	36
Cholesterol (mg)	0
Sodium (grams)	.5

Fresh Artichoke Filled With Baby Scallops

Poached artichoke filled with marinated scallops and surrounded with an array of shredded colorful vegetables
$8.25

APPROXIMATELY

Calories	253
Protein (grams)	33.4
Fat (grams)	3
Carbohydrates (grams)	.39
Cholesterol (mg)	.06
Sodium (grams)	1.7

FIGURE 13-3 Although most restaurants choose not to provide nutrient values on the menu, some present them with distinction. *(Courtesy Hyatt Hotels Corporation)*

their healthful qualities. Often the items are simply listed under a heading in one portion of the menu:

FITNESS FARE
"The selections below only taste indulgent!
...They are low in sodium, fat, cholesterol, and calories."

Symbols are a popular method of communicating to health-conscious consumers (Fig. 13-5). A heart, asterisk, apple, or another fitting symbol is placed beside menu items to identify them as low-fat, low-salt, fresh; the symbols are explained in a footnote or legend. Critics of this method say it is too confusing to guests, but when the footnotes are used sparingly and are explained plainly and clearly, they are readily understood. The American Heart Association (AHA) has achieved wide recognition for its heart symbol as a welcome indication that menu items meet AHA dietary guidelines.

Footnotes also can be used effectively alone to convey helpful nutrition information, for example, that lean beef is used in all beef recipes or that foods are salted only lightly in the kitchen.

Dietary Practices and Food Sensitivities. Certain diet-conscious consumer segments will look for menu information on vegetarian dishes or natural or organically grown foods. Some wish to avoid items they view as unsafe, such as certain food additives and "imitation" or artificial foods. Foodservices that cater to these markets should provide assurance that the operation is aware of their desires and should supply sufficient menu description in these areas to guide selections (Fig. 13-6).

Inquiries about ingredients may seem frivolous to some, but millions seek such information because they are on medically prescribed diets. They need clear, before-the-purchase information on menu item contents. They check the ingredient list on the foods they buy at the supermarket as part of their effort to manage their diet. Going out to eat is made more accessible when the information they need is available. This large market includes those with diabetes and other inborn errors of metabolism, those with disorders of the intestinal tract (e.g., ulcers), liver, kidney, gallbladder, and heart diseases, and those with food intolerances.

Food intolerance, including food allergies, is discussed more fully in Chapter 15. An estimated 5% of Americans have one or more sensitivities to food, consumption of which may lead to such symptoms as gastrointestinal distress, skin rashes, and obstructed breathing. Common foods associated most frequently with hypersensitivity reactions include milk and its products, eggs, fish and shellfish, nuts, legumes, wheat, and certain food additives (e.g., monosodium glutamate and tartrazine, a yellow dye). It is crucial for safety, ethical, and legal reasons that communications for sensitive persons be truthful and unambiguous. An Arizona hotel was found liable when a woman who had a severe intolerance to soybeans became ill after consuming the "seafood salad." Since soy-based imitation crabmeat was used along with real seafood, calling it "seafood salad" violates both the practice of truth in menus and meaningful menu item communications for concerned persons. The presence of soy should have been indicated clearly on the menu or by a staff member.

Substitutions and Special Requests. As discussed with menu planning, health-conscious guests frequently prefer low-fat cooking methods, sauces served on the side, and substitutions of lighter products (sauces, side dishes, salt substitute). Such options can be extended by using any of the formats discussed above or by a note on the menu headed "We will be happy to bake, poach or broil any fried entree if you so request." The food and beverage director of the O'Hare Hilton backs up such a statement on the menu with well-trained waitstaffers who offer alternate preparation methods, saying, "If we have pan-fried trout and the customer loves trout but can't eat fried foods, we'll prepare it a different way."

A menu footnote specifying available menu item *substitutions* can be a straightforward way to offer guests flexibility in customizing their meals. One nation-wide seafood chain notes on the menu that any diner is welcome to substitute items from a generous list of options to replace the side dish usually offered. Positioned near the bottom of the menu, the list recently included baked, mashed, or fried potatoes, baked beans, steamed rice, rice pilaf, cottage cheese, fresh tomato slices, and unsweetened apple sauce.

Few operations can allow *carte blanche* on menu modifications. One should give serious thought before placing an invitation on the menu such as, "If you have

"Waist Not, Want Not"*
An Example of a Nutrition Information Brochure from Denny's, Inc.

For guests who are counting calories, Denny's offers a large number of menu items with 550 calories or less. Because many calorie conscious individuals are on a diet of 1500 calories per day, 550 calories represents approximately one-third of a day's limit.

Diabetic exchange information is now included here for our guests who monitor their diet based on exchange groups.

General

The values used to calculate the per-serving content of foods and/or meals in this pamphlet are based primarily upon information obtained from USDA Handbook No. 456 and from nutritional information supplied by food manufacturers. These values are only as correct and complete as the information available. Every effort has been made to ensure that this information is as accurate as possible. Denny's does not, however, guarantee its accuracy or its suitability for any specific, medically imposed diet.

Denny's menu is subject to change without notice, and not all of the menu items listed may be served at all times or in all restaurants.

For further information related to the nutritional content of our menu items, refer to our other three brochures, "Salt Away," "Dine to Your Heart's Content," and "For Sensitive People," or write to us at our Research Center:

Denny's Inc., Research Center
14256 East Firestone Boulevard
La Mirada, CA 90637

Substitutions

We offer our guests the following low calorie alternatives:

Use of	In Place Of
Low calorie syrup	Regular syrup
Juice of a lemon wedge	Prepared salad dressing, tartar sauce
Dash of vinegar	Prepared salad dressing
Fruit, fruit juices or sherbet	Heavy, rich desserts
Iced tea or diet cola	Regular soft drinks
Sugar substitutes	Sugar

Restrictions

If you are counting calories, you may wish to avoid the following high-calorie foods:

- Deep fried foods
- Foods cooked in added fat
- Added fats and/or sauces (e.g., butter, margarine, mayonnaise, gravies, salad dressing, creamers, etc.)
- Foods with hidden fats (e.g., cheese, bacon, avocadoes, etc.)
- Condiments such as ketchup, mayonnaise, sugar, creamer, crackers, and jelly are not calculated in the values listed in this pamphlet unless specified otherwise.

Denny's Menu Items with 550 Calories or Less

Hamburgers	Diabetic Exchange	Approx. No. of Calories
Dennyburger	2½ bread, 4 meat, 1/3 veg., 2½ fat	537

Salads		
Chef's Salad—Regular	5½ meat, ½ veg., 1½ fat	388
Mini	3½ meat, ½ veg., 1 fat	244
Garden Salad	¼ meat, ¼ veg.	57
Albacore Tuna Salad—Regular (¾ c)	3½ meat, ½ veg., 1 fruit, 5 fat	515
Mini	2 meat, ½ veg., ½ fruit, 3½ fat	325
Fresh Fruit Salad	3 fruit, 3 fat	282
Cobb Salad	2½ meat, ½ veg., 3 fat	289
Salad Trio	4 meat, 1 veg., ½ fruit, 4 fat	470

Sandwiches		
Ham & Swiss Cheese	2 bread, 3½ meat, ½ veg., 3½ fat	496
Hot Turkey	2½ bread, 2 meat	285
Grilled Bacon, Cheese & Tomato	2 bread, 1 meat, ½ veg., 5 fat	450
Sliced Turkey	2 bread, 2 meat, ½ veg., 4 fat	445
Albacore Tuna	2 bread, 1½ meat, 3 fat	407
Bacon, Lettuce and Tomato	2 bread, ½ veg., 7 fat	542
Grilled Cheese	2 bread, 2 meat, 4 fat	454
Hot Open-Faced Seafood Sandwich	2 bread, 3 meat, ½ veg., ½ fat	409

Entrees		
Petite Top Sirloin	½ bread, 4 meat, ½ veg., ½ fat	296
Shrimp & Steak	1½ bread, 5 meat, ½ veg., 1½ fat	462
Golden Fried Shrimp	2 bread, 3 meat, 3 fat	476
Fish-in-a-Basket	2 bread, 3 meat, 2½ fat	416
Chicken Cacciatore	2½ bread, 4½ meat, 2 veg., 1 fat	527
Dijon Herb Chicken	4½ meat (herb moderation)	273
Chicken Fillet Strips	1 bread, 4 meat, 1 fat	362
Stir Fry Chicken	4 meat, 1 veg., 4 fat	435
Halibut	4 meat, 4 fat	412
Seafood Stir Fry	3 meat, ½ veg., 5 fat	424
Lemon Chicken	4½ meat, 3 fat	503

Sides	Diabetic Exchange	Approx. No. of Calories
Green Beans	1 veg.	20
Peas	1 bread	63
Corn	1 bread	67
Oriental Vegetables	1 veg.	27
Italian Vegetables	1 veg.	50
Applesauce	1 fruit	42
Sliced Tomato	½ veg.	10
Rice Pilaf	2 bread	164
Baked Potato	2 bread	167
Mashed Potatoes	½ bread	44
French fries	2 bread, 2 fat	288
Roll	1 bread	59
Herb Toast	2 bread, 1½ fat	235
Blueberry Muffin	3 bread, 2½ fat	348
Pickles	free in moderation	23
American Cheese	½ meat, ½ fat	50

Senior Citizens' Specials		
Grilled Ham	2 meat, ½ fat	120
Roast Turkey with gravy	1½ meat, ½ bread, ½ fat	120
Fried Chicken	1½ bread, 3 meat, 2½ fat	278
Fish Fillet Dinner	1 bread, 2 meat, ½ fat	208
Grilled Cod	2½ meat, 5½ fat	394
Pork Chop	3 meat, ½ fat	185
Senior Citizens' Omelette	4½ meat, ½ veg., 4½ fat	460

Desserts		
Cantaloupe (half)	1 fruit	82
Grapefruit (half)	½ fruit	40
Ice Cream, vanilla (1 scoop)	1 starch, 2 fat	164
Mixed Fruit	½ fruit	47
Sherbet (1 scoop)	1 starch	114

Breakfast		
Low Cholesterol Breakfast	1½ bread, 1 meat, 1 fruit, ½ veg., 3 fat	422
Senior Starter with bacon	3 bread, 2 meat, 1 fruit, 2 fat	472
Three-Egg Omelette, plain	5 meat, 4 fat	397
Three-Egg Omelette, made with Egg Beaters and margarine	3 meat, 1 fat	225
Pancakes	3 bread, 1 fat	272

Breakfast Sides	Diabetic Exchange	Approx. No. of Calories
Bacon	4 fat	174
Buttermilk Biscuit with butter and jelly	2 starch, 1 fruit 3 fat	342
Cantaloupe (half)	1 fruit	82
English Muffin with butter and jelly	2 breads, 1 fruit, 2 fat	332
Grapefruit (half)	½ fruit	40
Grits with butter	1½ bread, ½ fat	116
Ham	2 meat, ½ fat	120
Hashed Brown Potatoes	2 bread, 1 fat	205
Hot Oatmeal with whole milk	1½ bread, 1 milk, 1 fat	259
Mixed Fruit	1 fruit	47
Raisin Bran with whole milk	1 bread, 1 milk, 1 fat	209
Sausage Links	2½ meat, 4 fat	320
Toast with butter and jelly	2 bread, 1 fruit 2 fat	316

Beverages		
Apple Juice, regular	2 fruit	72
Chocolate Shake	2 starch, ½ milk, 2 fat	330
Regular or Decaffeinated Coffee, black	free	3
Grapefruit Juice, regular	2 fruit	60
Hot Tea, plain	free	less than 1
Iced Tea, plain	free	1
Nonfat Milk	1 milk	88
Orange Juice, regular	2 fruit	67
Tomato Juice, regular	½ fruit	35
Vanilla Shake	2 starch, ½ milk 2 fat	330
Whole Milk, large	1-1/3 milk, 2 fat	219

Figure continued on next page.

*This version lists available low-calorie substitutions, and the approximate calorie and food exchanges for menu items.

Figure 13-4 continued.

"Salt Away"*
A Second Example of a Nutrition Information Brochure from Denny's, Inc.

For guests concerned about their sodium intake, this pamphlet contains a listing of Denny's menu items with 1,100 mg of sodium or less. This amount is consistent with recommendation of the Food and Nutrition Board of the National Academy of Sciences[1], which estimates that a "safe and adequate" sodium intake is about 1,100 to 3,300 mg per day for an adult. As an additional service, we also offer a salt substitute, which is available upon request from your server.

General

The values used to calculate the per-serving content of foods and/or meals in this pamphlet are based primarily upon information obtained from USDA Handbook No. 456 and from nutritional information supplied by food manufacturers. These values are only as correct and complete as the information available. Every effort has been made to ensure that this information is as accurate as possible. Denny's does not, however, guarantee its accuracy or its suitability for any specific, medically imposed diet.

Denny's menu is subject to change without notice, and not all of the menu items listed may be served at all times or in all restaurants.

For further information related to the nutritional content of our menu items, refer to our other three brochures, "Waist Not, Want Not," "Dine to Your Heart's Content," and "For Sensitive People," or write to us at our Research Center:

Denny's Inc., Research Center
14256 East Firestone Boulevard
La Mirada, CA 90637

Restrictions

The following foods are typically high in sodium and should be limited if you are on a sodium-restricted diet:

Condiments such as soy sauce, Worchestershire sauce, pickles and olives

Spiced salts such as onion salt, garlic salt or celery salt

Cured or processed meats such as bacon, ham, hot dogs, etc.

Cheese

Sauces and salad dressings

Soups

Snack and convenience foods

Please note that we do *not* salt our French fries before serving.

Condiments such as ketchup, mayonnaise, sugar, creamer, crackers and jelly are not calculated in the values listed in this pamphlet unless specified otherwise.

Denny's Menu Items with 1,100 mg of Sodium or Less

Hamburgers[2,3]	Approximate mg of Sodium
British Burger	712
Dennyburger	428
Dennyburger with cheese	631
Patty Melt	903
Denny's Combo (with salad)	475

Salads & Lighter Fare[4]	
Mini Chef's Salad	817
Mini Albacore Tuna Salad	616
Albacore Tuna Salad	942
Garden Salad	32

Sandwiches[5]	
Philly Cheese Steak	520
Albacore Tuna Salad	741
Turkey Salad	1,097
Bacon, Lettuce and Tomato	763
Grilled Bacon, Cheese, Tomato	984
Sliced Turkey	979

Entrees	
Denny's New York Steak	286
Grilled Liver and Onions[5]	809
Stir Fry Chicken	148
Top Sirloin Steak	238
Halibut	397
Shrimp and Steak	621
Hearty Shrimp and Steak	911
Golden Fried Shrimp	672
Hearty Golden Fried Shrimp	1010
Dijon Herb Chicken	1183
Chicken Fillet Strips	396
Chicken Fried Steak	1065
Sirloin Tips and Mushrooms	1020

Senior Citizens Specials[6]	
Chicken Fried Steak	1,020
Fried Chicken (wing and breast)	1,074
Deep-Fried Cod Fillet (includes tartar sauce)	1,042
Sirloin Tips	864

Sides[7]	Approximate mg of Sodium
Applesauce	1
Baked Potato with butter	213
Breaded Zucchini	369
Coleslaw	176
Cottage Cheese	230
Green Beans	160
Italian Vegetables	175
Mixed Fruit	1
Oriental Vegetables	230
Peas	341
Sliced Tomatoes	3
Mashed Potatoes with butter	228
Mashed Potatoes with gravy	300
French fries (we do not salt our fries)	49
Onion Rings	1,054
Garden Salad with bleu cheese dressing	763
Garden Salad with Thousand Island dressing	536
Split Pea Soup (bowl)	794
Vegetable Beef Soup (bowl)	891
Dinner Roll	165
Butter	204
Margarine	90
Rice Pilaf	655
Cacciatore Sauce	258
Barbecue Sauce	446
Tartar Sauce	146
Chicken Gravy	258
Au Jus	262

Breakfasts	
No. 2 Two Egg Breakfast plain, with buttered toast and jelly	1,016
Low Cholesterol Breakfast	636
French Toast	444
Plain Omelette with sliced tomatoes, buttered toast and jelly	670
Senior Starter with bacon, buttered toast, and jelly	834
Senior French Toast	272

Breakfast Sides	
Bacon	586
Buttermilk Biscuits with butter and jelly	836
Cantaloupe (half)	33
English Muffin with butter and jelly	332
Grapefruit (half)	1
Grits with butter	569
Ham	1,076
Hashed Brown Potatoes	387
Hot Oatmeal with whole milk	496
Mixed Fruit	1
Raisin Bran with whole milk	281
Sausage Links	1,048
Toast with butter and jelly	458

Desserts	Approximate mg of Sodium
Chocolate Shake	135
Hot Apple Pie a la mode	453
Ice Cream	53
Sherbet (1 scoop)	8
Vanilla Shake	125

Beverages	
Apple Juice, regular	2
Cola, regular	13
Regular or Decaffeinated Coffee, black	2
Grapefruit Juice, regular	1
Hot Chocolate	180
Hot Tea, plain	32
Iced Tea with lemon wedge and 1 package of sugar	59
Lemonade	2
Nonfat Milk	127
Orange Juice, regular	1
Tomato Juice, regular	344
Whole Milk, large	168

Footnotes

[1] Food and Nutrition Board of the National Academy of Sciences. Washington, D.C.

[2] For jumbo size of these burgers, add 36 mg. of sodium.

[3] The pickle spear is not calculated into these values. One spear is approximately 283 mg. of sodium.

[4] Roll, butter and garnish are calculated into these values, but dressing is not. An order of Thousand Island dressing is 427 mg of sodium. A dash of vinegar or the juice of a freshly squeezed lemon wedge provide low sodium alternatives. Add 80 mg. of sodium for each package of crackers.

[5] Calculated with two rolls and butter, green beans and mashed potatoes ordered with margarine.

[6] Teriyaki glaze is not calculated into these values. An order of glaze is approximately 2,494 mg. of sodium. In other words, if you are watching your sodium intake, do not use the teriyaki glaze which is served on the side.

[7] Add 80 mg. of sodium for each package of saltine crackers.

[8] Calculated with salad, roll, butter, vegetable, French fries and garnish. Dressing is not calculated. An order of Thousand Island dressing is approximately 427 mg. of sodium.

FIGURE 13-4 Brochures prepared by Denny's Inc., help guests make informed menu choices.

*A guide to controlling sodium while enjoying Denny's menus. Approximate sodium content of items with 1100 mg sodium or less, plus sodium guidelines and notes, comprise this available leaflet. *(Courtesy Denny's, Inc.)*

a special preparation request, please let us know and whenever possible we will be pleased to accommodate." This can be good in encouraging patrons to suit their desires, but operators must realize that when guests respond to such an open invitation (and they *will)* they do not expect to be refused because their request is troublesome or costly to fill.

CAFE SANDWICHES

We will gladly serve your Cafe Sandwich on any of our homemade breads with any of our dressings. Our breads are baked fresh daily from scratch in our own bakery and are available to take home from our Markets.

Authentic Sourdough · Croissant
● Whole Grain Wheat · Double Twist Roll · New York Kaiser

● Smoked Turkey Breast on whole grain wheat, with Lingonberry Cumberland sauce.
Served with Jicama Salad 4.95

White Albacore Tuna Salad on sourdough with Chesapeake dressing. Served with Jicama Salad 4.95

Chicken Tarragon with toasted almonds and orange slices on our croissant.
Served with Dilled Cucumber Salad. 6.50

★ The American Cafe—thinly sliced rare roast beef on our croissant with orange horseradish dressing
Served with Dilled Cucumber Salad 5.95

The Eiffel—rare roast beef with homemade country pate and seasonal mushrooms on our croissant
with buttermilk dressing and Lingonberry Cumberland Sauce. Served with Dilled Cucumber Salad 5.95

● The New Californian—fresh guacamole, havarti cheese, sprouts, tomatoes and cucumbers on
whole grain wheat with creamy herb dressing. Served with Dilled Cucumber Salad 4.95

Maryland Crab Salad on sourdough. Served with tomato slices and Lemon Broccoli. 7.50

New York Club—triple-decker of country bacon, turkey, ham and tomato on whole grain wheat with
Chesapeake dressing. Served with Caraway Corn Slaw 5.95

★ Smoked Salmon and Maryland Crab Salad layered on whole grain wheat with cucumber dill
dressing. Served with Lemon Broccoli. 7.50

★ Trio of Sandwiches—Rare roast beef, Chicken Tarragon and Albacore tuna salad. Each on an onion-
poppyseed roll with creamy herb dressing. Served with Jicama Salad 5.95

HOT SANDWICHES

★ The AMCAF *Burger*—mesquite-grilled chicken breast with bacon strips, lettuce and tomato on a
grilled New York Kaiser, with Teriyaki sauce. Served with Caraway Corn Slaw 4.95

● Mesquite-Grilled Chicken Breast on toasted whole wheat, with creamy herb dressing. Served with
Jicama Salad 4.50

★ New Orleans Jazz—smoked ham, fresh steamed asparagus (in season) or broccoli, and melted Swiss
on our double twist roll with buttermilk dressing. Served with Jicama Salad 5.25

Georgetown Reuben—corned beef, Caraway Corn Slaw, and melted Swiss on toasted sourdough
with Chesapeake dressing. Served with Jicama Salad 5.95

Smoked Roasted Pork with homemade barbecue sauce—hickory and applewood smoked, thinly
sliced on toasted sourdough. Served with Caraway Corn Slaw 5.95

Our dressings are served on the side and any may be substituted on your sandwich

Orange Horseradish · Cucumber Dill · Chesapeake
Lingonberry Cumberland · Buttermilk ● Creamy Herb

BEVERAGES

Orange or Apple Juice freshly squeezed	1.95	Lemonade or Freshly-Brewed Iced Teas	1.25
Pepsi, Diet Pepsi, Ginger Ale glass .95 mug	1.25	Iced Coffee	1.25
Milk	.95	Iced Cappucino	2.50
Naturally Sparkling Water	1.25	Espresso Float with vanilla ice cream	3.50

● = Lower in salt, cholesterol, sugar and fat
★ = House Specialty

FIGURE 13-5 Symbols can be used effectively to communicate to patrons the healthful qualities of menu selections.

MANAGING THE MARKETING MIX FOR NUTRITION-CONSCIOUS GUESTS

For foodservice decision makers, marketing might be defined as finding what present and potential guests want and need, then selling the *right* products in the *right* form to the *right* people at the *right* time in the *right* place at the *right* price, to meet objectives of the seller.

In preparing and placing effective informative or persuasive materials, and in all other communications with customers concerning the healthful-foods program, the particular *characteristics of nutrition-oriented guests* must be kept foremost in mind. Chapter 11 shed light on the research that is helpful in identifying these consumers and their desires. This section outlines activities for marketing special menus to them.

Activities used by managers in selling products fall into four categories called, collectively, "the four Ps of the marketing mix": *product, promotions, place,* and *price* (Fig. 13-7). (Some include a fifth P, packaging. We see this as very significant and have chosen to portray it as a component of the others.) To tailor the marketing mix most advantageously to a healthful-foods menu, consideration must be given to the applications of each of the four Ps.

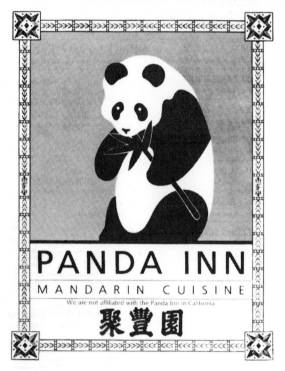

We do not allow the use of MSG in our cooking as a health precaution.

As another health precaution, we fry in low cholesterol vegetable oil and use only freshest meats and vegetables to attain the most nourishing results.

Now you can finally enjoy your meal knowing that it is healthful as well as delicious.

FIGURE 13-6 On the back of the Panda Inn menu is a clear message that management cares about guests' health, their possible food sensitivities (MSG), and their overall dining experience. *(Courtesy Panda Inn, Las Vegas NV.)*

The Product: Product, Service, and Image For Sale

It may seem obvious that an operation's product is its food, menu, and healthful-foods program, but in most cases, what people really buy is much more. Perhaps what they think their money pays for is food, but at different times, what they are seeking to satisfy is a desire for a *quick* but *nutritious* lunch or a *romantic* dinner rendezvous without the usual rich foods or a place that welcomes *youngsters* and reliably offers healthful foods kids enjoy.

While the elements of the marketing mix explained below bear on the program's success, they mean nothing without the right product to back them up. The program and menu must be appropriate and the foods very appealing. Simply stated, foods should taste good and be very satisfying—worth coming back for. It is better to sell quality of product than to try to sell the concept of "its good for you." The healthful elements should be implicit in the excellence of the offering as an added attraction.

Quality, reputation, trust: these words relate to aspects of an operation's image, which can be another selling point. For example, as an image-enhancing move, new owners of the Big Boy chain of family restaurants removed the chubby logo figure in 1988 after decades of service, because management felt that he put off fitness-conscious guests they want to attract.

Healthful-food patrons typically are image conscious, and seek quality products and services. These guests expect cleanliness and pride, qualities that can be displayed even to persons viewing the exterior of the operation through cues such as crisp signage, well-kept building and grounds, even paint colors (e.g., deep green with white suggests freshness). A pleasant, theme atmosphere usually is attractive to this market segment, so it is another part of the product and image that can be promoted. Atmosphere encompasses qualities such as decor, noise level, type of clientele, and type and pace of service.

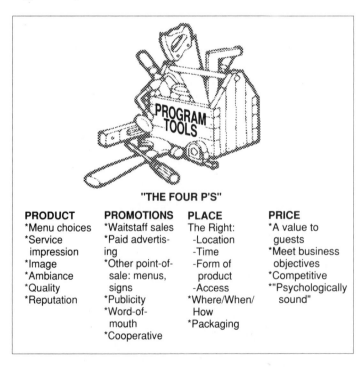

"THE FOUR P'S"

PRODUCT	PROMOTIONS	PLACE	PRICE
*Menu choices	*Waitstaff sales	The Right:	*A value to
*Service	*Paid advertis-	-Location	guests
impression	ing	-Time	*Meet business
*Image	*Other point-of-	-Form of	objectives
*Ambiance	sale: menus,	product	*Competitive
*Quality	signs	-Access	*"Psychologically
*Reputation	*Publicity	*Where/When/	sound"
	*Word-of-	How	
	mouth	*Packaging	
	*Cooperative		

FIGURE 13-7 The marketing mix toolbox.

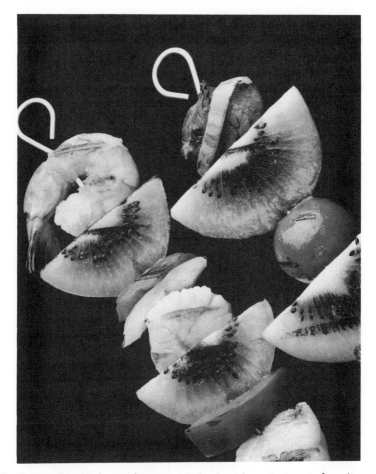

FIGURE 13-8 Eye-catching and appealing presentation is an important part of service.

The way the program's healthful *menu items* complement and enhance the overall menu and the operation's image can be important to the program's success in two ways: it should broaden the base of persons interested in visiting, and it can avoid any perception that the menu is split between good and bad foods.

Opportunities abound for selling the products through creative presentation, including plate arrangement, accompaniments, garnishing, and service flair. Santa Fe Restaurant, a large independent featuring southwestern American cuisine, never fails to sell a dining room full of fajitas after the first sizzling order comes to the table, and is set up in a customized, foot-high, candle-heated rack, accompanied by five bowls of assorted vegetables and sauces. The kiwi kabob in Figure 13-8 is another good example of using the idea that "we eat first with our eyes"; given the spotlight, these tempting foods sell themselves.

Service is an integral part of the product, as is obvious in the word *foodservice*. Is it *service* or *product* to offer decaffeinated coffee or salt substitute or to offer to broil certain menu items listed as fried? Consistently high-quality service repeatedly ranks at the top of the list of patrons' reasons for choosing one restaurant over another when dining out. Even when the food is good, if the service is poor, usually the lasting impression is of a bad experience: the food suffers from "guilt by association." Caring employees and thorough, ongoing training are required to maintain the level of service needed to win patrons and retain their loyalty.

Service desires more specific to patrons of healthful-foods programs include requests for the availability of nonsmoking dining areas (see Fig. 13-9); easy to understand information about menu items to guide informed selections on healthful food choices (e.g., how they are cooked), nutrition-related substitutions for menu ingredients or preparation methods, and a waitstaff sufficiently knowledgeable about nutrition to answer basic menu questions accurately. Finally, in some cases patrons (particularly those over age 50) often prefer for aesthetic reasons to have their food served on crockery or other durable ware rather than on disposable ware.

As you can see, the product is a blend of tangible and intangible features and impressions. The bottom line is how the promise of the food, the menu, the image, and the service elements appear to guests. They all come together to create an impression and to confirm or change an image. In the minds of healthful-food patrons, it is all product.

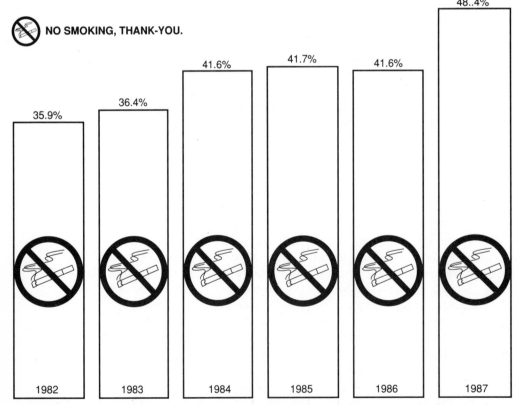

NO SMOKING, THANK-YOU.

1982	1983	1984	1985	1986	1987
35.9%	36.4%	41.6%	41.7%	41.6%	48..4%

FIGURE 13-9 Restaurant patrons' desire for a smoke-free dining place is on the rise. This graph depicts the percentage of patrons who feel others' smoking is an irritant when they dine out.

Promotion: Getting The Word Out

The terms "marketing" and "promotions" are sometimes mistakenly used interchangeably. Actually, promotions are just a (major) branch of the marketing tree that has many thriving sub-branches. Sometimes called the "communications mix," the foodservice promotions mix encompasses all the techniques used by the food-service industry to inform, influence, and create an image of products (including service) for the public. This image is based on messages that are both concrete ("The food tastes good") and conceptual ("The staff is concerned with health here"). The extent of the promotion program is usually governed by budget, as programs, especially those involving television time, can be very costly, but a good program need not be expensive. Here are some of the healthful-foods marketer's main opportunities in promotions.

Personal Selling. Before the competitive need arose to apply the marketing concept, personal selling was the only promotional tool required and used. Through direct face-to-face communication between seller (waitstaff) and patron, information was exchanged and the sale was made. Today, while service staff have a chance and responsibility to inform, assist, and often, to "sell" guests, their work is apt to be supported by many other promotional messages, such as TV ads.

In some settings, personal selling is used to influence guests and lead them to make certain selections. Usually the idea is to use "suggestive selling" to induce patrons to trade up; to spend more than they otherwise might have because they are persuaded to select more items or higher priced ones. The wait person can ask, "May I bring you a large orange juice with your cereal?" or "We also offer special breakfasts featuring whole grain breads, fresh fruit, and low-fat yogurt." Suggestive selling is easily overdone; patrons know when they are being manipulated, and the strategy can backfire. When it is used thoughtfully in a manner that expresses responsiveness to usual health-food wants, the technique can be a positive promotional force that serves patrons better.

The skill, technique, and ultimate success of the personal sales force in marketing healthful foods depends on the soundness of programs for hiring, training, and motivating the staff. After all, these employees represent *the customer contact* and will represent the product as much as, or more than, that wonderful recipe or that $2 million building.

Paid Advertising. Another offshoot of the marketing mix promotions branch is paid advertising. For smaller foodservices this might include buying advertisements in local newspapers or on radio, distributing coupons door-to-door, sending direct mail to neighboring zip codes, or leasing sign space on a billboard or taxicab. Larger firms and franchises often combine those strategies with campaigns using product branding and more costly media such as TV and national magazines. They place their advertising carefully, selecting particular media and programs whose audience characteristics are similar to those of existing and targeted nutrition-conscious patrons.

Sampling. A promotional technique that lends itself well to nutrition-oriented programs is sampling—giving guests and would-be guests a free taste of an actual product or recipe. For example, offering luncheon guests a sample of a featured fruit shake in a wine glass is a way to introduce new taste opportunities. Something as simple as providing a bread basket with both whole wheat and white rolls can work similarly but has far less flair. In addition to in-house sampling, guests may also be given a chance to taste foods at community fairs, cooking demonstrations, and similar public events. The challenges of sampling the healthful menu items are that: it can be expensive to provide the ingredients and labor, predicting needs may be difficult (e.g. if the offer were promoted publicly), those who sample should be persons who are likely to be near the restaurant (or a chain member) in the future, and, even if the chef had a bad night, the sampled product and service *must* taste good and be right or the promotion will backfire. Still, sampling can be a valuable promotional tool. It is risk-free to guests and can melt the initial resistance patrons sometimes have to less familiar foods or to those they may first perceive as being "for health nuts."

Point of Sale. A great deal of communication takes place at or near the place and time of the foodservice transaction. These are point-of-sale messages. Such messages communicate not only facts—what is for sale and how much it costs—but also impressions—the restaurant's style, level of sophistication, neatness, and cleanliness. Point-of-sale pieces should have appropriate copy, photos, or other graphics to attract the attention of guests, create a desire for what is featured, and ultimately, produce increased sales. Included in point-of-sale promotions (other than personal selling) are such printed items as the menu itself, menu-related signs inside the operation, clip-ons, table tents, special posters, recipes and flyers, the product wrap, take-out packaging, and even imprinted napkins. Verbal messages, such as greeting (and parting) at the door or comments while seating patrons, are other opportunities to influence guests near the point of sale.

It might seem that such items are minor or that they convey only a small portion of the message of the establishment, but this is not true. Such gestures can go a long way in promoting an image. Consider the way a menu is layed out or even the way it is handed to a patron. All point-of-sale impressions need to enhance the overall image of marketing good-tasting, healthful foods. This is an image logically associated with surroundings that demonstrate the foodservice operators' concern about the well-being of their patrons and about the pleasurable quality of the food and the dining experience.

Publicity. Another factor in promotions is good publicity, including public relations. Good press and a positive image are all important. Rather than paying for an advertisement that everyone knows is simply the company beating its own drum, public relations are enhanced by being associated with good things and by making a conscientious effort to have this connection publicized in the media (radio, newspaper, etc.) or communicated to target segments in a way that appears unbiased. It is not a paid message. For a recent American Dietetics Association Annual Conference, several area restaurants teamed together to send a welcome announcement to the conferees, complete with a giant fruit basket. The restaurateurs included in the bounty a list of the healthful-foods features on their menus along with the name and address of each operation. It made a good impression, was good for business, and was the proper approach to a known market segment that would be likely to try foods at these operations.

There are many additional ways to get the name and image of an operation in front of the market. Having the chef demonstrate how to make low-calorie entrees or sauces is an example that local clubs and even TV stations often clamor for. Another idea is to sponsor a contest among restaurants in which the most appealing meals meeting limit standards for calories, cholesterol, and fat, are awarded prizes and gain media exposure. It is important to have the contest judged by newsworthy people, such as the mayor of the city and spouse, a local newspaper columnist, a dietitian, a popular local celebrity, etc. This can earn good press and bring attention to specific operations.

Operators also should join in civic enterprises and participate in civic clubs whose members and missions are concerned about health, quality-of-life, community promotions, and similar issues. It might be wise to sponsor a little-league team and even to supply them with a healthful meal after some games. Putting on a free holiday meal for a disadvantaged group also can generate publicity. Earning good will in this way can cost very little and is often as effective as much more costly publicity programs or paid advertisements.

Publicity is a tricky part of the promotions mix because it is seldom controllable. It is not like buying air time for a radio message of one's choosing. The press may feel the publicity attempt is not newsworthy and may not use it or may bury it where few people see it. Or, a major news event may preempt the story.

Endorsements. An *endorsement* from a respected, well-known person or organization is a way to favorable publicity for a healthful-foods program. The endorser typically would agree to lend his or her name, written quote, voice, and perhaps photo to recommend or support the program or elements of the program. Health professionals and those associated in a positive way with fitness and sports are obvious candidates for the role of endorser, especially if they are already patrons and they volunteer their praise. These persons frequently are in a position to counsel others on food choices and likely would be pleased to know of a restaurant with a healthful-foods program which they could also recommend to their patients or clients. Other professionals may be sought and won over to the program, but endorsements work only if the spokesperson projects genuine enthusiasm for the program. There are a number of professional people in the health-related fields who make good endorsers, including:

- **Physicians**. Cardiologists, (heart specialists), internists, and family practice physicians ordinarily are among the most knowledgeable and interested in nutrition. One who writes a newspaper column especially could provide positive exposure.
- **Dietitians and Nutritionists**. They often act as counselors and advisors who help people with their diets. The healthful-foods menu should be sent to the nutrition professionals in local hospitals and clinics for use as a teaching tool with patients. It can serve as a "working" promotional piece.
- **Fitness and Sports Specialists**. Whether it's dance or yoga, marathons or mountaineering, credible specialists are concerned with health, as are the

persons they instruct or coach. Many also provide nutrition information as part of training programs.
- **Others**. Certain public health associations, such as the AHA, lend their names to restaurant programs that comply with their guidelines.

Word-of-Mouth Advertising. A subtle but powerful element of the promotions mix is word-of-mouth advertising—personal opinions passed from one person to another. It is often shaped by the other marketing mix components. In a 1987 survey, *nearly two thirds of foodservice respondents* agreed that the single *most influential consideration in choosing to visit a new restaurant is the recommendation of a friend or family member.* * Trading on this idea are such promotional tactics as two-for-one meal specials, the use of endorsements, celebrity spokespersons, restaurant reviews, and even sampling. Each is aimed at getting one person to persuade others of the desirability of a given experience. It can be a challenge to have word-of-mouth work in the operation's favor: the saying goes that one person who has a good experience *may* recommend the establishment to one associate, but after a bad experience, the same person will spread the word to between five and nine other persons. Good news travels fast, but bad news travels faster!

Place: The Right Place, Time and Form.

The third P of the marketing mix is place. Obviously, a product is not much good to a patron if it is not available where, when, and in the form wanted. A key part of the place objective in foodservice marketing is to identify the target market in conjunction with available sites; that is, where to locate the operation. As in buying a home, the three top considerations for property value may well be location, location, and location. The "place mix" decision can have long-range effects. It is much harder to move a restaurant and win over a new customer base than to change prices or replace menu items. Marketing intelligence information is vitally important here. The right concept for a certain city may be the wrong concept if the operation is not located near the appropriate neighborhood or thoroughfare, or even if it is on an inconvenient side of the street for targeted commuters. Place also has to do with access and form: can guests *get to* the menu items (hours of operation, drive-throughs) and are the products in the desired form (finger foods, packaged to go)? Desirable place considerations continue to be greater access and convenience features such as rapid service, drive-through, and delivery. The take-out food market is among the fastest-growing areas, while eat-in dining has reached a plateau. Making place work may mean preparing items for immediate consumption, as well as preparing and packaging items for "heat and serve" enjoyment at home or at the office. Fast food restaurants have had success with bulk packaging of take-outs: busy working parents have expressed interest in the availability of affordable healthful food packaged family-style to serve at home. Supermarketers are especially responsive to the expanding demand for individual meals for the nutrition-conscious with their frozen "light" dinners. Crystal-ball gazers predict that in the future we will have microwave oven (and freezer?) components in our home entertainment consoles, and, within the decade, microwave ovens in our automobiles. But even today, a

*"Tastes of America", *Restaurants and Institutions* December 9, 1987, vol. 97, 326, p. 84.

tremendous untapped market appears to lie in busy two-career families who own microwaves. (One working mother says her daughter has no concept of an oven roast, because they never cook. Says she, "I'm considering turning my kitchen into a den"!)

The Price is Right.

The fourth P of the marketing mix, price, is very important in influencing buyer behavior and response to the product and the eating experience. Establishing menu prices unquestionably affects buyer behavior, but pricing basics go back to the objectives and image of the establishment as well. Like so many aspects of marketing, pricing involves a good deal of general business knowledge and psychology. Thus, lower prices do not necessarily mean higher sales volume and do not always increase profits. Rightly or wrongly, quality-conscious patrons often avoid items with lower prices, either because they anticipate low quality or because expensive items have an elusive quality called "snob appeal."

In any commercial foodservice, prices *overall* need to be within reason so that expected total sales are sufficient to cover costs and also to meet goals for profit, volume, and market share. Patrons have expectations about prices, and an establishment should gear its price range to those expectations.

For healthful-foods, patrons usually will accept somewhat higher prices than those for comparable menu items with no special emphasis. As can be seen from Table 11-7, some nutrition-oriented segments tend to be more willing than patrons in general to pay for what they want. They recognize that extra costs and care may be needed to serve their needs. They *do* expect a good experience for their dollar, but with that modern "I am worth it and can afford it" attitude, they appear to have few reservations about paying a little more when they have reason to anticipate a pleasant dining experience.

Value remains important however, as some people have a resistance to "diet" foods, believing they will pay a lot for a little food. It is true that food costs may be lower for low-calorie fare owing to the modest portion sizes, but labor costs may offset this. What does the patron think is the value of the product offered? The price must be right for the value image. Patrons are not interested in what it costs an operation to produce an item. They are interested in getting something at a price that represents the value they see in the item, including service, and ambience. It is a delicate business.

Cooperative Marketing Efforts

Several related strategies supplement the four Ps for marketing healthful foods. Cooperative cross-marketing might be thought of as: "You scratch my back, I'll scratch yours." For example, a Denver-based wellness center noted the growing frequency with which members were dining out. The program's dietitians began working to assist local restaurants in offering menu items in keeping with the U.S. Dietary Guidelines for Americans. The center could then recommend cooperating restaurants to clients. By conforming to the center's program, the restaurants stood to gain more business: in turn, the restaurant programs provided the center's clients the potential of having better diets. Both earned good will for their effective outreach. This type of cooperative marketing is a natural for many independent operators, because it can promote a synergistic relationship (the whole is greater than the parts alone) between the healthful-foods program and other organizations and agencies that have health- and fitness-conscious guests.

Private and community-based wellness programs and health maintenance organizations (HMOs) are proliferating because many businesses today are seeing the productivity costs of health problems. They initiate wellness programs in an attempt to educate, screen, monitor, and encourage employees to have healthier lifestyles. This makes good economic sense. It is noted that 70% of lost work days are due to lifestyle-related problems. Employees with poor health habits have 25% higher health costs, are 85% more likely to miss work, and are twice as likely to limit the amount of work they perform on the job. The National Institutes of Health estimates that decreasing the fat intake of the average American diet by even 10% would save 100,000 lives per year from heart attacks, a statistic of interest to employers and employees.

Other examples of diet and lifestyle issues are how regularly people eat balanced meals or snacks; how close weight is to the published standards; what people eat for the first meal of the day (bran cereal, fruit, candy, coffee only?); and the average intake of nutrients compared to the RDA and dietary goals, over time.

As a career note, managers of corporate foodservice operations may be asked to participate in conducting a company-sponsored wellness effort. Some have modified their menus and recipes, added more fresh items, and made information available on selections from the executive dining and cafeteria menus, and even for the vending machine foods. Managers also may be asked to provide a person to prepare simple nutrition handouts, screen for special dietary needs of employees, monitor weights, participate in health fairs, and even give talks to groups on food-for-health fundamentals. Posters to draw attention to certain foods and to reinforce healthful-foods concepts also may be a part of the program.

Other cooperative possibilities that help to deliver the operation's message to healthful-food patrons are tie-ins with clinics, weight control centers, other diet plans, and health and fitness organizations, including clubs. The foodservice might offer some menu choices recommended by the center, plan, or club, in exchange for referrals from these programs and for mention in their member publications. In such an arrangement, the newspaper advertisement for an executive fitness and spa center may also include a note (or coupon, discount, etc) on the executive fitness breakfast available at a nearby restaurant. The restaurant cooperates by conforming to the healthful-food needs of members, and may even include featured specials and point-of sale marketing information about the executive fitness center and spa. Independent foodservice operators should take the initiative in working with area health-oriented centers to incorporate sought-after nutrition qualities into the menu.

Co-marketing is a final marketing tool that might be used to share costs with another organization. Some food producers or distributors will pay a percentage of menu printing costs for operations that name their brand on the menu. Rather than listing "assorted cold cereals," cereals might be listed by brand if companies that own these brands will contribute to printing costs.

The Real seal featured in an advertisement directed at foodservice operators (Fig. 13-10), is an example of a co-marketing partnership available to any foodservice operation using dairy foods that conform to common government standards. These operators have the opportunity to enter into a licensed agreement through the American Dairy Association for permission to display the symbol on menus, table tents, or signs. The Real Seal, recognized by millions as signifying quality, can be seen on thousands of menus and menu communications nationwide (e.g., Domino's Pizza uses the symbol on their pizza packaging for their cheeses.). The benefits to the operator can include free or inexpensive merchandising aids for dairy products as well as the image boost of assuring guests that this operation is concerned with quality and uses "the real thing," not imitations.

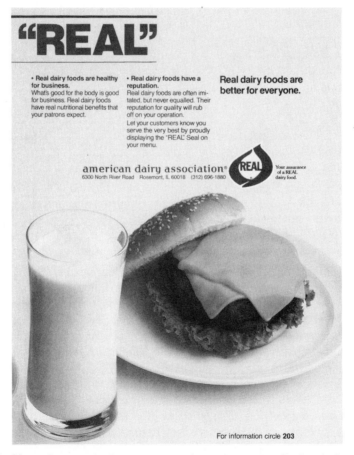

FIGURE 13-10 Often other organizations are prepared to cooperate in a foodservice's selling efforts for mutual benefit. Above, the American Dairy Association offers their "REAL"® Seal deal. The "REAL" Seal is a registered trademark of the United Dairy Industry Association.

There are many ways to form a mutually beneficial cooperative partnership, so remaining alert and working out possibilities may pay handsome dividends.

PROGRAM ROLL-OUT: BEFORE, DURING, AND ONGOING

Planning the Details of the Program Roll-Out

Having considered menu item communications and the marketing mix essentials in preparation for training and for program roll-out, it is time to produce or to deliver for design and reproduction any needed printed materials for the menu, for employee training, for other promotions, and for any other anticipated needs. Timing is important, as always: lay-out, paste-up, and printing can take weeks.

As mentioned in Chapter 11, the nutrition program planning and implementation checklist (e.g., the PERT diagram) should be used as a reference *throughout* the development of the program. Just prior to roll-out, a very *thorough review* should be undertaken to ensure that all elements of the checklist (complete with any changes or detours) have been addressed and are at an adequate level of readiness. The individual who is reviewing should make no assumptions but should, to the extent possible, personally check on each item, from the whereabouts of the program's recipes to the level of staff familiarity with the program. When plans and goals have been set, and paths and standards established to reach them, one has a blueprint for assuring that important activities are not overlooked, that various projects in separate areas are progressing according to schedule (and if not, why not), and that the varied projects will come together as envisioned and on time. To lessen the chances of a rocky or interrupted start, the program should not begin until the review indicates that all necessary elements are in place.

Program Roll-out

The announcement and roll-out of the program, its initial phase, is perhaps its most vulnerable time. An important element of getting off to a smooth start is being certain that staff is well-acquainted with the program and is prepared and equipped to carry it out (see Chap. 14). There is a particular need to be sure that the program is well-coordinated between back-of-the-house and front-of-the-house personnel. Employees might be brought together for at least one brief meeting to review and ensure that staff understand the program and the roll-out plan, and that the two groups are motivated to work as a team for program success.

As mentioned in the discussion of menu planning, it is good to have a test period to try out or sample some ideas and items for patrons in order to gauge their acceptance and to ease into production. This is done prior to investing in printing, training, and other program components. It can be very helpful as a "dress rehearsal," and can provide a foretaste of "the roll-out" when selected of these recipes are to be produced and served regularly.

Careful planning means that arrangements will be in place to introduce and begin the program at a given point in time in a way that befits the operation. It is recommended that a program begin simply, without high-pressure selling or fanfare, and that it grow gradually. The roll-out of a healthful-foods program may range from the quiet addition of a daily special introduced by a waitstaff member to the full promotional fervor of an open house, complete with billboards, celebrity guests, and contests. Once the recipes, testing, marketing, training, and other facets of the program have been fitted into place, the roll-out might amount simply to making the program benefits available to guests.

Fine Tuning for Success

Follow-through is *not* just getting a plan started. The requirement also is that it receive close checking and supervision, and through this, opportunities and problems should be identified and proper adjustments made quickly, when called for. The start-up period especially is a time when management and supervisory staff need to devote considerable time to the plan. This is part of the evaluation of the plan components and their effectiveness. Now management learns how solid the planning and early implementation procedures were, and how well the staff was prepared. Not everything is going to go perfectly. A contingency plan should be devised to provide for a graceful and inconspicuous withdrawal from the program for the time being if results are profoundly disappointing. But if management and the supervisory staff are ready to act promptly to correct minor "glitches," the program should thrive.

Measuring Success

According to objectives set at the program's outset, standards should be in place for measuring how well the program is doing. A manager who knows the score can be assured whether the program is succeeding and can use information gathered to plan for changes or to point to further answers needed.

Traditional management financial reports provide performance feedback and may include such information as an analysis of the type and number of each nutrition-oriented menu item sold and its popularity in comparison to other menu items; dollar sales and the proportion of total dollars contributed by each item's sales; dollar gross profit (sales minus food cost); and the proportion of total gross profit contributed by each item. A variety of menu analysis techniques are available to guide managers in using such information to help fine-tune the marketing mix (e.g., make changes in the menu, prices, promotions). While each analysis method gives valuable feedback, each provides different answers, and none replaces the need to watch for deviations from standards and forecasts.*

In the ongoing effort to keep a finger on the pulse of the program and to measure its success, management should be certain that an intelligence system is functioning to provide accurate and timely information to them that reflects the status of the program and possible opportunities for its improvement. Included in this system are both feedback and a continuing conscious review of the items involved in the checklist that was used to develop the nutrition-oriented foods program. Some feedback will

*For a discussion of menu analysis techniques, refer to Kotschevar: *Management by Menu, ed 2,* pp 171-194. New York: John Wiley and Sons, 1986.

trickle in randomly, but a well-rounded view of operations requires a more formal system for collecting needed information (e.g., opinions, statistics, observations) about a variety of topics (e.g., menu selections, dollar sales, guests' health concerns). Our industry and our diners are dynamic: their constantly changing and shifting demands require that providers remain alert and that the program be considered evolutionary, not static. As a simple example, in the early 1980s, the NRA found that the greatest health concern of many patrons was salt. Today "freshness" and "no additives" have replaced it atop the list; and salt has moved down. What about tomorrow?

Much can be learned from feedback provided by personnel. A short formal or informal discussion with service personnel at the end of a shift can provide information on volume, guest requests and comments, and suggestions to smooth service. Patron comments also can be important feedback. When comment cards are available in the dining room, a way must be provided for guests to drop off or mail the cards *to management*, rather than to waitstaff, to prevent "screening" by employees. Asking for patron comments about a menu item can be helpful, but it can encourage a degree of pickiness (in *any* program). Such comments are most useful when a few responses occur repeatedly.

Other feedback is provided by such indicators as repeat orders and repeat visits—or a lack of them. Plate waste can indicate recipe, production, portioning, or accompaniment problems. In this area it may be best for each individual operation to devise ways in which meaningful feedback can be gained in a cost-effective way, utilizing the resources available in the facility.

SUMMARY

For a successful nutrition-oriented foodservice program, a well-targeted menu plan should be supported by planning and implementing meaningful menu communication and marketing elements.

Offering a single menu for regular and more healthful selections is recommended; using a second menu to list nutrition-oriented program selections separately can detract from the overall operation and the program. Menu item communications to patrons should indicate specifically, accurately, yet simply, the healthful qualities of selections. The message should allow flexibility in operations and should "fit" the operation's image in tone and substance. Neither health claims nor dietary advice should be included.

Four information categories for menu communications are (1) general descriptions (e.g., whether food is fresh or canned); (2) nutrition (e.g., the calorie or fat range); (3) dietary practices and sensitivities (e.g., presence of ingredients commonly associated with food intolerance); and (4) substitutions and special requests (e.g., availability of low-fat side dish options). Studies show that only a small proportion of restaurants list nutrient values on the menu, but it is common to see menu subheadings indicating calorie range or symbols with footnotes to indicate healthful-foods program items.

The marketing mix consists of the four Ps—product, promotion, place, and price. The product includes menu items and their presentation and also the quality and impression of service. Promotion includes personal selling by dining room staff, paid advertising, sampling, point-of-sale devices (such as menus and signs) and publicity (including public relations, endorsements, and word-of-mouth advertising). Having products where, when, and in the form guests want them is the place aspect of the marketing mix and represents a major opportunity for operations that can market healthful foods "to go". The fourth element, price, embraces the many business and consumer considerations that must be figured in when setting prices of menu items.

Joining forces with other organizations, such as food manufacturers or fitness centers, in cooperative marketing efforts can increase marketing muscle and decrease expenditures.

Prior to roll-out of the program, a thorough review of the plan checklist should be made; the program should be introduced only when all preparations are complete. Printed materials must be produced, employees prepared, and program announcement plans set.

When the day comes for the roll-out, it is recommended that the program start simply with little fanfare and be allowed to gather strength gradually. Managers must be extra alert in the early, most vulnerable period of the program, checking closely on the need for corrective measures in menu, training, and marketing plans. Feedback from employees and guests, sales statistics, and a variety of other sources should be consulted frequently to establish whether the operation is on target in reaching identified market segments and in attaining the performance goals of the program.

Chapter Review

1. What types of information should patrons be provided about program menu selections?
2. Menu item communications to patrons may come from waitstaff. What are two other ways to provide information to guests?
3. Why is it recommended that, when an operation offers both, the menu for nutrition-oriented selections be included on the menu along with the regular fare?
4. List and explain the eight guidelines discussed for writing menu copy.
5. Make up a menu description for a tuna salad that provides the information items referred to as "general" (see Table 13-3).
6. The calorie evaluation of the shrimp salad recipe reveals that it provides 350 calories per serving. If calories are to be listed on the menu, what formats are suggested? Why might it be poor practice to list the salad as having "350 calories"?
7. Referring to Figures 13-4 A-D, explain how Denny's has chosen to respond to the health-related needs of guests.

8. Discuss the types of information guests may seek on dietary practices and food sensitivities. If this is too complex to be included in the menu, how else might it be communicated to patrons?

9. Why is it usually inadvisable to state on the menu, "We will gladly oblige your special menu request. Just ask." Compose a statement that expresses a willingness to be flexible without overextending the foodservice.

10. How would you define *foodservice marketing*? Now turn to the definition in the chapter and compare your response.

11. In marketing healthful foods, why is it unwise to stress to patrons that, above all else, certain items are "good for you"? What should be emphasized? How might the good-for-you concept be included in a more subtle way in the promotions mix?

12. Name the four elements of the marketing mix and briefly describe each. Why are they considered the tools of marketing management?

13. Beyond food itself, explain what people may actually be seeking in a restaurant's product. Why is service a part of the product?

14. How can image be used as a part of the healthful-food product to make selections more attractive to patrons? Why is it so important that the program's menu is congruent with the operation's overall image?

15. Distinguish between marketing and promotion. What is the function of the promotions mix?

16. As a type of promotion, how can the waitstaff help to market healthful-foods?

17. To promote a new "Heart's Desire" appetizer, describe two types of paid advertising and two different types of publicity one might exploit. How is publicity different from paid advertising?

18. A printed menu is perhaps the most obvious point-of-sale promotion piece. Besides what is being offered and how much it costs, what other message might be delivered by a printed menu? How? Name other point-of-sale tools that might be used in a take-out promotion for "fresh pineapple juice coolers."

19. What is an endorsement? For a healthful-foods program, why is it important that the person doing the endorsing be well-respected and involved with a field relevant to health? How can a good endorsement support a positive chain of events through word of mouth?

20. The place portion of the marketing mix directs efforts to have products where, when, and in the form they are wanted by the target market. List as many place-mix considerations as you can for planning to market a breakfast health shake to motorists traveling eastbound to a 9:00 AM work assignment.

21. How can price be used as a marketing tool with healthful foods? In your opinion, why is pricing considered such a delicate business?

22. Describe the purpose of a wellness program within a company office complex. What might be expected of foodservice management within the company (e.g., the employee cafeteria or vending center)? How might a commercial foodservice located near the complex market their healthful foods program to attract wellness program participants?

23. One way to amplify marketing efforts and to reduce costs in a healthful foods program is to work with other organizations in co-marketing. Describe how the marketing effort could be boosted in each of the following instances: (1) featuring FIT FOOD brand breakfast cereals on the menu; (2) contacting the Dairy Council for recipes; (3) tying in promotions with a nearby fitness center.
24. What do you think are primary considerations when preparing to announce and promote a new fitness fare program among patrons?
25. Now assume the program begins at dinner tonight. In your imagined operation, how will patrons be made aware of the program? How do operations and marketing efforts differ tonight from last night?
26. Why is it important to measure success? Why must standards and objectives be in place for determining how well targets are being hit?
27. Describe several sources of feedback and the types of insight each might provide about the program.

Chapter 14
Preparing Employees for Program Success

Chapter Goals

- To emphasize the role of well-trained employees in program success.
- In the program context, to amplify the importance of communications.
- To identify training responsibilities of management and trainers.
- To provide a dual framework for evaluating training needs: the needs of employees and the tasks required for program success.
- To provide a resource for building an ongoing nutrition-oriented training program, including suggested formats, types of instruction, specific topics, and program evaluation.

"The taste of the roast depends on the handshake of the host."

–Benjamin Franklin

Such vintage wisdom rings with renewed meaning today as competition builds and the expectations of consumers for healthful foods and good service escalate. Capable, trained personnel, true human resources, are the ones who carry the ball; they determine whether or not guests receive that handshake.

Train we must. Authorities who have studied successful and unsuccessful healthful-foods programs agree that the most common cause of failure is lack of adequate planning and staff training. According to National Restaurant Association (NRA) figures, between 1988 and the year 2000, 2.5 million persons will join the 8 million now employed in the foodservice workforce, generating the largest number of new jobs of any industry. A quality training program to meet the needs of this important, growing, dynamic workforce is an investment that can continue to pay off for both employer and employee. This chapter discusses development and implementation of training programs that prepare employees throughout the operation to effectively carry out healthful-foods program activities for which they are responsible.

The objective of the training program is to inform and to develop employee attitudes, knowledge, and skills specific to the program (Fig. 14-1). *"Knowledge training"* could include menu item information a waitstaff member needs in order to respond knowledgeably to guests' questions. Much of the information that must be communicated to program employees in knowledge training relates to policies and procedures (e.g., free refills for spilled drinks); and to the qualities of food products

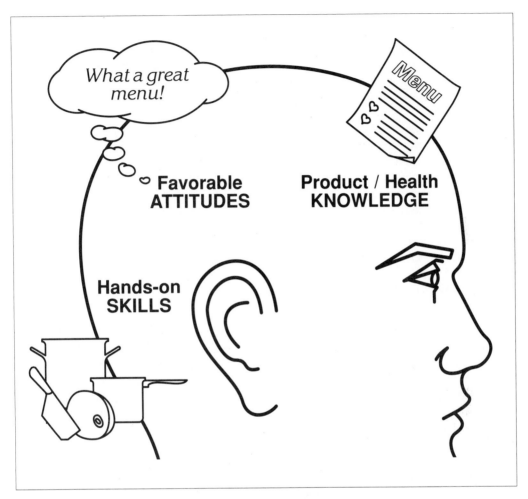

FIGURE 14-1 Main Training Thrusts—Attitudes, knowledge and skills needed for the healthful foods program must be developed in employees according to the role of each.

of significance to targeted guests (the vegetable soup contains no meat broth). *Skills training* refers to the "how to" of hands-on tasks and techniques (the proper way to clean salad greens). An employee with the attitude that the healthful-foods menu is just extra fuss is a candidate for *attitudinal training*. The objective is to foster a new perception of the program (e.g., "Because I can assist these guests in having a pleasant dining experience, my work is appreciated, and my job will be secure.").

MANAGEMENT'S RESPONSIBILITY

Management has the responsibility to see that employees are informed adequately about the healthful-foods program and that they have the necessary attitudes, knowledge, and skills to carry out their related responsibilities in line with program goals. Proper informing of employees must occur about the fitness fare program if employees are to understand the goals of the program, have some of the basic facts, know how to go about interpreting the program, and understand how to put it into operation in the "real world." It is up to management to provide clear goal orientation, ongoing motivation, and responsive supervision and direction to keep the program progressing as planned.

Management also must provide needed supplementary resources to implement the program, especially trainers, training materials, facilities, money, and employee time. Relabeling certain menu items as healthful and then neglecting to provide some general training is a recipe for frustrated employees and disappointed guests. Management must be committed and should be totally involved in ongoing planning and training efforts; the degree of this managerial dedication can be an indicator of potential program success. Training modules for healthful-foods programs mesh perfectly with quality foodservice employee training programs for procurement, production, and service that meet the needs of the operation's entire menu.

THE COMMUNICATION LOOP
A TRAINING IMPERATIVE

Although the need to understand the dynamics of communication is not unique to nutrition management in foodservices, it is a training essential. Training and its objectives rely on complete, two-way communication (Fig. 14-2). The traditional communications elements are *the sender, the message, the receiver*, and *feedback*. Breakdown at any point can result in misunderstandings, hard feelings, confusion, and regrettable mistakes, both among employees and between employees and guests.

The *sender* must send the *appropriate* message of the right length and form at the right place and time. Thus, if a waitstaff member calls to the cook to "hold the bacon" and the cook consults only written checks for menu modification requests, the sender has used the wrong form of communication and trouble results. Next, the *message* must be complete, unambiguous, accurate, and undistorted (e.g., by a noisy kitchen). For example, a menu planner who asks that the purchasing person buy some "vegetable fats" should not be surprised if what is purchased is hydrogenated shortening. If the planner wants *polyunsaturated oil* (or nonhydrogenated vegetable oil), then that should be specified. The *receiver* must actually take in (not ignore) and accurately interpret and comprehend the message. During instruction on changing a familiar task, for example, as in a training session on new types of guest requests to be accommodated on menu items, trainees may simply "tune out," thinking they already know what to do. Or, if they do not understand the terms used in the lesson, learning may be impossible. They did *not receive*. *Feedback* is the final link in the loop. It is here that the sender learns whether the message got through and whether it is was received as intended. This step is not automatic and must be cultivated by sender and receiver alike. In training, this can take several forms:

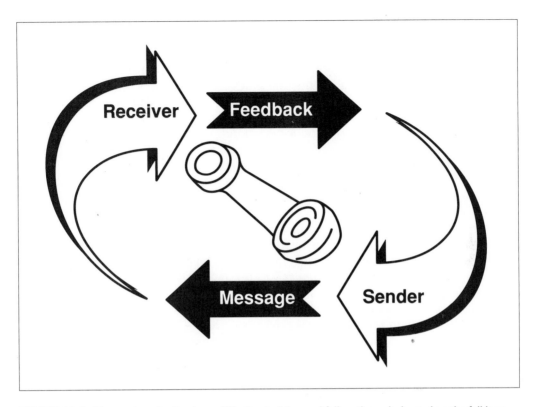

FIGURE 14-2 The communication loop: Effective training and follow-through depend on the full loop.

1. asking questions of the receiver to hear the response (e.g., "What would you say to a guest who asked for a suggestion for a low-fat breakfast item?")
2. asking the receiver to state the message as he or she understands it (e.g., "From what we have just discussed, how would you say that storing these fresh melons will be different from storing the canned fruit?")
3. role playing, with trial and practice activities.

About the Trainer: Who is to Train?

Some operations have a special full-time training staff which uses regional or national centers or travels from unit to unit, but in general, this is practical only for large multiunit operations. In smaller operations, the trainer may be the manager, assistant manager, head supervisor, chef, cook, steward, maitre d', captain, or any combination. It is a mistake to assign training to someone just because that person knows the job; the trainer also must know how to train (i.e., must have at least an ability in two-way communication and a working understanding of what it means to comprehend and learn the subject matter the trainee needs to know). For this reason, training the trainer often should include instruction in effective teaching. On the other hand, someone who is a good teacher may be not be appropriate as a trainer for every subject or skill. Also consider the trainer's actual knowledge of and level of commitment to the program. *Assuming* that a chef knows how to identify or develop a low-fat recipe, for example, is a common error. The same is true for the manager who leaves program planning and all training up to a chef who, understandably, may be ignorant of nutrition, or may not wish to make the necessary changes in recipes that he or she developed and regards as personal property. For optimal learning, the trainer should have the confidence of trainees concerning his or her ability in relevant topic areas (namely planning, handling, producing, and/or serving *healthful* foods for targeted guests).

Motivation Strategies. Trainers need first to get the attention of the trainees, to develop a desire to learn and to win a willingness to cooperate. Proper motivation of the trainee is a key to adequate learning. Trainees must *want* to learn; they must be motivated to learn, and this should be done at the start of be training. A positive reason may be management's appreciation of a well done job, a pat on the back, or other praise. Favorable recognition is a powerful motivator. No reinforcement is more effective than a specific, deserved, and sincere acknowledgment. Trainers and managers (and fellow employees) should not fail to reward desired behavior with praise. Guest feedback to waitstaff members of their enjoyment of a meal is another motivator when a program is meeting guests' needs. Each of us has a psychological need to have our efforts recognized, and timely praise can provide powerful positive reinforcement that lets trainees know that their efforts are valued and that they are noticed. The usual result is that praised behavior is repeated more frequently, and employees come away with a stronger feeling of self-esteem for being part of the team and of pride in their work. To achieve this outcome, it is important that praise be given, if it is deserved, at the time it is deserved and that it be given evenhandedly; that is, without bias or oversight. It should also be specific, rather than a general "nice job, there". Here is an example of potentially motivating praise: "Judy, the bride herself just told me that the asparagus appetizers were especially delicious. She's right. What an excellent job you did training and working with your pantry team to perfect the low-fat recipe we developed. Thank you."

Waitstaff also can be motivated by better tips from impressed patrons. A sales incentive system for obtaining orders for fitness fare might be worked out at the beginning of the program to boost waitstaff promotion of the program. But when such sales competitions allow only one winner, the result is often a single employee who wins repeatedly, which can be demotivating to other waitstaff members.

About the Trainee

The trainee's background, intelligence, desire to learn, attentiveness, and willingness to cooperate are some of the principal factors that influence the learning process. Adding to the complexity is the fact that different people learn at different rates. Some may have an aptitude or particular confidence, say, in sodium-free cookery but may seem almost backward in their ability to grasp cash control essentials. It is also very common to encounter employees who are semi-literate or functionally illiterate (though pictures on product labels and recipes can serve as a universal language). Because of these variations, it may be necessary to adapt the training format to accommodate different types of topics, and topics of varying levels of difficulty, and to schedule separate sessions involving different individuals or groups. Effective trainers must shape the learning process and formats around such factors.

TRAINING FORMATS: TYPES OF TRAINING PROGRAMS.

In general, any one of four training formats or a combination might be chosen as a way of packaging and delivering training (Fig. 14-3).

On The Job Training (OJT)

OJT probably is the most common form of training in foodservices, largely because it is quick, available, and inexpensive. The trainee begins working right away and is able from the beginning to take on some of the workload, ideally while receiving guidance from more experienced workers. A nickname for a poorly implemented OJT program is "the magic apron treatment." The tongue-in-cheek message is that employees seem expected to "magically" know all about what and how to perform

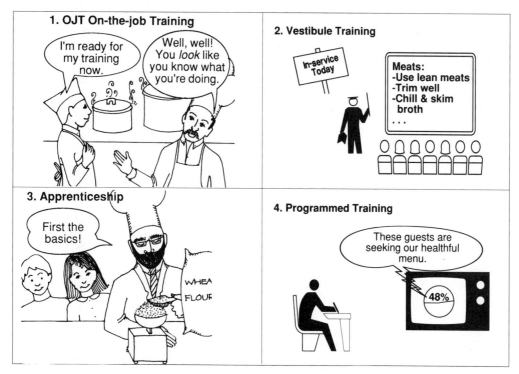

FIGURE 14-3 Four training formats.

their jobs as soon as they don their uniforms and *look like* employees. For the healthful-foods program, using OJT exclusively probably is a weak choice; the trainee does learn by doing and observing, but without purposeful instruction, the learning may be inaccurate. Further, such OJT could force the trainee to struggle unnecessarily, making discouraging and guest-alienating mistakes.

Apprenticeship Training

Apprenticeship training is sometimes used to train a person in all aspects of a specialized skill by starting out at the bottom rung of the functions ladder and moving in successive steps to the highest level, the journeyman. In foodservices it is more a European approach, and is most often used to train cookery specialists: the apprentice spends years assigned to various experts and becomes involved in all the related tasks, from the most basic to the most elaborate. It is described here to emphasize that OJT is *not* the same as an apprenticeship, which has far greater content, scope, duration, and employee development payoff.

Vestibule Training

Vestibule training usually takes place in a classroom-like setting. It can take a variety of forms—lectures, demonstrations, simulated work situations, laboratory experiments. It often occurs before the trainee starts the job, but it may be a later enhancement. Examples of relevant vestibule training opportunities that may already be available in the area include "Train the Trainer" seminars to develop trainers (often at NRA and other foodservice shows including many state restaurant conferences); adult education courses in such areas as cooking for special health needs; seminars through hospital foodservice departments and by local vendors of commercial healthful-foods products; and college courses in nutrition and foodservice management.

Programmed Training

Programmed training is a self-paced, often self-administered, program in which trainees have available reinforcement or corrective information as they progress toward a training goal. Flashcards—cards with questions on one side, the answers on the other—are an example of an early programmed training medium. While interest slumped for many years, with the advent of computer-aided learning, and videotape, a growing number of operations are using computers and especially VCRs to develop programmed training "modules" (courses). The TGI Friday's restaurant chain uses videotaped segments to orient employees to the organization and to instruct them in many aspects of their assigned roles. Employees take a written test following each segment. In the nutrition-oriented foods program, after initial implementation a videotape could be produced to inform new employees of the program, and eventually, tapes also could be made to teach healthful foods policies and procedures, specific product knowledge, and skill training. Reports from those who are using these technologies are that they make training more interesting, more consistent in what is communicated, and, because the materials are available and well-accepted, managers are more inclined to implement (rather than gloss-over) training programs. Also, once the materials are produced, training is less costly because a live trainer need not be present for instruction. This approach is sometimes criticized as lacking a personal touch, but it is not a problem if the manager or trainer touches base with the employee regularly for questions, feedback, and support. The majority of employee response has been very positive.

TRAINING PREPARATION

In setting up a program to inform and train, it is advisable to first take an overview of what training is needed of various employees and to think about how this all can best be accomplished. What skills and information are needed should be defined. For many programs there will be little change from normal procedures, so little specialized training will be needed. One of the best approaches is to keep it simple. While it might be desirable to have employees who are as well-informed as dietitians, this is neither possible nor necessary; however, the rudiments should be understood.

Preparation for the instruction portion of the training program can be approached in three steps: assess the training needs, prepare the training plan, including timetable, and ready the required teaching aids and resources.

Assessment of Training Needs

Managers must be involved in determining what attitudes, knowledge, and skills (AKS) employees need to develop. Unfortunately, what training provides is information; yet what we try to cultivate with on-target training programs is AKS which we can evaluate on the basis of employees' performance. With the need to bridge this gap in mind, assessing the AKS training needs and preparing a *job list* are the first steps in understanding *what* an employee in a given position needs to be trained to do. The employee must perform these tasks in order for operations to proceed effectively and efficiently, both within that employee's area of functioning and in other operations this particular job could influence. From the job list is prepared the *job breakdown*, which tells *how* each task on the job list is to be performed. It also should specify the *performance standards*, a description of the expected quality level for doing each job. Table 14-1 provides a sample job breakdown for several steps in scrubbing potatoes, as it might be written for a healthful foods skills training manual. A well-prepared *job breakdown* becomes a trainer's list of AKS training needs.*

Writing A Plan

A training plan and timetable are the next preparation step; when possible they should be developed from the job breakdowns of involved trainees. While the knowledge and skill components of AKS can be derived from the job breakdown, the trainer must identify and plan how to articulate the desired attitudes in a way that encourages their adoption by employees. (Attitudes for the employee scrubbing

*For more information on training and preparations, see Forrest LC Jr: *Training for the Hospitality Industry.* The Educational Institute of the AH&MA, 1982.

potatoes could include: "My role is an important part of a team effort. I'm proud that guests ask for my potatoes because they're good for them.") Key points of the training plan should be written out. This may be done merely to serve as a reminder and a safeguard against omitting needed points and inconsistent communication. Writing the plan also can help clarify objectives and organize the teaching into one or more appropriate formats to encourage interest, accurate learning, and retention.

In planning the timetable, determine how much AKS is expected of which employees and how soon, how long training will take, when employees are available, and what training resources are available.

TABLE 14-1
Job Breakdown:
Pre-preparation of Baked Potatoes for the Healthful Foods Menu

What to do	How to do it	Additional information
1. Brush	a. Set up a tub of water, the potatoes to be cleaned, and obtain a stiff brush, a paring knife, a 5-gallon container and a 2-gallon container. b. Discard soft and foul-smelling potatoes. c. Using a stiff brush, vigorously scrub entire potato surface. d. Use water as necessary until the potato is thoroughly scrubbed.	a. Perform this at the pantry sink; tools are in adjoining drawer; tubs are on shelf below. b. Leave none, because they will taint those remaining. c. A small bit of the potato skin will be removed in this process.
2. Rinse	a. Plunge potato into water tub, brushing until all traces of dirt and debris are disposed of.	It may be necessary to change the water for this step.
3. Remove blemishes	a. Using a knife, cut out blemishes in potato surface. b. Potatoes with over one-tenth of the surface cut are to be placed in a storage bin and taken to the pantry for potato salad.	a. Cut as shallow as possible, but as deep as necessary. b. Guests do not expect many cuts in their baked potato.
4. Rinse	Repeat step #2.	
5. Store	Place in 5-gallon storage container and deliver to the sous chef.	
6. Clean	Thoroughly clean the tub, brush, and knife, using _____ (cleaning product).	Be certain to clean the drain trap in the sink and to clean the floor, if soiled.
7. Put away	Return all tools	See 1a for where to return items used.

Gathering Training Aids

Having all teaching aids and resources ready before training begins allows the training to move along more smoothly and reduces the likelihood that training will be interrupted or not completed. Needed resources include trainers and training programs, money, materials, facilities, personnel, and time. Include resources required to teach the involved elements and any required for activities. If the training takes place on the job, the workplace (equipment, ingredients) should be set up precisely as the employee is expected to maintain it.

In choosing teaching and learning aids, strive for trainee involvement and keep in mind that people learn by hearing, seeing, and doing, and the best learning occurs when all three are involved. Many people believe that people forget what they hear, remember what they see, and understand what they do, so allowing the trainee to *do* may be the most effective type of training, especially in manual skill.

INSTRUCTION

Most foodservices skill jobs can be taught efficiently and well by using the four-step instruction method outlined below. In it, the trainee hears about, sees, and does the job, while in addition, is participating in two-way communication for training clarification, reassurance, and other feedback.

Four Steps in Skill Instruction

Prepare the trainee, present the job, have the tryout of performance, and follow through. The specific steps for each are as follows:

I. Prepare the trainee.
　1. Put the trainee at ease.
　2. Explain the job and why it needs to be done a specific way.
　3. Arouse a desire to succeed in the job.
II. Present the job.
　1. Explain and demonstrate the job one step at a time.
　2. Tell why and how.
　3. Stress key points.
　4. Instruct clearly and patiently.
　5. Give everything you will want back, but no more.
III. Tryout performance.
　1. Have trainee do the job.
　2. Have trainee tell why and how, stressing key points.
　3. Correct errors or omissions as they are made.
　4. Encourage trainee.
　5. If necessary, repeat Step II and continue until trainee has mastered the job.
IV. Follow through.
　1. Put the trainee on his or her own.
　2. Encourage questions.

3. Check frequently to see how the job is being done.
4. Let the trainee know how she or he is doing.

TRAINING PROGRAM EVALUATION

An important element to build into any training program is an evaluation of how effectively the *training* is being done. Training is done to obtain desired behaviors. Were they produced? If not, why not? What was the mistake? How is it corrected? Mistakes must be corrected. It is advisable also to see that the program stays on course. Best results occur if training materials and content are kept up to date and fresh. Because changes are needed for any program, it is necessary to set up an adequate system of communication and feedback.

WHEN TO BEGIN TRAINING

Once menu implementation gets under way and recipe testing begins, the staff usually will know that a new program is being considered. At this point, management should announce the program, giving enough information to generate interest and a feeling of involvement but not so much as to compromise the flexibility of the program. Additional information can be provided later, as management feels it is appropriate, in order to maintain a properly informed staff. When the menu and recipes have been finalized, training preparations should be well under way. Planning for training lead time is important: the training outlined below definitely needs to be implemented *prior to* the launching of the healthful-foods service, but if it takes place weeks or months before, the staff may forget what they learned and lose interest.

WHO TO TRAIN AND TOPICS FOR TRAINING

With training principles and suggested structure in mind, we now turn to the specifics of who to train and what to teach. Blended or layered with other foodservices training will be topics of special interest to healthful-foods program employees in both the back of the house (the kitchen and offices) and the front of the house (where the guests are). Table 14-2 furnishes a training matrix to be used as a guide in determining probable training needs. In this training matrix, the stages presented in the top row represent activities for which responsible employees may require training to prepare them to "deliver" the promises of the menu. Listed in the left column of the matrix are topics and subtopics that comprise general categories of training needs within the healthful-foods program. These topics, in turn, correspond to activity responsibilities in the top row.

Decisions must be made on who and what to train, and the depth and breadth of detail must also be defined for different topics and for different groups. Table 14-2's legend describes the depth of detail likely to be called for in training for a particular topic with a given responsible employee. For example, there is a 1 in the matrix cell at the intersection of the Preparation column and the Menus, Recipes row (with its nutrition focus). This suggests that persons responsible for preparing healthful foods should receive training in careful handling and manipulation as it relates to foods' nutrient values; training that prepares them to apply their understanding.

Table 14-2 can be a useful tool in thinking through who, what, and how much to train, but it is only a tool; training needs are not universal. Different foodservice operations vary in their healthful foods emphasis and in their organizational structure. Even more widespread is the variation among operators in their reliance on employee training. It is possible to simplify procedures and to minimize or de-emphasize the need for healthful foods training, at least at the service site. These strategies include centralizing purchasing decisions as a means to overcome product and ingredient confusion; using a greater proportion of pre-processed healthful food products; and adopting a firm policy of accommodating only limited special menu requests.

Training Topics For All Employees Involved In The Program.

Numerous topics from Table 14-2 are relevant for *all* employees involved in the healthful foods program. If these topics are covered in orientation sessions for groups of employees with diverse responsibilities, the information might be very general. If, instead, orientation and training groups consist of persons with similar roles (e.g., all production personnel), much more detail and explanation might be provided for training topics they all need to learn, which others do not require.

The Program. Every employee involved in operations needs to know what the healthful-foods program and menu are and what they involve. They should be informed of the program objectives and of patron demands behind the decision to start the program.

The Menu and Components. Ideally, all employees should understand the healthful characteristics of the menu, selections, but this may be too advanced for some. So detail-oriented training may be limited to that pertaining only to an individual employee's responsibilities. Depending on the menu offerings, most employees should understand broadly what is (and what is not) a menu selection that can be called low-calorie, low-fat, low-cholesterol, low-sodium, or to understand any other selection description the menu lists. Employees likely will be hearing such terms frequently when the program starts. It also may be desirable to know the health benefits associated with each; e.g., low-cholesterol for heart and blood vessel concerns. Even this basic association between recipes and patron objectives can enhance the training effect by lending purpose and pride to employees' program activities. The descriptive copy on the menu also needs to be understood, to alert employees throughout the operation to product qualities that could be influenced by activities for which they are responsible (e.g., rotating stock so that it is fresh).

A general knowledge of the nutrient consequences of certain ingredients may be appropriate for employees in preparation activities. They may need to understand that there are important differences, and which products are used for a given menu item (e.g., *skim milk* rather than whole milk lowers calories, fat, and cholesterol).

TABLE 14-2
Training Matrix for a Healthful Foods Program

Match-up the Responsible Employee (top row), with the Program Topic (left column).
(See legend, below, for using #'s 1-4 inside the matrix.)

Program Topic:	Example Training Subjects:	Employees Responsible for the Activities of:			Production			
		Menu Development	Purchase/ Receive Foods	Store/ Issue Foods	Prepara- tion of Foods	Tempera- ture Treatment	Hold for Service	Serve Guests Food
The Program: Overview and Rationale	• What the healthul foods program involves; • Why we are doing it; program objectives; • Who the program is for; • When and How the program begins.	1	2	2	2	2	2	1

Menu and Recipes	• The program menu: What, and for whom;
	 • Why and how items are different and special
	 • Relationship with (any) existing menu;
	 • Basic understanding of guest health concerns (e.g. cardiovascular disease);
	 • Basic understanding of menu content and terms, examples;
	  low-calorie low cholesterol
	  low fat vegetarian
	  low saturated fat cookery alternatives
	  low sodium/salt fresh
		1	2	2	1	1	2	1

Managerial Input	• Commitment to program and training; • Assignment of responsibilities; • Delicate nature of "birthing" phase; • Motivation: What is in it for each of us; • The fact that care and accuracy MATTER; • Appreciation of employee support;	1	1	1	1	1	1	1

Table continued on next page.

TABLE 14.2 (continued)

| Program Topic: | Example Training Subjects: | Employees Responsible for the Activities of: | | | Production | | | Serve Guests Food |
		Menu Development	Purchase/ Receive Foods	Store/ Issue Foods	Prepara- tion of Foods	Tempera- ture Treatment	Hold for Service	
Guest-Sensitive Policies and Procedures	• Importance of clean, sanitary facilities; • Delicacy in promoting the "healthful" image; • What to say (menu and features . . . facts); • Accommodation of guests' "special requests"; • Problem resolution (for guests).	1	4	4	2	2	2	1
Marketing and Feedback	• Notice of upcoming plans, changes; • Updates on promotions directed to guests; • Importance of and techniques in communicating feedback.	1	3	3	3	3	3	1

Legend:

The scope and the level of detail in training employees should be appropriate to their ability and their program responsibilities. Although programs vary, the numbers in the matrix above are suggestions; the numbers correspond with the numbered training objectives below. The training objectives are ranked from most extensive to least extensive:

Training should:
1. prepare the employee to use information, tools and techniques; to carry-out, to "do".
2. support the employee and help explain duties.
3. provide an involved feeling, and answers to basic questions.
4. provide awareness. Actual training may be unnecessary.

Managerial Input. Management's training input is critical. Appropriate persons must be assigned roles in the program's success and be motivated to carry them out. It should be emphasized that employees will be receiving training for their roles and that their care and accuracy truly can make a difference in meeting guests' expectations and assuring menu accuracy.

All personnel should understand at the start of the program that it is at a critical stage, and that good effort is needed to make it succeed. While the operation of the healthful-foods program is somewhat different from the regular program, it is not so different that it cannot, with everyone's attention, be solidly incorporated into the overall function's plan. It must *not* be made to appear as an appendage, but as part of the whole. Overselling or overemphasis should be avoided because the first few days are so critical. (The Chinese don't even announce a birth lest evil spirits learn the child is there and destroy it at its most defenseless time.) While patrons should be made aware that the program is there, the entire staff should perform as if it were a routine but important addition.

Guest-Sensitive Policies and Procedures. Program guests tend to expect at least a moderate level of special request accommodation. They seek food that is fresh and consistently high quality, and access to truthful, relevant information about foods' healthful qualities. Cleanliness and hygienic practices are especially important to the health-conscious. The grooming and behavior of all employees visible to guests should convey wholesomeness.

Marketing and Feedback. Relevant marketing efforts definitely need to be a component of ongoing training and communication updates. Nothing can short-circuit a promotions program faster than failing to inform and update employees. From purchasing to cashiering, imagine the program impact of failing to communicate to employees about distributing a special introductory coupon for the *Light Delights* menu: stock shortages, confusion, and ill will among employees, management, and guests surely would result. Involved employees should be made aware of related news such as forthcoming menu changes, availability of new nutrition fact sheets, and of paid or unpaid media exposure, and each should be trained in the responses expected of him or her.

It also is advisable to encourage and "walk through" simple alternative methods that any employee can use to provide feedback about the healthful-foods programs (e.g., a verbal report, a form, an anonymous note). Employee feedback can be the first line of meaningful comments for smoothing operations and for relaying guests' attitudes, opinions, and desires. It should be used as valuable market intelligence for shaping a successful healthful-foods program.

Training Directed to Back-of-the-House Employees

The Chef. In the back of the house, the chef should be perhaps the best informed on the needs of the program. She or he also should be brought in early for planning and implementation. It may be an error to assume that chefs understand the objectives for program recipes at the outset. This may not necessarily be the case. Further, chefs frequently are uncomfortable at first when they try to restrict "flavorful" or rich ingredients like salt, cream, eggs, and butter. Suggestions for using herbs, reductions, and modest quantities of traditional ingredients can convince the chef of the abundant opportunities for creativity with the program, and can dispel possible feelings of loss of control.

Purchasing, Receiving, Storing, and Issuing. When necessary, a training emphasis for employees involved in purchasing should be ingredient and product specification qualities. They should understand precisely what to order for program recipes, menu accompaniments (e.g., low-calorie Italian salad dressing), and items that must be available to accommodate guests' special requests. Those responsible for product receiving need to be able to distinguish whether or not delivered goods are acceptable (e.g., fresh, or whole-grain, or skimmed). Those involved in product storage and issuing will require an emphasis on preserving nutrients through maintaining items at their proper temperature and humidity levels, and through correct packaging for storage or transport. They should be thoroughly familiar with preventive techniques against bacterial, physical, and chemical contamination.

Production: Pre-Preparation, Temperature Treatment, Holding. One of the most important training objectives to accomplish in preparing production personnel for the program is a positive attitude that includes willingness and a desire to see the plan succeed. These personnel especially need to know why things must be done in specific ways, and why another way is wrong. Workers who understand patrons' desires for healthful food and how the menu can satisfy them are more apt to comply. Training for the attitude that their actions matter is a very important factor in engaging the production department's support.

In developing product knowledge, materials, recipes and product specifications can be used as guides for assessing and meeting the training needs of these employees. It is wise to go over carefully who will take part in the production of planned dishes. Stress points that are critical to proper preparation. Emphasize nutrient preservation, especially the effects of heat and excess water on some nutrients. Clarify again the need to ensure that items described as low-calorie, low-fat, low-cholesterol, and so on, reach the patron "as described." Show how improper handling and recipe changes can undermine the healthful-foods program goals. Unless employees understand the importance of adhering to recipes and the consequences of seemingly innocent alterations, the program goals easily can be defeated. For example, employees may try to "enhance" the low-salt recipe for broccoli casserole by adding soy sauce, prepared mustard, or soup mix concentrate instead of the sodium-free ingredients the recipe calls for, any of which could make the casserole no longer truly low in sodium.

Training for new products, methods, and procedures adopted with the healthful-foods program also must be provided to enable employees to properly meet program requirements. It does not just *happen*. In this vein, instruction may be necessary to introduce new equipment, new products, or new handling requirements or to bring about a procedural change. An example of a likely change is to delay food pre-preparation in order to reduce the time prepared food is held ("sits") prior to service, in order to maximize quality and nutrient retention.

Portioning and plating per individual recipe has special significance in the healthful foods program and should be a mainstay of production employee training. If menu copy states portion weight, volume, or count, or assigns the menu item a nutrient value category, such as light or low-calorie, such claims must be upheld. From the meat cutter portioning 4-ounce fish fillets, to the employee portioning pasta and ladling the marinara sauce, production persons are involved in exactly how much of an item guests receive.

Pre-preparation. In training employees with responsibility for food pre-preparation, extra attention should be given to providing clear detail and follow-up feedback on each job, because often these workers are unable to make the desired interpretation about specifics from general instructions. Using the four steps of instruction, based on a detailed job breakdown of each task can be an effective way to reinforce *how*, and *how not* to perform the involved manual tasks.

Persons involved with vegetable and fruit preparation may begin to work more with fresh, rather than frozen or canned, produce. What are they expected to do with it? What are the expectations for washing, peeling, soaking with chemicals, use of cutting tools, cutting procedures, and timing of work? Because the potential for nutrient quality is so excellent for products such as salads, which are served fresh, special emphasis should be given to preserving their freshness and nutrients. Employees also need to be alerted to guest's special request accommodations, both those anticipated to be routine, such as serving salad dressing or sauces on the side, and those that may be less common but that the foodservice intends to fulfill.

Preparing healthful menu items that contain red meat, poultry, fish, and shellfish may require training employees in new ways of portioning them and trimming all fat possible. They may need to be trained in the skinning of poultry and in techniques to minimize the fat content of certain soups, sauces, gravies, and other foods based on meats. Training should also review the need to adhere to the standardized recipe ingredients, and, for example, while cooking or plating, not to add any type of fat other than that listed in the recipe.

Temperature Treatment. Cooking, chilling, and freezing have the potential of both enhancing and destroying healthful qualities. The chef and other production employees need to understand the vulnerability of nutrients and how they, personally, can protect nutrients in items they work with through proper techniques. They need to understand the effects of different cooking methods on menu claims (e.g., that a low-fat item should be broiled, baked, or poached *as stated in the recipe*).

Holding. Unless a food intentionally is aged or fermented, holding it only detracts from its quality. Production personnel need to be aware of the damage to nutrient value and edible quality caused by letting foods sit for unnecessarily long periods of time. Training could include production schedule changes and reduction in recipe batch sizes to avoid excessive holding time.

Dishing Up. Training for portioning and plating menu items for service should smooth operations by ensuring that each item's presentation makes a positive impression on the guest. Sometimes these activities are the responsibility of back-of-the-house employees; sometimes, as often is the case for salads, service personnel may perform the task. Training for the responsible persons should include detailed instruction on portion control, arrangement, and standards. The recipe should be ready at hand for reference and should describe clearly the menu item portion size including just how to measure (e.g., serve one half cup rice, using #8 disher scoop). The arrangement of foods on serviceware and proper garnishing also should be detailed to guide employees in consistently and accurately crafting a visual feast for guests. Some operations find it effective to provide photographs near the service landing of properly turned out menu items. Training also should include instruction on the appropriate accompaniments and condiments for healthful-foods menu items, especially when they differ from the usual (e.g., if polyunsaturated margarine is used in place of another product). Directions should indicate how to set up for and serve special requests. Thus, if salad dressing is served on the side, what serviceware is needed and where should it be placed? Or if a guest asks to have chicken skinned and broiled instead of fried, consider indicating its plating as a separate item, since the broiled version might be served to best advantage on a smaller plate and with different accompaniments.

Some foodservices use checkers or expediters, employees who can be instrumental in coordinating production with the next stage, service. Their work is to assure that menu items are prepared, portioned, plated, assembled, and otherwise packaged properly. This is the last check before the food leaves the production area, so in any operation *some* employee should be accountable for a final verification at this crucial point, whether it is the cook, a checker, or a waitstaff member. It is here that foods that are identified as not being ready or suitable for service are stopped. (The alternative is that the *guest* must deal with the error.) Stopped orders should be returned to the appropriate production person for correction.

Training Directed to Front-of-the-House Employees

Many employees—management, hostpersons, food and beverage waitstaff, cashiers, and support personnel such as buspersons—come in contact with guests in the front of the house, in the parlor, lounge, or dining room, on the serving line, or at the cashier's station. Those front-of-the-house employees who interact with guests on a frequent or regular basis concerning the operation and menu are one of the most important factors in the success of a fitness fare program. They convey an image, they inform, and they sell. To the guest, these employees may represent the program itself; they communicate the handshake of the host. The attitudes, knowledge, and skill they display in their association with guests actually may constitute a major part of the guests' perception of the program.

Front-of-the-house employees need the general staff training content of the *program goals* and *menu* overview, and they should receive additional detailed training in particular program areas, depending on their responsibilities. For example, hosts may benefit from a sound understanding of the program, menu items and promotions. Cashiers may need to be very familiar with those points, as well as with techniques to elicit feedback from guests and policies for responding to complaints or problems.

Staff training for front-of-the-house employees branches into two distinct areas: Product knowledge (menu item content and preparation), and service that is "tuned in" to the healthful foods program patron. One goal of trainers should be to equip servers (and others who might be in the position to interact with guests) to have the AKS to explain the purpose and the menu of the healthful-foods program in positive (not indifferent or negative) and accurate terms.

Product Knowledge. Waitstaff in particular need to be able to respond to patrons' questions about menu items relating to diet and health. Effective waitstaff training programs range from the three-day orientation carried out by Jerome's, a "fresh food" restaurant in Chicago, to half-day formal ones provided by major hotel programs (which supply each employee with menu training kits), to those that rely solely on daily consultation with the chef covering meals on the menu for each shift.

For programs with a set or limited-cycle (rotating) menu especially, it is a good idea to provide trainees with a copy of the healthful-foods menu during their training, giving them a chance to follow an explanation of each main item and to gain a working familiarity with menu items and key points. Supplemental information such as brochures, labels, or print-outs of nutrient values, also should be reviewed with employees, taking care to advise which are available to guests, how they might be used in the event of guest inquiries, and where they are stored (Denny's flyers for interested guests were presented in chapter 13). Producing a fact sheet for employees also can be the first step in gathering information for materials to make available to inquiring guests.

Fact Sheet Facts. A useful menu fact sheet for waitstaff is easy to understand and provides needed information for each individual menu item. It might be a booklet that profiles each menu item according to the types of information of interest to targeted nutrition and health issues (weight control, sodium restriction). Regardless of its form, the fact sheet's purpose is to assist service staff in familiarizing themselves with the obvious and less obvious aspects of menu items and to prepare them to meet the needs of program patrons. Guests have their own needs and ways of filtering information, so not everyone receives the same message from the menu or newspaper advertisement or other source, whether because it is not sufficiently descriptive or because the patron overlooked the message. Guests often want further information or clarification. Thus, even if preparation, major ingredients, and cooking methods are given in the menu copy, waitstaff may be asked to explain or elaborate. When appropriate, it also can be important to train employees in what is *not* in a product: (e.g., for vegetarians or persons with a food intolerance). Table 14-3 sets out typical guest questions about healthful-foods menu selections. It could be very helpful to include answers to such questions in the fact sheet or other training materials.

Fine Tuning Waitstaff Product Knowledge. When any new items are added to the menu, it is wise to sample them to waitstaff, allowing questions and discussion time to clarify recipe or nutrition aspects of probable interest to target patrons. Pre-meal sampling, or at least a pre-shift briefing by the chef or manager also can help build team spirit among employees. Enthusiasm for the program items, in turn, can enhance the sales efforts of service persons. Guests *will* ask, so employees also should be prepared to describe what a menu item resembles or what familiar food item is similar to this one in taste and appearance. Guests may ask waitstaffers, "Is

TABLE 14-3
Examples of Questions Waitstaff May Encounter.

General
   Available substitutions and special accommodation for ingredients/preparation
   Are these vegetables fresh? Frozen? Locally grown?
   How large is the order?
   What is its composition?
   How is it cooked?
Focus on Fat, Cholesterol, and/or Calories
   Are low-fat or skim dairy products used in this recipe? Milk? Cheese?
   What type of fat is used in cooking and food preparation?
   What type of margarine do you offer?
   What cut of meat is used for this menu item? Lean? Trimmed?
   Is the poultry skin removed? Before or after cooking?
   Are egg yolks part of this recipe?
   In what range is this for calories, fat, cholesterol?
Other Nutrition and Diet Concerns
   About how much sodium does this contain?
   Is the fruit preserved or prepared in heavy syrup?
   Do you have whole grain bread, waffles, sandwich buns?
Food Practices or Sensitivities
   Does this dinner contain milk, wheat, eggs, nuts, soybeans, shellfish?
   Is artificial sweetener, flavor, color, or other imitation substance used in this recipe?
   Does this contain MSG or other additives?
   Is the meat, fruit, vegetable organically grown?

it fresh? Do *you* like it?" or even "What do *you* suggest from this light menu?" If you were a waitstaffer faced with such questions, wouldn't you feel more involved and more inclined to promote the program if you had had the opportunity to sample the food and have *your* questions answered?

Servers need not overstress the healthful foods menu to patrons. Training should emphasize the need for quality in the products, and should strive to cultivate pride in the program. The new menu items should be introduced simply to guests, who should then be left to study the menu in peace, allowing them to make selections based on their own judgment about the healthful benefits of certain items and of the promise of a quality dining experience.

The matter of special requests and substitutions must be discussed so that waitstaff know how and to what extent they are to be accommodated. Staffers need to be familiar with the policy stated on the menu, such as availability of substitutes for menu accompaniments or statements; e.g., "We do not salt any foods in our kitchen." Emphasize to trainees what accommodations can be made and how to refuse or modify a request diplomatically. Remind staffers not to make nutrition claims or give health advice. They should politely provide patrons only with facts, such as an item's preparation method or the type of fat used.

Attentive Service. The *product knowledge* needs of service persons was discussed above, but training in at least one broad area of service AKS could further increase the ability of employees to serve guests' healthful-foods wants and needs. In addition to noticing how food was placed on the plate or carried to the table, guests respond to whether or not the service truly is tuned in to them. A positive attitude and timely, accurate, and courteous service are essential in almost any service setting, but *attentiveness to guests*, cultivating them, not merely processing them, is particularly important in a healthful-foods program, because opportunities are so great for enhancing patrons' enjoyment of their dining experience.

The emphasis in this training is developing in employees the interest, ability, and willingness to place themselves in the position of the guest, thinking, "If I were this person, how would I like to be served?" This does *not* mean that waitstaff should try to second-guess patrons or impose their feelings on guests, but it does mean being aware and sensitive, and following through. For example, consider that many persons on special diets prefer that their special menu needs be met inconspicuously. Attentive service can be something as thoughtful, yet ultimately simple, as an employee quietly offering to serve potatoes without gravy to a guest who appears to be concerned about fats but perhaps hesitates or forgets to make a special request.

Waitstaff and cashiers need to be taught and encouraged to take advantage of their unique opportunity to hear directly from guests about their experiences with the healthful-foods menu, menu items, and service. It goes without saying that complaints will be part of the feedback, so training staff to interpret, acknowledge, defuse and attend to legitimate sources of complaint should be part of building a responsive and strong healthful-foods program. Following the meal, the cashier might ask, "Did you enjoy your meal? Did you try any of our fitness fare food?" If the patrons did, the next question might be, "What did you like best about it?" A parting remark might be, "Come back soon and we will have some new items for you to try. It was a pleasure to serve you."

Service employees should be trained to sense problems and to know what to do to try to correct them. It might be desirable to call the manager or someone else who can discuss with the patron what was wrong and decide what can be done about it. An offer to have the patron return to have a complimentary meal might be appropriate.

Attentive service employees can pick up all sorts of clues about guests—from age to style of dress—that could help them sense how to accommodate their needs. Attentiveness means constantly looking ahead to see how best to make the guest's experience a more pleasant one. The Four Seasons hotels express this proactive approach with style and dignity in Figure 14-4.

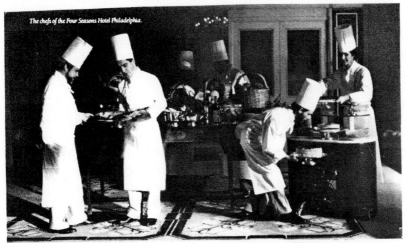

A Good Hotel Reacts To Your Requests. A Grand Hotel Anticipates Them.

A grand hotel should be judged not simply by how quickly it responds to your requests, but by how few requests you find it necessary to make in the first place.

Thus, at Four Seasons, we devote an enormous amount of time to anticipating precisely what the changing needs and desires of our guests are likely to be.

Our exclusive Alternative Cuisine menu selections, for example, were developed in anticipation of the growing number of people who've become careful about calories —yet no less discriminating about taste.

We also recognize that while business travellers generally want to eat in a city's best restaurants, they don't necessarily want to leave the hotel to do so. Which is why you'll find 4-star restaurants in all our hotels.

And we realize that the rigors of business travel often dictate irregular hours. So we offer 24-hour room service —with food prepared by our highly acclaimed chefs.

But the Four Seasons philosophy of anticipating needs rather than reacting to them extends considerably beyond the kitchen.

We've anticipated, for instance, that many people don't want travel to disrupt their daily routines—which is why we provide jogging maps and workout gear in all our hotels, and health clubs in many of them.

And since many of our guests prefer to travel with only carry-on luggage, we offer overnight pressing and shoe shining, so whatever you bring will look fresh in the morning. And we furnish our rooms with bathrobes, hair dryers and other essentials that might not fit into a single overnight bag.

We've anticipated all this and more because at Four Seasons we staunchly believe that a grand hotel should adapt to its guests. Not the other way around.

Four Seasons Hotels

UNITED STATES
Austin (1987)
Boston
Chicago
The Ritz-Carlton
Dallas/Las Colinas
The Mandalas
Las Colinas Inn and
Conference Center,
Four Seasons Fitness
Resort and Spa
Houston
Four Seasons,
Inn on the Park
Los Angeles (1987)
New York
The Pierre
Newport Beach
Philadelphia
San Antonio
San Francisco
The Clift
Seattle
The Olympic
Washington, D.C.
CANADA
Edmonton
Montreal
Ottawa
Toronto
Yorkville,
Inn on the Park
Vancouver
UNITED KINGDOM
London
Inn on the Park
Call (800) 268-6282
or your travel agent

© 1986 Four Seasons Hotels, Ltd

FIGURE 14-4 "A good hotel reacts to your requests. A grand hotel anticipates them." *(Courtesy The Four Seasons Hotels Limited)*

SUMMARY

The development and implementation of quality training programs is essential in preparing employees to produce and to serve nutrition-oriented fare. A lack of sufficient or appropriate employee training in Attitudes, Knowledge, and Skills is one of the most common causes of failure in such programs. Management commitment can be shown in well-defined program goals and by support in the form of dollars, time, competent trainers, facilities, and materials. Employees should be well prepared and motivated to carry out their portion of the food program activities, and quality performance is maintained by program components coupled with management's motivation, supervision, evaluation, and leadership.

Throughout the training effort, the communications loop comes into play. For a message to be transmitted meaningfully, the *sender* and *receiver* must be tuned in to one another and the *message* and *feedback* components themselves must be comprehensible and interpreted as intended.

Because all trainees have different aptitudes, intelligence, and interest in learning, shaping training formats to their needs can be effective. The relative merits of four formats are outlined: on-the-job training, apprenticeship, vestibule training, and programmed training. Skill training instruction in general should include a focus on the trainee, on the job, and on the trainee's job performance. Preparation for training involves assessing the training program needs and setting the specific AKS for each activity. A plan and timetable should be developed and all teaching aids and resources prepared.

Training should begin when the nutrition-oriented menu is taking shape. Topics to be communicated to *all* employees involved include the program's purpose, the menu and related health basics, individual assignments and incentives, the marketing plan, and feedback mechanisms.

People in the back-of-the-house, who are involved with purchasing and storing should gain fluency in nutrition-related specifications and food handling facts. It is especially important to attain the support of the production persons and the chef. They must develop the nutrition know-how to police and preserve nutrients throughout the pre-preparation, temperature treatment, and other pre-service and portioning processes.

Front-of-the house trainees may need to have a more detailed understanding of the menu as it relates to the diet and health desires of patrons. They may benefit also from training in being attentive to the subtle indicators of the nutrition-oriented guests' food and service wishes.

Chapter Review

1. Why is the development of a nutrition component for foodservice training programs referred to as an investment?
2. Within a healthful-foods program, give an example of each of the following to be addressed in the employee training program: a. attitude, b. knowledge, c. skill.
3. What responsibilities for employee preparation rest with management?
4. Describe the four parts of the communication loop. How might a trainer determine whether communication was accurate and complete?
5. Discuss the qualifications of one who should and one who should not train.
6. Why is motivation a prerequisite to effective learning?
7. How might production persons be motivated to learn about and cooperate in preparing healthful foods? Describe a different type of motivator for service personnel.
8. Discuss how a person's background and level of readiness to learn would make a difference in how training about proper portioning might be carried out.

9. Name and briefly describe each of the four types of training formats discussed.
10. Briefly compare and contrast the pros and cons of the above formats in terms of learning effectiveness, cost, and time required.
11. What is a job breakdown? How can it be assembled? How does it relate to the overall job list of an employee?
12. Why should key points of a training plan be written down?
13. Using the four steps in training instruction, describe how a trainee might be taught to store leftovers properly through hearing, seeing, and doing during the lesson.
14. What types of questions should be investigated in evaluating training programs?
15. Referring to Figure 14-2, for each responsibility (column heading), suggest one main topic of foodservice nutrition training that employees might need.
16. In your own words, why should all involved employees be informed about the nutrition-oriented program and menu?
17. Why is it so important that employees be "sold" on the program?
18. Should employees in the back of the house be informed about program advertising? Why or why not?
19. Is it safe to assume chefs understand nutrition or that they automatically support the program? How might the chef's cooperation be earned?
20. Prepare a list of nutrition-related training topic needs for those in purchasing, receiving, storing, and issuing.
21. Imagine that you are reviewing a standardized recipe with three new cooks. How could you use the recipe to explain the nutrition-related handling points?
22. Why is it advisable to show production employees how improper handling or recipe changes can change or ruin healthful qualities of foods?
23. Why are ingredient measuring and recipe portioning such significant training topics for a nutrition-oriented program? What instructions might be included in thorough portioning instructions?
24. What is the role of a good checker or expediter?
25. In general, what should be contained in a menu fact sheet for waitstaff? What is the purpose of the fact sheet?
26. How would you train the waitstaff in a family restaurant to introduce the nutrition-oriented program without overstressing it?
27. In service, what is meant by "attentiveness to guests"? Describe the difference between processing a guest and giving attentive service.

Chapter 15
Serving Special Dietary Needs of Guests

Chapter Goals

- To define common meanings of the term "diet" in various contexts.
- To distinguish between the usual emphases in serving guests' dietary needs within health care facilities and outside this setting.
- To indicate the dietary management needs of persons with diabetes.
- To outline how foodservices might meet the dietary needs of those on diabetic, sodium-restricted, and residue-control diets.
- To explain the purpose and composition of dietary recommendations for persons with gastrointestinal ulcers.
- To examine the common misconceptions about hypoglycemia.
- To identify the common sources of food intolerances and allergies.
- To suggest ways to protect guests from "sensitive" substances.
- To present the diet needs of vegetarians, and to provide recipe and menu suggestions.

DIETS AND FOODSERVICES

When the word "diet" comes up in casual conversation, a food plan for calorie control might spring to mind; such is the way we so often use the word. Actually, diet can describe the food and drink regularly provided or consumed, so whatever a person eats constitutes that person's diet. Another definition of diet is the focus of this chapter, "the kind and amount of food prescribed for a person or animal for a special reason." That reason could be weight control or it could be to combat a tendency toward high serum cholesterol, among many other possibilities.

Diet recommendations might be made by dietitians and other health practitioners to patients or to a patient's physician. A formal *diet prescription* is given only by a physician. Of course, informal diets of all types are self-prescribed. People may use diet plans made available through credible persons or health-related agencies, or they may rely on something they adopted from what could be an inappropriate source, such as a popular magazine or a well-meaning but naive friend. In this chapter we review the characteristics and menu requirements of a variety of diets, some of which may be followed on a physician's orders and some of which may be embraced for other reasons.

There are countless diets, some simple and some quite complex. Some foodservices, such as hospitals, and those of other health-related institutions, may have to be concerned with many formal ones, but most commercial foodservices do not. When a facility must meet formal dietary needs, professionals should be available to see that the requirements of a specific diet are followed.

The farthest a commercial foodservice might go toward providing healthful foods is to provide foods in the low-calorie, low-sodium, low-fat, and low-cholesterol categories. Some few may go farther, but not much. They just are not equipped to do more. Nevertheless, persons on more strictly controlled diets as discussed in this chapter often eat in commercial operations, and their dietary needs usually can be accommodated when a sound healthful-foods program is in place.

The material in this chapter represents a review and application of some material discussed in earlier chapters, but here the organization is around a particular subject, and there is a more inquiring slant on specific health problems and, in some cases, more detail. The therapeutic value of eating or avoiding certain foods and of their particular nutrients or characteristics are discussed. Since many foodservices serve the general public—all kinds and categories of people—some patrons inevitably will need special foods. It is good for foodservice personnel who serve these guests to have some idea of what these diets are. Also, knowing why a particular diet is called for can inform decisions about carrying out guests' requests. Personnel can then be effective in meeting patrons' needs. Not every person in every foodservice operation must know how to plan, prepare, and serve such diets, but all benefit from having some general information that increases their awareness and understanding.

HEALTH CARE PRESCRIPTION: NUTRITION MANAGEMENT

This book is directed to managers in all types of foodservice operations who wish to offer more healthful foods. In reference to diets, it is appropriate to look inside the health care industry foodservice segment. Health care differs from other food services in its formality and in the fact that dietary planning may be compulsory. In a hospital, convalescent center or related setting, rather rigid procedures must be followed for prescribed diets. Only a physician knows a patient's medical condition and problems, thus only the physician prescribes a diet. In prescribing the diet, the physician may consult with a dietitian or other professional. A diet is a prescription in the same way that a medication or treatment is. In a health-related facility, any diet prescription should be a part of the patient's written medical record, and the physician should sign the diet order, whether to begin, modify, or discontinue the diet. Physicians should review records periodically, making comments and considering changes.

Health care facilities have manuals that describe the purpose of various kinds of diets and which menu items conform to these standards. Menus may provide common needs of hospital patients (e.g., various levels of solid food, sodium, or fat) or medical conditions (e.g., cardiac, postsurgical). Patients or residents receive and select from a menu that offers only foods that meet their needs.

Health care diets usually, but not always, are planned by dietitians. Individual doctors may personally design diets and instruct the foodservice to use theirs rather than ones from a traditional diet manual, and although they do not have to, many operators will comply. In some cases where there is only a part-time consulting dietitian arrangement, someone other than a dietitian plans menus to meet patient needs. In such a situation, the consulting dietitian checks patients, menus, and meals from time to time to see that menus conform to proper dietary standards.

DIETS SIGNIFICANT TO COMMERCIAL FOODSERVICE PATRONS

A significant number of patrons of commercial foodservices have dietary prescriptions or recommendations from health care professionals. Most revolve around weight control, cardiovascular problems or precautions, diabetes, gastrointestinal disorders, and in a positive light, nutrition for health. The expanding portion of the guest market composed of seniors is a particular challenge—and opportunity—for foodservice managers. The American Dietetic Association reports that about 85% of older person have one or more chronic, potentially debilitating diseases and could benefit from nutrition services. Up to half of all seniors have clinically identifiable nutrition problems. Promotion of a well-conceived nutrition-oriented menu can offer these guests more choices and can win the foodservice more business and good will.

Under most circumstances, diets outlined for specific persons should be nothing more than a customization of the foods needed to obtain their normal nutritional needs. Most diets are accommodated adequately with everyday food products. The principles of more formal therapeutic diets involve a prescription for balancing—or for highlighting modifications in—one or more of the following: *energy*, or calorie value; *nutrients* (carbohydrate, protein, fat, vitamins, and minerals), and/or *textures or seasoning*, as in the amount of fiber included. Whether in health care or in a commercial restaurant, the final and critical step is still to suit the principles of the "right foods" to the tastes of the guest. The meal or snack must be appealing and the food must taste good.

Nutrition management for meeting many important dietary needs of guests has been discussed in the foregoing chapters, and so will not be repeated here. We specifically refer the reader to the noted sections of the indicated chapters for guidance in accommodating guests with the dietary or menu wants or needs at left:

Common dietary myth	See Chapter 2
Fiber or residue-management	See *complex carbohydrates* and *fiber* in Chapter 4
Fat-controlled or low-cholesterol	See Chapter 6
Calorie-controlled	See Chapter 7

Iron-deficiency anemia,   See Chapter 9
Sodium sources   See Chapter 9

Diabetic Diets

One in every 20 Americans has or will develop diabetes.* An immensely complicated disease, (likely a group of disorders which have in common low blood sugar) diabetes is still incurable; it is a leading cause of blindness in the United States. The hormone, insulin (produced in the pancreas) is required to keep the body's blood sugar (serum glucose) level within proper limits. Diabetes can result when the pancreas does not produce enough usable insulin or when the body does not use what is produced efficiently. Body cells "starve" from lack of their major fuel, glucose. And when there is too much or too little sugar in the blood, the vital water-electrolyte and acid-base balances in the body are disturbed.

About 15% of diabetics must take insulin daily to sustain life. Usually those who become diabetic later in life can control their blood sugar level entirely through careful control of their diet. Since 85% of diabetics are not insulin dependent, sound diet therapy remains the foundation of managing diabetes. A healthful-foods program can fit with the needs of conscientious diabetes patients perfectly. The Dietary Exchange System (Appendix B) originally was developed in a joint effort of the American Diabetes Foundation and the American Dietetic Association as a tool for counseling diabetics in food selection. The use of the Exchange System in energy-balance diets is set out in Chapter 7.

Each diabetic has specific needs, and each has an individual diet plan. People have different thresholds (the ability to hold sugar in the blood) and respond differently to insulin and other drugs. A diabetic's meals should be spaced so there is a slow, steady release of energy tailored to the insulin that is present or taken. The steady release of energy from food becomes part of the treatment. For instance, an evening snack might be desirable to abbreviate the overnight fast.

Until a few years ago, the diabetic diet recommendations called for severe restriction of all carbohydrates, but more recent research indicates that this is not necessary. Today it is believed that a normal proportion of calories from carbohydrates (50-66%) is appropriate, but that they should consist primarily of starch and other complex carbohydrates rather than refined sugars. Some studies show that fiber helps make the rise in blood sugar more gradual, another factor in favor of including complex carbohydrates. Table 15-1 provides a look at the types of simple selections a woman who has diabetes might make at a restaurant if she also wishes to manage calories for weight control. Many non-insulin-dependent diabetics are overweight, so calorie control is particularly important for them. For this reason and because diabetics are susceptible to cardiovascular disease, the proportion of fat in the diet should be low (25 to 30%).

As you can see, the diabetic diet is a model of a prudent, moderate-calorie, moderate-fat diet, and it can be served readily, with "ordinary " food. With the exception of sugar-free beverages and artificial sweetener packets, there is no call to use special "diabetic" or "dietetic" foods. Besides, such foods often are costly and

*Williams SR: *Nutrition and Diet Therapy*, ed 5, p 564, St. Louis, Mosby College Publishing, 1985.

may be perceived as more gimmick than good. A food labeled dietetic or diabetic is not necessarily low in sugar or calories. It may simply be low in sodium, for example. Or, it could refer to the fact that the product contains a substitute sugar that is used by the body much as sucrose is, such as sorbitol or another sugar alcohol—products with calorie levels similar to table sugar. Only an alert, informed reading of the label will tell, but the product probably is not necessary.

Simple, fresh, and nonrich snacks, entrees, and dessert foods often are welcomed by diabetics (among other guests). For example, while they usually must forego apple pie, a piece of fresh fruit served stylishly can allow the diabetic to enjoy

TABLE 15-1
Possible Food Selections from a Typical Commercial Menu for a Diabetic Concerned about Weight Control

Breakfast	Calories	Carbohydrates (grams)
Grapefruit, 1/2	46	12
40% bran flakes, 3/4 cup	90	23
Low-fat milk, 1/2 cup	45	6
Poached egg, 1	81	—
Whole wheat toast, 1 slice	75	13
Breakfast Total	337	54
Lunch		
Consomme, 1 cup	5	trace
Whole wheat melba toast, 2 pieces	34	7
Large fresh fruit plate (pineapple, strawberries, peach, seedless grapes, apple, banana)	144	36
Cottage cheese, (1% fat), 1 cup	162	6
Hard roll, whole wheat	75	13
Lunch Total	420	62
Dinner		
Oysters, (Eastern), 4 raw with 1.5 fluid ounces cocktail sauce	72	10
Spinach mushroom salad w/oil-free vinaigrette	25	4
Chicken, broiled, 1/2 breast w/o skin (3 ounces)	142	trace
Carrots, fresh, sliced, cooked 1/2 c.	24	6
Bread, cracked wheat, 1 slice	66	13
Cantaloupe, cubed, 1/2 cup	24	6
Milk, skim 1 cup	86	12
Dinner Total	439	51
Total for the day	1196	167

Percent of carbohydrate for the day's intake is approximately 56%
From Leveille, et al. *Nutrients in Foods* Cambridge, MA: The Nutrition Guild, 1983.

dessert with others at the table. Also, insulin-dependent diabetics, who must distribute their food intake throughout the day, may look on the menu for wholesome appetizers, mini meals, and snack foods, like skim milk and fruit, that fit into their regimen.

Sodium-Restricted Diets

High blood pressure is an incentive for some 60 million Americans to be concerned with moderating sodium intake. Hundreds of thousands of Americans are medically *required* to limit the sodium in their diets, owing to kidney or heart disease or high blood pressure.* In addition, to "avoid too much sodium" is among the Dietary Guidelines directed to all Americans. Recall that the main source of dietary sodium is table salt (sodium chloride) and that sodium makes up about 40% of the combination (see Chap. 9). In developing recipes and menus, foodservice planners can accommodate the needs of a large proportion of sodium-restricting diners by providing menu selections and information that fits in with their need to limit sodium to approximately three grams or less daily. While more severe sodium restriction sometimes is prescribed, it is doubtful that guest demand would be sizable enough to make the effort of providing it worthwhile.

"No Added Salt". Mild sodium restriction (2 to 3 grams sodium). As described by the American Heart Association, in this commonly prescribed diet, salt may be used lightly in cooking, but no added salt is used at the table. Foods such as pickles, olives, and sauerkraut preserved with salt are excluded, as are cured meats such as ham, bacon, frankfurters, corned, chipped, and smoked meat, and similarly processed fish. Heavily salted foods are out also, including crackers, snack chips, salted popcorn, and nuts. Salt-rich condiments to omit include bouillon cubes, catsup, prepared mustard, Worcestershire and soy sauce, and garlic, onion, and celery salt. Exclude mono*sodium* glutamate (MSG), meat sauces, and meat tenderizers, and, except for low-sodium types, cheese and peanut butter. Limit quick breads made with baking soda or powder. The diet is easy to remember as "the no added salt diet." Aware foodservice menu planners and employees can readily meet these needs with few or no special ingredients, but knowledgeable planning is a must.

Residue-Control Diets

The cellulose in fruits, vegetables, grains, and a few other substances bring bulk into the digestive system, aiding digestion and absorption of nutrients. Since bulk or fiber is not digested but leaves the body in the feces, it often is called "residue." The intent of a diet rich in fiber is to avoid or combat problems such as digestive irregularities, diverticulosis, or other gastrointestinal problems. Abundant intake of certain fibers also is believed to reduce the risk of colon cancer and other types and to be useful in nutrition therapy for diabetes and elevated cholesterol levels.

As much as 20 to 30 grams (about 1 ounce) or more of dietary fiber is often recommended daily, (but *too* much can interfere with nutrient absorption). A diet containing plenty of bran, nuts, leafy vegetables, fruits, whole grains, corn, and legumes is high in fiber. Highly refined carbohydrate foods should be limited. Usually

*The Council on Renal Nutrition; National Kidney Foundation Letter, New York, May, 1986.

any diet that follows the Basic Four Plan with the addition of some good fiber-rich foods meets the goal. At least 6 to 8 cups of fluid should be a part of this plan.

Some people may need to *limit* the amount of fiber in the diet because fiber may irritate the digestive tract. A strict *low-residue* diet requires straining foods such as fruit juice, cream soups, and cooked fruits and vegetables. Tender or ground lean meat, fish, or poultry, young cheeses, and eggs are advised. Whole-grain cereals, breads, nuts, legumes, spicy and fatty meats and any frying preparation usually would be restricted, milk being limited to 2 cups, according to tolerance. An intermediate level of residue control might permit all but highly fibrous peeled vegetables and fruits and allow more flexibility in other areas, according to needs and tolerances.

Diets and Ulcers

On a worldwide basis, an estimated 10% of the population is affected by peptic ulcer disease and its consequences. It can occur at any age, but most frequently crops up between the ages of 35 and 55. Peptic ulcer is the general term for a lesion in the central portion of the gastrointestinal tract—the lower esophagus, the stomach, and the first portion of the duodenum. Most peptic ulcers are duodenal (located where gastric contents empty into the duodenum and are very concentrated). Some duodenal ulcers are not painful, ("silent ulcers"). Stomach (gastric) and esophageal ulcers are less common; a gastric ulcer usually is associated with stomach pain two to three hours after eating.

The stomach and alimentary tract are lined with *mucous* cells (the lining is called *mucosa*), which secrete *mucous* fluid that protects the mucosa from harsh digestive juices and enzymes. Many of the mucosal cells are capable of replacing themselves rapidly, and the fluid acts as a protective agent. But when digestive agents become too abundant or acidic, or when tissue protection processes fail, the lining of the digestive tract can erode as if it were being digested; the result is a painful inflammation, or sore, called an ulcer.

Ulcerated areas can become so deteriorated that an entire digestive tract wall area is eaten through, causing a hole, a "perforated ulcer"; such lesions sometimes require surgical repair. Bleeding from ulcers can cause anemia from loss of iron in blood.

A hiatal hernia (an outpouching of the esophagus where it joins the stomach) can act much like an ulcer. Food can get caught there or can back up from the stomach (reflux) and cause irritation. Tight clothing around the stomach also can contribute to reflux.

The exact cause of gastrointestinal ulcers is not fully understood, but evidence points to a possible genetic link and to the involvement of an imbalance between two factors: the amounts of gastric acid and pepsin secreted and the resistance of mucosal tissue to these secretions.

Much of the misunderstanding surrounding diets for peptic ulcer and related gastrointestinal disorders probably reflects a need to update the public's understanding. Major advances in medicine for ulcer sufferers have ushered in a modern approach with a liberal diet. To those familiar with earlier "ulcer diets", the new approach may seem incongruous with the bland regime that, in the past, generally was recommended.

At one time ulcer therapy called for a diet that excluded foods containing fiber and those that allegedly formed gas. Earlier diets called for major restrictions in foods considered to be acidic (such as citrus) limited spices, herbs, and condiments, and required that foods only be boiled, steamed, or otherwise cooked without added fat or flavoring. Only very tender meats, poultry, and fish were allowed, and the diet generally was built around such bland fare as refined grain products, eggs, soft cooked vegetables, and milk. This approach proved to be ineffective and unnecessary. Today the ulcer victim's diet is more mainstream, with accommodations to both the healing needs of the tissue and the individual's food intolerances, preferences, and habits. Their diet needs often are readily met through the same menu planning considerations used for other nutrition-conscious guests.

In today's diet for a peptic ulcer, good food sources of dietary fiber have proved to be beneficial, not harmful. The gas-forming tendency of foods is difficult to predict and is highly variable from one person to another. So-called gas-forming foods are not categorically restricted unless they actually bother a given ulcer sufferer. The ban on many acidic foods and herbs, spices, and condiments was lifted because researchers noted no significant change in gastric acidity or ulcer irritation when these foods were eaten. There are exceptions, however; ulcer victims should restrict *alcohol, coffee, tea, and cola beverages* (whether or not caffeinated), *chocolate, cocoa, chili powder,* and *red and black pepper.* Milk is no longer believed to act as a protective coating for the intestinal lining, but since any form of fat tends to suppress gastric secretion, this might explain the soothing influence claimed for whole milk. As a source of needed nutrients for health and healing it certainly deserves a place in the diet.

In addition to the restricted items named above, a modern diet for a peptic ulcer usually calls for others, with the limits set according to the tolerance of the individual. This avoidance list might include fried foods, including meat, vegetables, and pastries; highly concentrated bases (for sauces, gravies, soups, etc.); highly-seasoned foods and condiments, especially those strongly seasoned with peppers, hot peppers, and pepper sauces; and nuts, coconut, and popcorn. Although this list may *seem* extensive, most persons with ulcers find that they have only minor limitations in choosing foods and recipes. Further, it is common today, as part of one's ulcer treatment, to take medications that reduce harmful gastrointestinal action and can lessen dietary restriction. Eating-style also can affect ulcer sufferers and may apply to those who have other gastrointestinal disorders. Food should be eaten slowly and chewed thoroughly, and to the extent possible, the eating environment should be relaxed. It is better to take small meals at frequent intervals than fewer large meals. The implication for foodservice planners is to include in the menu accommodating snacks and meals of modest size and to make them available throughout the day.

MISUNDERSTOOD CONDITIONS, WITH DIETARY NOTES AND CLARIFICATION

Diets that allegedly combat low blood sugar, food allergies, ulcers, and dozens of other conditions are easy to come by in scores of popular magazines but are apt to be outdated or merely sensationalized fiction (i.e., fraud). And many people are confused about whether they even *have* such a condition if they have not seen a physician. In this section, we set out to clarify what is involved in certain medical conditions and then to place in perspective whether or not a particular diet might actually be needed, and finally, what the purpose and composition of any needed diet is in light of the condition (or of symptoms that mimic the condition).

Hypoglycemia

When too much insulin is produced and the blood glucose level becomes low, a condition develops called hypoglycemia (literally, below normal sugar in the blood). Too little insulin can cause too much glucose to accumulate in the blood, and this is called hyperglycemia ("hyper" meaning too much).

Many nondiabetics claim to have hypoglycemia, but medical authorities tend to dismiss most such claims as merely temporary symptoms—anxiety and nervousness, hunger, fatigue, headaches, weakness, and heart palpitations. Medical authorities *disagree* with the lay public's view that hypoglycemia causes mental depression, radical mood swings, or criminal activity and that it is associated with an excessive amount of sugar in the diet.

Professionals identify two types of hypoglycemia. *Reactive* hypoglycemia occurs after a meal and usually affects persons who have diabetes or are recovering from abdominal surgery. *Fasting* hypoglycemia usually develops after long periods without adequate food (including poor eating habits), but can also be caused by several common drugs, by alcohol, or by organic disorders. Other authorities hold that a type of hypoglycemic reaction is stress related; that stress increases production of insulin, which then causes a drop in the blood glucose level.

There is continuing disagreement on how to diagnose hypoglycemia. The lay public tends to believe that if the symptoms are there, so is the disease. On the other hand, traditional medical diagnosis of a body's ability to "handle" glucose (as the major breakdown product of digestion) has been the oral glucose tolerance test. After a short fast, the subject consumes a beverage containing 75 to 100 grams of glucose. (Recently, testing may be begun when the patient is experiencing symptoms.) Then, blood glucose is measured every 30 minutes for several hours to determine how well the insulin works to keep the blood glucose level within the normal range. If one tests "normal" on this test, and most *do*, physicians usually rule out hypoglycemia as a cause, regardless of symptoms. The symptoms of hypoglycemia are also those of other disorders, so anyone who suspects hypoglycemia is wise to have a medical exam.

Possibly because it also is known as "low blood sugar", some people incorrectly try to treat hypoglycemia by eating large doses of concentrated sweets. A modest amount may counteract a hypoglycemia attack, say a glass of fruit juice, but if too much sugar enters the bloodstream abruptly, a large load of insulin will be produced to manage the blood sugar, and soon there will be too much insulin, leading again to low blood sugar. The blood glucose level can swing wildly up and down if the person eats carelessly (Fig. 15-1). Others attempt to self-treat hypoglycemia with a very low-carbohydrate, high-protein diet; then the body must struggle to secure enough glucose to maintain a moderate blood sugar level.

Whatever the results of a test for hypoglycemia, persons who say they experience the symptoms often benefit from following the dietary treatment recommended for persons medically diagnosed with it. There is no risk or cost in trying it.

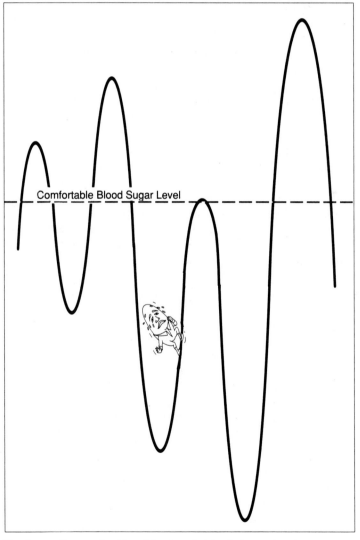

Comfortable Blood Sugar Level

FIGURE 15-1 Careless eating can lead to wild swings in blood glucose level.

A sound approach is to develop a habit of eating six meals daily; regular, frequent, and relatively small meals. Caffeine, alcohol, and concentrated sweets are to be avoided; even milk's sugar troubles some. According to tolerance, foods selected should be rich in complex carbohydrates including fiber, and low in refined sugar products. Protein should be a mainstay in mini meals and snacks because it is converted to glucose at a moderate rate. Including some fat in each meal can further prolong digestion, helping to avoid feeling empty between meals. Thus a fitting snack might be whole grain crackers, cheese and a small piece of fresh fruit.

Food Intolerance and Food Allergies

Patrons may need to avoid certain foods because they have a food intolerance or allergy. Despite claims to the contrary, genuine food allergy reactions in adults are relatively uncommon. This is because a great many so-called food allergies are really intolerance reactions to foods and food additives. A food *allergy* includes a hyper-sensitivity reaction that can be shown to be caused by an allergen, a substance in food, usually a protein, that stimulates the immune system to respond (sometimes violently) in the same way certain people react to pollens or insect stings. A food *intolerance*, on the other hand, is an unfavorable response to food that does not involve the immune system. A food intolerance might arise from spoiled food, from physiological problems such as a genetically based enzyme deficiency (e.g., lactose intolerance), from interactions of drugs with a food, or from reactions to foods that affect metabolism.

How many people have adverse reactions to food is unknown, but those with food intolerance reactions are believed to far outnumber those with food allergies. We have described various food intolerances throughout the nutrient sections of this book, so in this section, we will take a closer look at food allergies in order to explore the myths and explore what is known.

Most of the signs and symptoms of food allergy involve the skin (itching, hives, eczema) or the gastrointestinal tract (vomiting, diarrhea, abdominal pain). Some persons suffer anaphylaxis, a severe and sometimes fatal systemic hypersensitivity reaction that follows contact with the causative agent. Symptoms involve the respiratory system (sneezing, wheezing, and, in the extreme case, throat constriction and suffocation), the eyes, and the cardiovascular system (irregular heartbeat, shock, collapse). Recent studies fail to demonstrate a significant relationship between diet (assuming it is nutritionally complete) and problems with the nervous system, muscles, joints, or behavior; so, symptoms such as headache, muscle and joint pain, arthritis, and hyperactivity do not appear to represent food allergy reactions.

Reports conflict but it is likely that about 90% of tested food allergy reactions are caused by only a few foods—milk, eggs, legumes, tree nuts, and wheat (Table 15-2). The most common sufferers (estimated incidence 1%) may be infants who consume cow's milk. (Some foodservices that serve families with infants offer infant bottles with a choice of cow's milk or nonmilk formula.) Other studies focusing on more severe anaphylaxis suggest that such reactions often are caused by fish and

TABLE 15-2
Foods Often Associated with
Hypersensitivity Reactions

Most Often
  Eggs
  Fish and shellfish (especially shrimp)
  Food additives
  Assorted coloring agents
  Monosodium glutamate (MSG)
  Sulfites
  Legumes, (in particular soybeans and peanuts)
  Milk and milk products (lactose)
  Nuts
  Wheat and wheat products
Less Commonly
  Bananas
  Barley
  Celery
  Citrus fruit
  Corn
  Melons
  Rice
  Tomatoes

seafood, particularly shrimp, and, to a lesser degree, by citrus fruit, melons, bananas, tomatoes, corn, barley, rice, and celery.

Diagnosing an adverse reaction to food can be painstaking. The cornerstone of diagnosis is a detailed patient history that may link the reaction to an event associated with the reaction and to food consumed there. The history is then investigated for clues that may distinguish responses that probably are not allergies from those that could be allergic reactions. The foods eaten and the symptom outcomes are the major clues.

If food allergy is suspected, the next step is usually an *elimination diet* that eliminates the more common foods associated with allergies (see above). Typically, the diet is followed strictly for two weeks, after which one food is added back to the diet for a period of several days to a week, followed by a second food, until the addition of a new food provokes a reaction that identifies it as the offending substance. This technique is not recommended for those with systemic anaphylaxis because of the risk involved in an allergic reaction. Further testing for confirmation can be performed by medical laboratory methods.

Whether the problem is food allergy or intolerance, the principal treatment is avoidance. This is why descriptive copy on menus or supplemental information about menu selection content (Chap. 13) can be so vital (Fig. 15-2). Once an offending food ingredient or additive has been identified, it should either be eliminated completely from the diet or controlled so that symptoms are avoided. The latter can be a difficult adjustment when the offending food is an excellent nutrient source or a favorite food. Milk is a good example. Intolerance to milk is widespread, even among adults. Some are allergic to the particular protein in milk, but lactose intolerance (inadequate ability to break-down milk sugar) is much more widespread. About 80% of humans are estimated to be lactose intolerant, particularly those of new world Indian, Black, Oriental, and Greek ancestry. Simple modifications in milk products offered on the menu can allow these persons to take advantage of the quality nutrients supplied by milk rather than eliminating it from their diets. Many persons who have an adverse response to drinking a large glass of milk because of lactose intolerance find that their systems can tolerate milk, cottage cheese, ice cream, and other dairy foods in small portions. Alternatively, many enjoy and readily can digest fermented milk products such as yogurt and acidophilus milk (in which the lactose has been changed to lactic acid).

The classic form of allergy treatment, in which patients get injections of allergens to become desensitized to specific substances, has not been shown conclusively to be helpful in the management of common food allergies.

CATERING TO VEGETARIAN DIETS AND ORDERS

Table 15-3 describes modifications of the Basic Four Food Plan that might be used as a guide in considering the special daily dietary needs for lacto-ovovegetarians (who consume eggs and milk) and vegans. Vegans (who consume no animal products) need to select food knowledgeably to obtain nutrients such as protein, calcium, and iron, otherwise supplied by milk and meat. Further, they may be advised to take supplemental vitamin B_{12}, as this nutrient is *not* contained in plant products.

Foodservice orders for vegetarian fare are on the rise (Figure 12-1). Orders come not only from dedicated vegetarians but often from nonvegetarians who simply find such dishes appealing, and from nutrition-oriented patrons who are interested in food that is flavorful, packed with fiber, and free from or low in animal fat and cholesterol. Vegetarian menu items range from the very newest "faux (imitation) foods" to meatless meals so unprepossessing they may once have been called soul food.

Faux foods for vegetarian meals *may* be considered imitations, but they are real food. Many are look-alike products made from vegetable ingredients. For example, soybean-based substitutes are available for such items as crab legs and

As a courtesy to our guests who suffer allergic reactions, this pamphlet lists those Denny's menu items that contain sulfites, monosodium glutamate (MSG) and lactose. All foods are listed, even the ones with small percentages of the possible allergen, to accommodate for various levels of sensitivity.

MONOSODIUM GLUTAMATE (MSG)

MSG is used as a flavor enhancer in food. It is sold in its pure form in the supermarket and has been used by the Chinese for centuries.

However, it is a potential allergen for some MSG-sensitive people, who react when large amounts are consumed on an empty stomach. Listed below are the products we serve that contain some degree of MSG:

- Croutons
- Roast Beef
- Sausage Patties
- Breaded Chicken Pieces
- Breaded Chicken Strips
- Battered Cod
- Breaded Shrimp
- Breaded Onion Rings
- Green Beans
  in butter-style sauce
- Italian-Style Vegetables
  in butter-style sauce
- Ranch Dressing
- Brown Gravy
- Chicken Gravy
- Country Gravy
- Au Jus
- Cacciatore Sauce
- Clam Chowder
- Split Pea Soup
- Chicken Noodle Soup
- Cream of Potato Soup
- Teriyaki Glaze

SULFITES

During the past year there has been an increasing concern over the use of sulfites in food, due to the possible negative effects they may have on sulfite-sensitive persons.

Sulfites are used primarily to preserve the whiteness and/or freshness in fruits and vegetables, as a preservative, and as a dough conditioner. It is a known fact that asthmatics are (generally) sulfite-sensitive, and should be aware of foods containing sulfites so that they may avoid them.

There are six compounds that are referred to as sulfites:

- Sulfur Dioxide
- Sodium Metabisulfite
- Sodium Sulfite
- Potassium Bisulfite
- Potassium Metabisulfite
- Sodium Bisulfite

It is our company policy to *not add or apply* sulfiting agents on premise to any menu item. We do not rinse our produce (salads, garnishes, etc.) with sulfites as they are prepared fresh. However, a few products used in our restaurants are known to contain sulfiting agents as the manufacturers of these products cannot produce an acceptable end product without sulfites as an ingredient. The seven Denny's products known to contain sulfites are:

- Breaded Shrimp
- Hashed Brown Potatoes
- Mashed Potatoes
- Stuffing
- Maraschino Cherries
- Lime Juice
- Beer and Wine

Presently, research and testing are under way to find suitable future alternatives to sulfiting agents.

LACTOSE

Lactose is the sugar found in mammals' milk, and is most frequently consumed by humans in the form of milk or milk by-products. Occasionally the powder form is used in the food manufacturing industry.

Some individuals are merely sensitive to lactose, while others—whose systems lack the enzyme lactase—are unable to digest lactose at all. The kind of sensitivity varies; some persons may have an allergic response after drinking 8 oz. of milk, others may respond similarly after eating the milk solids found in butter or margarine.

Due to these varying sensitivities, the foods listed below include everything served at Denny's that contain lactose in its pure form, as well as in the form of whey, milk, milk solids, and nonfat dry milk.

- Brown Gravy
- Country Gravy
- Chicken Gravy
- Au Jus
- Clam Chowder
- Chicken Noodle Soup
- Chicken Fried Steak
- Chicken Strips
- Breaded Shrimp
- Real Cream Topping
- Saltine Crackers
- English Muffins
- Hushpuppies
- Special K
- Waffles
- Onion Rings
- Zucchini
- Green Beans in
  butter-style sauce
- Mashed Potatoes
- Hot Chocolate
- Cacciatore Sauce
- Coffee Creamer
- Corn Muffins
- Fudge Brownies
- Chocolate Cake
- Apple Cobbler
- Custard Pie
- Cheesecake
- Carrot Cake
- Italian-Style Vegetables
  in butter-style sauce
- Buttermilk Biscuits
- Ice Milk
- Sherbet
- Milk
- Skim Milk
- Ice Cream
- Buttermilk
- Butter
- Cheese
- Cream Cheese
- Cottage Cheese

GENERAL

The foods and/or meals listed in this pamphlet were selected based upon the information obtained from our manufacturers. These lists are only as correct and complete as the information available. While every effort has been made to ensure that this information is as accurate as possible, Denny's does not guarantee its accuracy or its suitability for any specific medically imposed diet.

Denny's menu is subject to change without notice, and not all of the menu items listed above may be served at all times or in all restaurants.

For further information related to the nutritional content of our menu items, refer to our other three brochures: "Dine to Your Heart's Content," "Waist Not, Want Not," and "Salt Away," or write to us at our Research Center:

Denny's Inc., Research Center
14256 E. Firestone Blvd.
La Mirada, CA 90637

FIGURE 15-2 "For Sensitive People" Some operators make available supplementary brochures for guests requesting menu information to avoid possible food sensitivities. *(Courtesy Denny's, Inc.)*

TABLE 15-3
A Food Guide for the Vegan

	Four food group plan for an adult vegan	Four food group plan for an adult (nonvegan)
Milk	2 servings soy milk fortified with calcium and vitamin B_{12}	2 servings
Fruits and vegetables	4 servings, including 1 cup dark greens for females (to help meet iron requirements). Seek vitamin C source daily and vitamin A source at least every other day.	4 servings, at least one rich in vitamin C, and a vitamin A source at least every other day
Grains and cereals	4 servings whole grain or en- riched products	4 servings whole grain or en- riched products
Protein-rich foods	2 servings (approx. 1 cup) protein rich foods. Minimum 2 cups le- gumes for females to help meet iron requirements. Use 1/4 cup as a serving for peanut butter.	2 servings

Adopted from Hamilton E, Whitney. and Sizer *Nutrition: Concepts and Controversies* 3 ed. St. Paul, MN., West Publishing Co., 1985.

veal cutlets. Such products can allow the menu planner to avoid cholesterol and animal fat and perhaps, to offer food at a lower price than might be possible with the actual animal products. They are not for every operation but may play a role.

A menu approach that is much more common than you might guess is to offer combinations of plant foods which, together, are complete because they are protein complements (Table 15-4). For instance, for legume-grain combinations, one might think of Mexican-American foods, coming up with such popular combinations as

TABLE 15-4
Vegetarian Diet Protein Complements*

Legumes (incl. tofu + peanuts)	+	Grains (wheat, corn, rice) or nuts and seeds, or brewer's yeast
Grains (Whole grain best: enriched acceptable)	+	Legumes, or sesame or sun- flower seeds, or brewer's yeast
Brewer's yeast	+	Whole grains (and corn), or legumes, or seeds and nuts
Any of the above	+	Even a modest amount of animal protein (e.g. grated cheese topping, diced pork as flavor ingredient, egg(s), milk in recipe, beef broth soup base.)

* For quality protein using little or no animal protein, combine the plant foods as shown, within selections for meals and snacks.

beans and rice, or beans and (wheat) flour tortillas or (corn) chips. Why combine certain plant foods with others? As mentioned in discussing protein value previously, the protein in most foods other than animal products is not complete. Incomplete proteins are deficient in certain amino acids needed by the body. These are called limiting amino acids because they limit the use the body can make of the other amino acids that are available in the protein. Recipe or menu complementarity results when the amino acid limits of one food are overcome by pairing that food with a food that has plenty of the needed amino acids.

The popularity of plant-food combinations is expanding with the growing sophistication of consumers and their knowledge about what constitutes a healthful diet. Their exposure to new cuisines through travel and visits to exotic restaurants (particularly those with an ethnic emphasis) also has helped win over many traditional meat-and-potatoes types to at least occasional meals that contain little or no meat. They may try black beans and rice, a famous New Orleans dish adopted from Cuba, or Japanese dishes in which rice and vegetables are the foundation of the meal, and bits of fish or/and animal food are used sparingly, almost as condiments. Table 15-5 provides some menu selections that may include little or no meat. This is only a beginning. What others can you think of for each combination that might appeal to patrons?

TABLE 15-5
Thinking Vegetarian: Protein Complement "Starter Kit" for Menu Ideas

With eggs and dairy products
- Omelette
- Souffle
- French toast
- Quiche Lorraine (plain)
- Custard casseroles and desserts
- Egg Foo Yung

With dairy products, no eggs
- Cereal and milk, rice pudding
- Toasted cheese sandwich or cheese pizza
- Cream of mushroom soup

With legumes and grains
- Peanut butter on wheat bread sandwich
- Red beans and rice, "Hoppin' John"
- Black-eyed peas and corn bread
- Boston baked beans and brown bread
- Refried beans and wheat or corn tortillas

Vegetables and grains
- Vegetable chop suey and steamed rice
- Lentil or barley and mixed vegetable soup

Other complements
- Sesame spread sandwich

From around the world
- Latin America: Beans, rice, grains and potatoes (with poultry, pork)
- The Orient: Rice and soybean products (also with fish)
- India, Mediterranean: Rice and local legume crops (with fish, lamb, etc.)

Some foods, like legumes, had to shed an undeserved negative reputation before they gained popularity. For a long time, legumes were underrated because they were often the mainstay foods of the poor, and they were believed to cause indigestion. Some people still think legumes are fattening, the fallacy of which is illustrated in Table 15-6. This table presents a list of protein foods ranked from the lowest calorie count to the highest. The portion size was determined by the amount of the given protein food needed to supply about 16 grams of protein. Of the nine items listed, the two legumes rate second lowest and fourth lowest in calories. With consumers more enlightened today about such controversies and about the delicious and healthful dishes that can be made with legumes, this food family has regained popularity in forms including garbanzo beans on salad bars, split pea, navy bean, and lentil soups, chili beans, baked beans, and even as tofu (soybean-curd) ice cream and yogurt, and as a base for many faux foods.

Some foods are good ingredients for "beefing-up" a recipe's protein level without using meat. Because carbohydrate foods often are the ones chosen to enrich with protein supplements, they can be especially appropriate for elderly persons, who tend to eat too little protein in favor of (less expensive) easy to eat carbohydrate foods. For lactovegetarians, nonfat dry milk crystals are easy to include in soups, breads, and certain beverages. When nonanimal ingredients are desirable, there are still choices. Brewer's yeast or nutritional yeast products are good meatless protein sources; each tablespoon provides about three grams of protein plus iron and B vitamins. Often brewer's yeast is an ingredient in high-protein baked goods, and it can be used in soups and casseroles. It is important that live forms of yeast such as that used for leavening bread not be used this way; only reputable brewer's yeast brands or nutritional yeast products. Soy flour can add considerably to the protein value of bakery products when used in place of some of the wheat flour. Peanuts, peanut butter, and pumpkin, squash, and sesame seeds can be regarded as meat substitutes, but other nuts and seeds may not because they bring with them the "baggage" of a high proportion of lipid, or fat.

TABLE 15-6
Protein Foods and their Calorie Comparisons:
Calorie-Contribution Ranking for Portions
that Provide 16 to 17 Grams of Protein

Food Item	Measure Per Item	Protein (grams)	Fat (grams)	Carbohydrates (grams)	Total Calories
Milk, skim	2 Cups	16	6	24	170
Lentils, cooked	1 Cup	16	1	39	210
Eggs, Large	2 2/3 eggs	16	16	3	213
Pinto beans, cooked	1 cup	16	1	50	262
Cheddar Cheese	2 1/2 ounces	16	21	1	265
Milk, whole	2 cups	16	16	22	300
Roast beef lean & fat	3 ounces	17	33	0	375
Peanut butter	1/4 cup	16	32	12	380
Almonds, chopped (shelled)	2/3 cup	16	47	17	517

From cooking with less salt, to developing meatless entrees, promoting menu selections that satisfy the desires and needs of potential patrons on common "diets" represents still another avenue of opportunity for nutrition-oriented foods program planners.

SUMMARY

The term diet can refer to a plan for the kind and amount of food an individual should take in for a given reason, such as weight control. A significant proportion of foodservice guests want the opportunity to select food for a particular diet that they are following for medical or personal reasons. When foodservice personnel are familiar with the characteristics and menu requirements of a variety of common diets, accommodating these guests through a nutrition-oriented foods program can be enhanced.

Providing foods appropriate to patients in health care facilities differs from serving people in the public setting. Only a patient's physician can prescribe or change a diet, and diet service is carried out in a structured way.

Most *diets* amount to careful selection from among usual foods in order to meet nutrition needs while attaining a specific health goal. More formal therapeutic diets involve planning appealing meals while balancing or modifying food elements that contribute energy (caloric value), nutrients (fat, protein, carbohydrate, vitamins or/and minerals) and/or texture or seasoning (fiber, spices).

Diets for diabetics should be individualized to manage each patient's personal need for blood glucose control. The Dietary Exchange Method of dietary management was developed for this purpose. Meals providing 50 to 66% of calories from (primarily complex) carbohydrates and 25 to 30% from fat are needed. Many diabetics also need to restrict calories.

There is much disagreement about the symptoms and diagnosis of hypoglycemia (low blood glucose). The diet recommendations for those experiencing the symptoms are to eat regular, frequent, small meals and snacks composed of foods very low in caffeine and refined sugars, with plenty of complex carbohydrates and protein, and enough fat to prolong digestion.

For sodium-restricted diets, the mild-restriction, or "no added salt," diet meets the needs of many diners and is practical for foodservice operations to offer. Sodium-rich foods are not served, salt may be used only *lightly* in cooking, and no salt is added at the table.

A diet rich in residue or fiber might be expected to combat digestive irregularities, while residue restriction may be called for if dietary bulk is irritating to the digestive tract.

A gastrointestinal ulcer is like an open sore in the membrane lining the stomach or intestine. According to individual tastes and tolerances, the ulcer victim's diet should provide plenty of fiber and should restrict fried foods and certain harsh substances.

Food allergies are relatively uncommon in adults, but they are only one type of food intolerance. Certain foods and substances frequently are associated with intolerance, and listing them on the menu or in supplementary information could protect guests from the misery of reactions. In turn, this can protect the establishment and good will.

The diet of a strict vegetarian should be planned to provide the nutrients usually supplied by meat and milk. Complete protein can be obtained with plant foods by combining sources of complementary proteins. Orders for meatless meals, which are also popular with nonvegetarians, are increasing.

Chapter Review

1. What are two definitions of the term "diet?"
2. What might influence someone to follow a diet plan?
3. What types of common diets (e.g., low-calorie) might be menued in a nutrition-oriented foods program in a commercial restaurant?
4. How does the emphasis on nutrition in a health care foodservice usually differ from that in a commercial restaurant?
5. A _____ is the only person who can formally prescribe a diet.
6. In formal therapeutic diets, a balance or modification is sought in one or more of what three food components?
7. What function does the hormone insulin perform?
8. Explain how diabetics may differ from one another in the insulin and diet therapy they require.
9. Describe in general the carbohydrate, fat, and calorie characteristics recommended for an adult diabetic's diet.
10. What could the term "dietetic" mean on a food label?
11. Approximately how many persons are estimated to have high blood pressure?
12. List the restrictions in a menu for a mild sodium restriction diet.
13. To what does the term residue refer in nutrition?
14. A diet high in residue, or fiber, may have what benefits? About how many grams of dietary fiber is recommended in a high-fiber diet?
15. What is a peptic ulcer?
16. Describe the recommendations for planning a menu for an ulcer sufferer.
17. What happens to the blood glucose level in fasting hypoglycemia? What can occur if concentrated sweets are eaten to combat the symptoms?
18. Describe the timing, portioning, and principal food categories included in the diet recommendation for those with symptoms of hypoglycemia.
19. Differentiate between a food allergy and other types of food intolerance.
20. About which common foods and substances might foodservice planners provide information for "sensitive" guests?
21. How does the Basic Four Food Plan for the vegetarian differ from that for the nonvegetarian? Why?
22. Name three foods or food types that are protein complements for grains (wheat, corn, rice, etc.) and describe a meatless dish that can be made from each.

Appendix A COMBINATION FOODS

Much of the food we eat is mixed together in various combinations. These combination foods do not fit into only one exchange list. It can be quite hard to tell what is in a certain casserole dish or baked food item. This is a list of average values for some typical combination foods. This list will help you fit these foods into your meal plan. Ask your dietitian for information about any other foods you'd like to eat. The *American Diabetes Association/American Dietetic Association Family Cookbooks* and the *American Diabetes Association Holiday Cookbook* have many recipes and further information about many foods, including combination foods. Check your library or local bookstore.

Food	Amount	Exchanges
Casseroles, homemade	1 cup (8 oz.)	2 starch, 2 medium-fat meat, 1 fat
Cheese pizza 🐟, thin crust	1/4 of 15 oz. or 1/4 of 10″	2 starch, 1 medium-fat meat, 1 fat
Chili with beans 🌾, 🐟 (commercial)	1 cup (8 oz.)	2 starch, 2 medium-fat meat, 2 fat
Chow mein 🌾, 🐟 (without noodles or rice)	2 cups (16 oz.)	1 starch, 2 vegetable, 2 lean meat
Macaroni and cheese 🐟	1 cup (8 oz.)	2 starch, 1 medium-fat meat, 2 fat
Soup:		
Bean 🌾, 🐟	1 cup (8 oz.)	1 starch, 1 vegetable, 1 lean meat
Chunky, all varieties 🐟	10-3/4 oz. can	1 starch, 1 vegetable, 1 medium-fat meat
Cream 🐟 (made with water)	1 cup (8 oz.)	1 starch, 1 fat
Vegetable 🐟 or broth 🐟	1 cup (8 oz.)	1 starch
Spaghetti and meatballs 🐟 (canned)	1 cup (8 oz.)	2 starch, 1 medium-fat meat, 1 fat
Sugar-free pudding (made with skim milk)	1/2 cup	1 starch
If beans are used as a meat substitute:		
Dried beans 🌾, peas 🌾, lentils 🌾	1 cup (cooked)	2 starch, 1 lean meat

🌾 *3 grams or more of fiber per serving,* 🐟 *400 mg or more of sodium per serving*

We often eat a combination of foods such as a stew, a vegetable soup, or a casserole dish, and these do not fit well into any one list but must be considered to have two or more different kinds of food in them from the various lists. Some examples of how exchanges are allocated for some of these combination foods is given:

Casseroles, homemade   1 cup (8 oz.)   2 starch, 2 medium fat meat, 1 fat
Cheese pizza, etc.

CEREALS/GRAINS/PASTA

🌾 Bran cereals, concentrated (such as Bran Buds,® All Bran®)	1/3 cup
🌾 Bran cereals, flaked	1/2 cup
Bulgur (cooked)	1/2 cup
Cooked cereals	1/2 cup
Cornmeal (dry)	2 1/2 Tbsp.
Grapenuts	3 Tbsp.
Grits (cooked)	1/2 cup
Other ready-to-eat unsweetened cereals	3/4 cup
Pasta (cooked)	1/2 cup
Puffed cereal	1 1/2 cup
Rice, white or brown (cooked)	1/3 cup
Shredded wheat	1/2 cup
🌾 Wheat germ	3 Tbsp.

DRIED BEANS/PEAS/LENTILS

🌾 Beans and peas (cooked) (such as kidney, white, split, blackeye)	1/3 cup
🌾 Lentils (cooked)	1/3 cup
🌾 Baked beans	1/4 cup

STARCHY VEGETABLES

🌾 Corn	1/2 cup
🌾 Corn on cob, 6 in. long	1
🌾 Lima beans	1/2 cup
🌾 Peas, green (canned or frozen)	1/2 cup
🌾 Plantain	1/2 cup
Potato, baked	1 small (3 oz.)
Potato, mashed	1/2 cup
Squash, winter (acorn, butternut)	3/4 cup
Yam, sweet potato, plain	1/3 cup

BREAD

Bagel	1/2 (1 oz.)
Bread sticks, crisp, 4 in. long x 1/2 in.	2 (2/3 oz.)
Croutons, low fat	1 cup
English muffin	1/2
Frankfurter or hamburger bun	1/2 (1 oz.)
Pita, 6 in. across	1/2
Plain roll, small	1 (1 oz.)
Raisin, unfrosted	1 slice (1 oz.)
🌾 Rye, pumpernickel	1 slice (1 oz.)
Tortilla, 6 in. across	1
White (including French, Italian)	1 slice (1 oz.)
Whole wheat	1 slice (1 oz.)

🌾 3 grams or more of fiber per serving

1. Starch/Bread List

Each portion in this list contains approximately 15 grams of carbohydrate, 3 grams of protein, a trace of fat, and 80 calories. If whole grain, the average is about 2 grams of fiber per serving but some may be higher. Foods with 3 grams or more of fiber per portion are indicated by a head of grain. Usually an ounce of bread or a similar product, a half cup of cooked cereal, grain, or pasta, or a cup of dry ready-to-eat cereal is a portion.

CRACKERS/SNACKS

Animal crackers	8
Graham crackers, 2 1/2 in. square	3
Matzoth	3/4 oz.
Melba toast	5 slices
Oyster crackers	24
Popcorn (popped, no fat added)	3 cups
Pretzels	3/4 oz.
Rye crisp, 2 in. x 3 1/2 in.	4
Saltine-type crackers	6
Whole wheat crackers, no fat added (crisp breads, such as Finn®, Kavli®, Wasa®)	2-4 slices (3/4 oz.)
Taco shell, 6 in. across	2
Waffle, 4 1/2 in. square	1
Whole wheat crackers, fat added (such as Triscuits®)	4-6 (1 oz.)

STARCH FOODS PREPARED WITH FAT

(Count as 1 starch/bread serving, plus 1 fat serving.)

Biscuit, 2 1/2 in. across	1
Chow mein noodles	1/2 cup
Corn bread, 2 in. cube	1 (2 oz.)
Cracker, round butter type	6
French fried potatoes, 2 in. to 3 1/2 in. long	10 (1 1/2 oz.)
Muffin, plain, small	1
Pancake, 4 in. across	2
Stuffing, bread (prepared)	1/4 cup

LEAN MEAT AND SUBSTITUTES

(One exchange is equal to any one of the following items.)

Beef: USDA Good or Choice grades of lean beef, such as round, sirloin, 1 oz.
and flank steak; tenderloin; and chipped beef 🧂

Pork: Lean pork, such as fresh ham; canned, cured or boiled ham 🧂 ; 1 oz.
Canadian bacon 🧂 , tenderloin.

Veal: All cuts are lean except for veal cutlets (ground or cubed). 1 oz.
Examples of lean veal are chops and roasts.

Poultry: Chicken, turkey, Cornish hen (without skin) 1 oz.

Fish:
All fresh and frozen fish — 1 oz.
Crab, lobster, scallops, shrimp, clams — 2 oz.
 (fresh or canned in water 🧂)
Oysters — 6 medium
Tuna 🧂 (canned in water) — 1/4 cup
Herring (uncreamed or smoked) — 1 oz.
Sardines (canned) — 2 medium

Wild Game: Venison, rabbit, squirrel — 1 oz.
Pheasant, duck, goose (without skin) — 1 oz.

Cheese:
Any cottage cheese — 1/4 cup
Grated parmesan — 2 Tbsp.
Diet cheeses 🧂 (with less than 55 calories per ounce) — 1 oz.

Other:
95% fat-free luncheon meat — 1 oz.
Egg whites — 3 whites
Egg substitutes with less than 55 calories per 1/4 cup — 1/4 cup

---

🧂 *400 mg or more of sodium per exchange*

Each portion of meat or equivalent in this list contains about 7 grams of protein. The quantity of fat and number of calories differs depending on the meat or equivalent chosen. The list is therefore divided into lean, medium-fat, and high-fat items. An ounce is an exchange giving, respectively,

Meat Item	Carbohydrate (grams	Protein (grams)	Fat (grams)	Calories
Lean	0	7	3	55
Medium-fat	0	7	5	75
High-fat	0	7	8	100

Meat items or their equivalents with 400 or more milligrams of sodium per exchange are indicated with a salt shaker.

MEDIUM-FAT MEAT AND SUBSTITUTES
(One exchange is equal to any one of the following items.)

Beef:	Most beef products fall into this category. Examples are: all ground beef, roast (rib, chuck, rump), steak (cubed, Porterhouse, T-bone), and meatloaf.	1 oz.
Pork:	Most pork products fall into this category. Examples are: chops, loin roast, Boston butt, cutlets.	1 oz.
Lamb:	Most lamb products fall into this category. Examples are: chops, leg, and roast.	1 oz.
Veal:	Cutlet (ground or cubed, unbreaded)	1 oz.
Poultry:	Chicken (with skin), domestic duck or goose (well-drained of fat), ground turkey	1 oz.
Fish:	Tuna ✒ (canned in oil and drained) Salmon ✒ (canned)	1/4 cup 1/4 cup
Cheese:	Skim or part-skim milk cheeses, such as: Ricotta Mozzarella Diet cheeses ✒ (with 56-80 calories per ounce)	 1/4 cup 1 oz. 1 oz.
Other:	86% fat-free luncheon meat ✒ Egg (high in cholesterol, limit to 3 per week) Egg substitutes with 56-80 calories per 1/4 cup Tofu (2 1/2 in. x 2 3/4 in. x 1 in.) Liver, heart, kidney, sweetbreads 　(high in cholesterol)	1 oz. 1 1/4 cup 4 oz. 1 oz.

✒ *400 mg or more of sodium per exchange*

HIGH-FAT MEAT AND SUBSTITUTES

**Remember, these items are high in saturated fat, cholesterol, and calories,
and should be used only three (3) times per week.**

(One exchange is equal to any one of the following items.)

Beef:	Most USDA Prime cuts of beef, such as ribs, corned beef 🐟	1 oz.
Pork:	Spareribs, ground pork, pork sausage 🐟 (patty or link)	1 oz.
Lamb:	Patties (ground lamb)	1 oz.
Fish:	Any fried fish product	1 oz.
Cheese:	All regular cheeses 🐟 , such as American, Blue, Cheddar, Monterey, Swiss	1 oz.
Other:	Luncheon meat 🐟 , such as bologna, salami, pimento loaf	1 oz.
	Sausage 🐟 , such as Polish, Italian	1 oz.
	Knockwurst, smoked	1 oz.
	Bratwurst 🐟	1 oz.
	Frankfurter 🐟 (turkey or chicken)	1 frank (10/lb.)
	Peanut butter (contains unsaturated fat)	1 Tbsp.

Count as one high-fat meat plus one fat exchange:

Frankfurter 🐟 (beef, pork, or combination)		1 frank (10/lb.)

🐟 *400 mg or more of sodium per exchange*

3 VEGETABLE LIST

Each portion in this list contains about 5 grams of carbohydrate, two grams of protein, and 25 calories. A portion normally contains 2 to 3 grams of fiber. Items that have 400 milligrams or more of sodium are identified by/a shalt shaker. A portion usually is a half cup of cooked vegetables, a half cup of vegetable juice or a cup of raw vegetables.

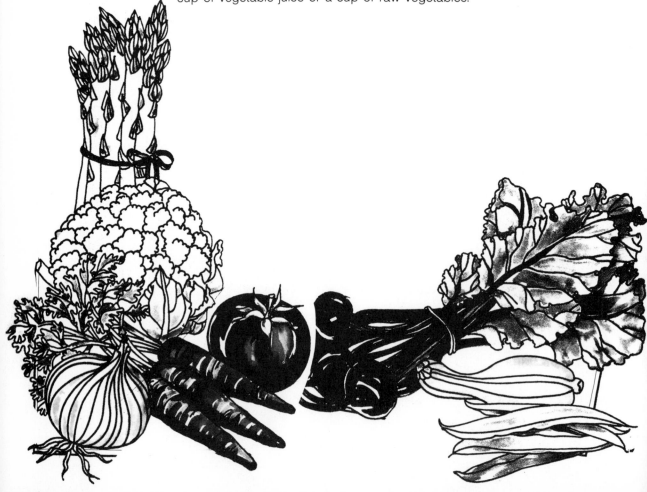

Artichoke (1/2
  medium)
Asparagus
Beans (green, wax,
  Italian)
Bean sprouts
Beets
Broccoli
Brussels sprouts
Cabbage, cooked
Carrots
Cauliflower
Eggplant
Greens (collard,
  mustard, turnip)
Kohlrabi
Leeks

Mushrooms, cooked
Okra
Onions
Pea pods
Peppers (green)
Rutabaga
Sauerkraut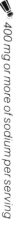
Spinach, cooked
Summer squash
  (crookneck)
Tomato (one large)
Tomato/vegetable
  juice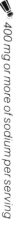
Turnips
Water chestnuts
Zucchini, cooked

Starchy vegetables such as corn, peas, and
potatoes are found on the Starch/Bread List.

For free vegetables, see Free Food List on
page 22.

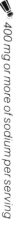 *400 mg or more of sodium per serving*

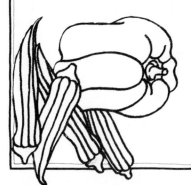

4

FRUIT LIST

E ach portion in this list contains about 15 grams of carbohydrate and 60 calories. A portion of fresh, frozen, or dry fruit has about 2 grams of fiber. Items with 3 grams or more of fiber per portion are indicated by a head of grain. Fruit juices, especially strained, contain very little fiber. The size of a portion is usually a half cup of fresh fruit or fruit juice and a quarter cup of dried fruit.

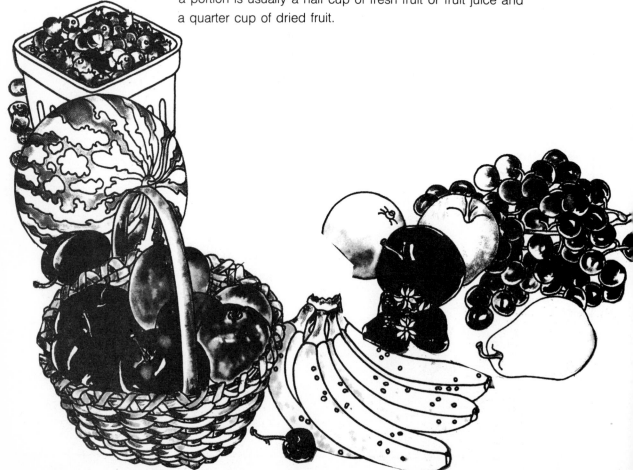

FRESH, FROZEN, AND UNSWEETENED CANNED FRUIT

Apple (raw, 2 in. across)	1 apple
Applesauce (unsweetened)	1/2 cup
Apricots (medium, raw) or	4 apricots
Apricots (canned)	1/2 cup, or 4 halves
Banana (9 in. long)	1/2 banana
🌾 Blackberries (raw)	3/4 cup
🌾 Blueberries (raw)	3/4 cup
Cantaloupe (5 in. across) (cubes)	1/3 melon 1 cup
Cherries (large, raw)	12 cherries
Cherries (canned)	1/2 cup
Figs (raw, 2 in. across)	2 figs
Fruit cocktail (canned)	1/2 cup
Grapefruit (medium)	1/2 grapefruit
Grapefruit (segments)	3/4 cup
Grapes (small)	15 grapes
Honeydew melon (medium) (cubes)	1/8 melon 1 cup
Kiwi (large)	1 kiwi
Mandarin oranges	3/4 cup
Mango (small)	1/2 mango
🌾 Nectarine (1 1/2 in. across)	1 nectarine
Orange (2 1/2 in. across)	1 orange
Papaya	1 cup
Peach (2 3/4 in. across)	1 peach, or 3/4 cup
Peaches (canned)	1/2 cup, or 2 halves
Pear	1/2 large, or 1 small
Pears (canned)	1/2 cup or 2 halves
Persimmon (medium, native)	2 persimmons
Pineapple (raw)	3/4 cup
Pineapple (canned)	1/3 cup
Plum (raw, 2 in. across)	2 plums
🌾 Pomegranate	1/2 pomegranate
🌾 Raspberries (raw)	1 cup
🌾 Strawberries (raw, whole)	1 1/4 cup
Tangerine (2 1/2 in. across)	2 tangerines
Watermelon (cubes)	1 1/4 cup

DRIED FRUIT

Apples	4 rings
Apricots	7 halves
Dates	2 1/2 medium
Figs	1 1/2
Prunes	3 medium
Raisins	2 Tbsp.

FRUIT JUICE

Apple juice/cider	1/2 cup
Cranberry juice cocktail	1/3 cup
Grapefruit juice	1/2 cup
Grape juice	1/3 cup
Orange juice	1/2 cup
Pineapple juice	1/2 cup
Prune juice	1/3 cup

3 or more grams of fiber per serving

6. Fat List

Each portion in this list contains about 5 grams of fat and 45 calories. Most are pure or almost pure fat but some may contain some protein or other nutrients. Check the label for the amount of sodium these various items contain.

5

MILK LIST

Each portion of milk or milk products in this list contains about 12 grams of carbohydrate and 8 grams of protein. Fat varies according to percentage of milkfat, and calories usually 100 also because of the fat difference. A portion of milk (one exchange) of the various kinds of milk or milk products provides.

Item	Carbohydrate (grams)	Protein (grams)	Fat (grams)	Calories
Skim or very low-fat	12	8	Trace	90
Low-fat	12	8	5	120
Whole	12	8	8	150

Skim or very low-fat milk

Skim milk	1c			
½% milk	1c			
1% milk	1c			
Low-fat buttermilk	1c			
Evaporated skim milk	½c			
Dry nonfat milk	⅓c			
Plain nonfat yogurt	8oz (1c)			

Low-fat milk

2% milk	1c			
Plain low-fat yogurt with added milk solids	8 oz (1c)			

Whole milk

Whole milk (3¼% milkfat)	1c			
Evaporated whole milk	½c			
Whole plain yogurt	8oz (1c)			

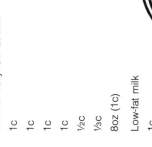

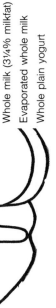

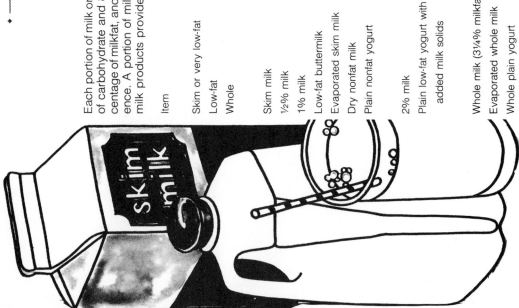

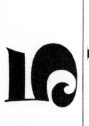

UNSATURATED FATS

Avocado	1/8 medium
Margarine	1 tsp.
Margarine, diet	1 Tbsp.
* Mayonnaise	1 tsp.
* Mayonnaise, reduced-calorie	1 Tbsp.

Nuts and Seeds:

Almonds, dry roasted	6 whole
Cashews, dry roasted	1 Tbsp.
Pecans	2 whole
Peanuts	20 small or 10 large
Walnuts	2 whole
Other nuts	1 Tbsp.
Seeds, pine nuts, sunflower (without shells)	1 Tbsp.
Pumpkin seeds	2 tsp.

Oil (corn, cottonseed, safflower, soybean, sunflower, olive, peanut)	1 tsp.
* Olives	10 small or 5 large
Salad dressing, mayonnaise-type	2 tsp.
Salad dressing, mayonnaise-type, reduced-calorie	1 Tbsp.
* Salad dressing (all varieties)	1 Tbsp.
Salad dressing, reduced-calorie	2 Tbsp.

(Two tablespoons of low-calorie salad dressing is a free food.)

SATURATED FATS

Butter	1 tsp.
Bacon	1 slice
* Chitterlings	1/2 ounce
Coconut, shredded	2 Tbsp.
Coffee whitener, liquid	2 Tbsp.
Coffee whitener, powder	4 tsp.
Cream (light, coffee, table)	2 Tbsp.
Cream, sour	2 Tbsp.
Cream (heavy, whipping)	1 Tbsp.
Cream cheese	1 Tbsp.
* Salt pork	1/4 ounce

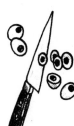

· *If more than one or two servings are eaten, these foods have 400 mg. or more of sodium.*

· *400 mg. or more of sodium per serving.*

FREE FOODS

A free food is any food or drink that contains less than 20 calories per serving. You can eat as much as you want of those items that have no serving size specified. You may eat two or three servings per day of those items that have a specific serving size. Be sure to spread them out through the day.

Drinks:
Bouillon 🧂 or broth without fat
Bouillon, low-sodium
Carbonated drinks, sugar-free
Carbonated water
Club soda
Cocoa powder, unsweetened (1 Tbsp.)
Coffee / Tea
Drink mixes, sugar-free
Tonic water, sugar-free

Nonstick pan spray

Fruit:
Cranberries, unsweetened (1/2 cup)
Rhubarb, unsweetened (1/2 cup)

Vegetables:
(raw, 1 cup)
Cabbage
Celery
Chinese cabbage 🌾
Cucumber
Green onion
Hot peppers
Mushrooms
Radishes
Zucchini 🌾

Salad greens:
Endive
Escarole
Lettuce
Romaine
Spinach

Sweet Substitutes:
Candy, hard, sugar-free
Gelatin, sugar-free
Gum, sugar-free
Jam / Jelly, sugar-free (2 tsp.)
Pancake syrup, sugar-free (1-2 Tbsp.)

Sugar substitutes (saccharin, aspartame)
Whipped topping (2 Tbsp.)

Condiments:
Catsup (1 Tbsp.)
Horseradish
Mustard
Pickles 🧂, dill, unsweetened
Salad dressing, low-calorie (2 Tbsp.)
Taco sauce (1 Tbsp.)
Vinegar

Seasonings can be very helpful in making food taste better. Be careful of how much sodium you use. Read the label, and choose those seasonings that do not contain sodium or salt.

Basil (fresh)
Celery seeds
Cinnamon
Chili powder
Chives
Curry
Dill

Flavoring extracts (vanilla, almond, walnut, peppermint, butter, lemon, etc.)
Garlic
Garlic powder
Herbs
Hot pepper sauce
Lemon

Lemon juice
Lemon pepper
Lime
Lime juice
Mint
Onion powder
Oregano
Paprika
Pepper

Pimento
Spices
Soy sauce 🧂
Soy sauce, low sodium ("lite")
Wine, used in cooking (1/4 cup)
Worcestershire sauce

🌾 3 grams or more of fiber per serving; 🧂 400 mg or more of sodium per serving

Each portion of food in this list contains 20 calories or less. One can have two or three portions of these foods a day without counting them as an exchange. Foods contributing 3 grams or more of fiber per portion are indicated as well as those with 400 milligrams or more of sodium per portion.

Appendix B
The Exchange Method

The Exchange Method divides foods into lists according to the similarity in their carbohydrate, protein, fat, and calorie yields. Thus bread and starch foods are grouped together in portion sizes to give approximately the same number of these nutrients and calories. A given number of exchanges often is recommended from each list each day, and individuals may select any of the foods in the list. The following gives the amounts of nutrients and calories from each portion in each exchange list.

Exchange List	Carbohydrate (grams)	Protein (grams)	Fat (grams)	Calories
Starch/Bread	15	3	Trace	80
Meat				
Lean	—	7	3	55
Medium-fat	—	7	5	75
High-fat	—	7	8	100
Vegetable	5	2	—	25
Fruit	15	—	—	60
Milk				
Skim	12	8	Trace	90
Low-fat	12	8	5	120
Whole	12	8	8	150
Fat	—	—	5	45

Recently, exchange lists have also been highlighting foods that give 3 grams or more of fiber per exchange (as desirable), and those that give 400 milligrams or more of sodium (as those to avoid). The six exchange lists follow; each contains representative foods and portion sizes per exchange.

APPENDIX B

The Exchange Method

The Exchange Method divides foods into lists according to the similarity in their carbohydrate, protein, fat, and calorie yields. Thus bread and starch foods are grouped together in portion sizes to give approximately the same number of these nutrients and calories. A given number of exchanges is allowed from each list each day and individuals may select any of the foods in the list. The following gives the amounts of nutrients and calories from each portion in each exchange list.

Exchange List	Carbohydrate (grams)	Protein (grams)	Fat (grams)	Calories
Starch/Bread	15	3	Trace	80
Meat				
Lean		7	3	55
Medium-fat		7	5	75
High-fat		7	8	100
Vegetable	5	2		25
Fruit	15			60
Milk				
Skim	12	8	Trace	90
Low-fat	12	8	5	120
Whole	12	8	8	150
Fat			5	45

Recently, exchange lists have also been differentiating between some foods that give 3 grams or more of fiber per exchange and those that give 400 milligrams or more of sodium. The six exchange lists follow; each contains a representative number of foods and their portion size per exchange.

1. Starch/Bread List

Each portion in this list contains approximately 15 grams of carbohydrate, 3 grams of protein, a trace of fat, and 80 calories. If whole grain, the average is about 2 grams of fiber per serving but some may be higher. Foods with 3 grams or more of fiber per portion are indicated by a head of grain. Usually an ounce of bread or a similar product, a half cup of cooked cereal, grain, or pasta, or a cup of dry ready-to-eat cereal is a portion.

2. Meat List

Each portion of meat or equivalent in this list contains about 7 grams of protein. The quantity of fat and number of calories differs depending on the meat or equivalent chosen. The list is therefore divided into lean, medium-fat, and high-fat items. An ounce is an exchange giving, respectively,

Meat Item	Carbohydrate (grams)	Protein (grams)	Fat (grams)	Calories
Lean	0	7	3	55
Medium-fat	0	7	5	75
High-fat	0	7	8	100

Meat items or their equivalents with 400 or more milligrams of sodium per exchange are indicated with a salt shaker.

3. Vegetable List

Each portion in this list contains about 5 grams of carbohydrate, 2 grams of protein, and 25 calories. A portion normally contains 2 to 3 grams of fiber. Items that have 400 milligrams or more of sodium are identified by a salt shaker. A portion usually is a half cup of cooked vegetables, a half cup of vegetable juice or a cup of raw vegetables.

4. Fruit List

Each portion in this list contains about 15 grams of carbohydrate and 60 calories. A portion of fresh, frozen, or dry fruit has about 2 grams of fiber. Items with 3 grams or more of fiber per portion are indicated by a head of grain. Fruit juices, especially strained, contain very little fiber. The size of a portion is usually a half cup of fresh fruit or fruit juice and a quarter cup of dried fruit.

5. Milk List

Each portion of milk or milk products in this list contains about 12 grams of carbohydrate and 8 grams of protein. Fat varies according to percentage of milkfat, and calories usually do also because of the fat difference. A portion of milk (one exchange) of the various kinds of milk or milk products provides:

Item	Carbohydrate (grams)	Protein (grams)	Fat (grams)	Calories
Skim or very low-fat	12	8	Trace	90
Low-fat	12	8	5	120
Whole	12	8	8	150

Skim or very low-fat milk

Skim milk	1 c
½% milk	1 c
1% milk	1 c
Low-fat buttermilk	1 c
Evaporated skim milk	½ c
Dry nonfat milk	⅓ c
Plain nonfat yogurt	8 oz (1 c)

Low-fat milk

2% milk	1 c
Plain low-fat yogurt with added milk solids	8 oz (1 c)

Whole milk

Whole milk (3¼% milkfat)	1 c
Evaporated whole milk	½ c
Whole plain yogurt	8 oz (1 c)

6. Fat List

Each portion in this list contains about 5 grams of fat and 45 calories. Most are pure or almost pure fat but some may contain some protein or other nutrients. Check the label for the amount of sodium these various items contain.

Free Foods

Each portion of food in this list contains 20 calories or less. One can have two or three portions of these foods a day without counting them as an exchange. Foods contributing three grams or more of fiber per portion are indicated as well as those with 400 milligrams or more of sodium per portion.

Combination Foods

We often eat a combination of foods such as a stew, a vegetable soup, or a casserole dish, and these do not fit well into any one list but must be considered to have two or more different kinds of food in them from the various lists. Some examples of how exchanges are allocated for some of these combination foods is given:

Food Item	Portion Size	Exchanges per Portion
Casseroles, homemade cheese pizza, etc.	1 c (8 oz)	2 starch, 2 medium fat meat, 1 fat

NUTRITION RESOURCES

Computer Nutrient Analysis

The firms listed below perform computerized nutrient analysis of recipes.

Computrition
21049 Devonshire Street
Chatsworth, CA 91311
818/341-9739
800/222-4488

DDA Software
P.O. Box 26
Hamburg, NJ 07419
201/764-6677

Health Development, Inc.
1165 West Third Avenue
Columbus, OH 43212
800/200-4630
614/294-2688 for Ohio residents

Data Control Information Service
347 Seneca Road
Hornel, NY 14843
607/324-5510

ESHA Research
P.O. Box 13028
Salem, OR 97309
503/585-6242

Larry Miller, Inc.
919 Hickory View Circle
Camarillo, CA 93010
805/484-1616

Nutrition Counseling Service
2444 39th Place, N.W.
Washington, DC 20007
202/338-7328

Health Management Systems
1409 Willow St., Suite 200
Minneapolis, MN 55403
612/874-9444

Nutriquest
Capital Systems Group, Inc.
1803 Research Boulevard
Suite 600
Rockville, MD 20850
301/762-1200

Practorcare
10951 Sorrento Valley Road
San Diego, CA 92121
800/421-9073
800/421-9074 CA residents

Federal Government Agencies

Below are departments in both the Department of Agriculture (USDA) and Department of Health and Human Services (DHHS) that develop nutrition materials for consumers. They will provide a publications list on request. Materials are available through U.S. Government Printing Office bookstores.

Food and Consumer Services
USDA
14th St. & Independence Ave., S.W.
Washington, DC 20250
202/447-7711

U.S. Government Printing Office
710 North Capitol St., N.W.
Washington, DC 20401
202/275-3050

Food and Drug Administration (FDA)
Office of Consumer Affairs
5600 Fishers Lane (HFE-88)
Rockville, MD 20857
301/433-3170

National Health Information
   Clearinghouse Office of
   Disease Prevention and Health
   Promotion
Public Health Service-DHHS
P.O. Box 1133

Human & Nutrition Information
   Service
6505 Belcrest Road
Hyattsville, MD 20782
301/436-7725

Washington, DC 20013-1133
800/336-4797
703/522-2590 for Metro
   Washington, DC residents

Trade, Health and Other Organizations

The American Dietetic Association
430 North Michigan Avenue
Chicago, IL 60611
312/280-5000

> The American Dietetic Association maintains a directory of consulting nutritionists that can be obtained by contacting the association. Your state and local dietetic association or local hospital may also help you locate a registered dietitian.

American Health Foundation
320 East 43rd Street
New York, NY 10017
212/953-1900

> The American Health Foundations is a nonprofit organization devoted to the prevention of disease and the promotion of good health. The Foundation's nutritionists have developed MENU MANHATTAN, a low-fat, low-calorie food concept for restaurants. The Foundation's nutritionists work with chefs and managers to implement MENU MANHATTAN on a fee-for-service basis.

American Heart Association
7320 Greenville Avenue
Dallas, TX 75231
214/750-5362

> The American Heart Association AHA has designed Eating Away From Home, a restaurant plan that features foods low in calories, fat, and cholesterol. The Heart Association's program is designed in a step-by-step fashion and includes manuals, recipes, a cookbook, and an instruction guide. Contact your local AHA affiliate or AHA headquarters in Dallas. AHA also publishes pamphlets about heart disease and diet.

Beef Industry Council
444 North Michigan Avenue
Chicago, IL 60611
311/467-5520

> Beef Lite Recipes, a series of calorie-controlled, quantity recipes, is available through the Beef Industry Council.

California Beef Council
551 City Boulevard, Suite A
Foster City, CA 94404
415/571-7000

> The California Beef Council has developed a set of low-calorie beef food-service recipes that are available to industry members.

Florida Department of Citrus
P.O. Box 148
Lakeland, FL 33802
813/682-0171

Florida's Department of Citrus has developed quantity recipes for nonalcoholic cocktails, salads, entrees, and desserts that are available free of charge to foodservice operators.

Idaho Potato Commission
P.O. Box 1068
Boise, ID 83701
208/334-2350

Spa Series is a collection of calorie-controlled, quantity recipes featuring potatoes that originated at California's Golden Door and other exclusive spas.

National Fisheries Institute
2000 M. St., N.W., Suite 580
Washington, DC 20036
201/296-5090

The Fisheries Institute has a collection of foodservice recipes for naturally nutritious fish. These recipes are appropriate for nutritious promotions.

National Livestock and Meat Board
444 Michigan Avenue
Chicago, Il 60611
312/467-5520

The Lighter Side of Beef, produced by the Livestock and Meat Board, is a collection of 13 light beef recipes that will appeal to your health-conscious clientele. Recipes are for light breakfasts, lunch and dinner entrees, and appetizers. The cost is 75 cents. To order, send a self-addressed, stamped envelop to: Box LSB, National Livestock and Meat Board.

Produce Marketing Association (PMA)
P.O. Box 6036
Neward, DE 19714-6036
302/738-7100

PMA's Food For You series includes foodservice recipes approved by the American Heart Association as well as purchasing and nutrition information on produce.

Rice Council of America
P.O. Box 740121
Houston, TX 77274
713/270-6699

The Rice Council offers a collection of light recipes that are low in calories, featuring rice. All the recipes yield 25 portions and the caloric content per serving.

The Rodale Food Consultants
33 East Minor Street
Emmaus, PA 18049
215/967-5171

The Rodale Food Consultants, a division of Rodal Press, Inc., consists of nutritionists, food technologists, chefs, chemists, and researchers. Their services include healthy food workshops, food service consultation, and recipe development and they specialize in creative, nutritious food.

Academic Organizations

This is a partial list of culinary schools and organizations that offer nutrition courses. Many junior community colleges that feature culinary programs are incorporating nutrition courses into their curriculums. Generally, these courses concentrate on the application of nutritional principles in a foodservice operation. Contact your local college or cooking school to determine if a whether nutrition course is avaiable locally.

American Culinary Federation (ACF)
P.O. Box 3466
St. Augustine, FL 32084
904/824-4468

The Culinary Federation has developed a nutrition course that is required for certification or recertification by the ACF. The nutrition course can be taken on a correspondence basis in twelve 90-minute tapes. Some ACF chapters have organized classes to teach the nutrition course.

Culinary Institute of America (CIA)
Hyde Park, NY 12538
914/452-9600

The CIA offers a number of continuing education courses for working professional chefs and cooks. Among these is a 5-day nutrition course that covers the fundamentals of cooking food reduced in calories, sodium, fat, and cholesterol.

Johnson and Wales College
Department of Continuing Education
8 Abbott Park Place
Providence, RI 02903
401/456-1120

The nutrition course at Johnson and Wales is introductory, concentrating on nutrient requirements, food sources of nutrients, and the effects of deficiencies. It is a three-credit course that can be taken during the week or on weekends.

The New York Restaurant School
27 West 34th Street
New York, NY 10001
212/947-7097
   Although a standard nutrition course is not offered, the New York Restaurant School offers courses like, "Low-Calorie Italian Cuisine" and "Low-
   Calorie Dessert Making," which vary from semester to semester.

Definitions of Food and Drug Administration (FDA) Label Terms

Dietetic, or diet: Food claiming to be dietetic or diet must either meet the requirements for low or reduced-calorie foods (see below) or be clearly intended
for a special dietary purpose other than weight control, such as "for low-sodium
diets."

Label: Graphic matter either on the food, its wrapper or container, or accom-
panying the food.

Light, or lite: The FDA has not defined these terms but interprets them to
describe a low- or reduced-calorie food. But, FDA acknowledges that light or
lite can refer to properties other than calories. The syrup in canned fruit is
described as light based on its density, whereas "light cream" describes fat
content.

Low-calorie: A low-calorie food must contain no more than 40 calories per serving and no more than 0.4 calories per gram (11 calories per ounce).

Reduced-calorie: A reduced-calorie food must be at least one-third lower in
calories than and otherwise nutritionally equal to its nonreduced counterpart.

Significant source: To be considered a significant source of a particular
nutrient, a single serving must provide 10% or more of the U.S. RDA of that
nutrient.

Sodium-free: Cannot contain more then 5 milligrams of sodium per serving.

Very-low-sodium: A low-sodium food must deliver not more than 140 milligrams of sodium per serving.

Reduced-sodium This represents a 75% reduction in usual sodium content.

Unsalted: This term applies to a product that has been processed without the
salt normally used. Good examples are unsalted potato chips and nuts.

APPENDIX C

NUTRITIVE VALUES
OF THE EDIBLE PART OF FOODS

(Dashes (—) denote lack of reliable data for a constituent believed to be present in measurable amount)

DAIRY PRODUCTS (CHEESE, CREAM, IMITATION CREAM, MILK; RELATED PRODUCTS)

Butter. See Fats, oils; related products, items 103-108.

Item No.	Foods, approximate measures, units, and weight (edible part unless footnotes indicate otherwise)	Grams	Water Per cent	Food energy Calories	Protein Grams	Fat Grams	Saturated (total) Grams	Unsaturated Oleic Grams	Unsaturated Linoleic Grams	Carbohydrate Grams	Calcium Milligrams	Phosphorus Milligrams	Iron Milligrams	Potassium Milligrams	Vitamin A value International units	Thiamin Milligrams	Riboflavin Milligrams	Niacin Milligrams	Ascorbic acid Milligrams
(A)	(B)		(C)	(D)	(E)	(F)	(G)	(H)		(I)	(K)	(L)	(M)	(N)	(O)	(P)	(Q)	(R)	(S)
	Cheese:																		
	Natural:																		
1	Blue—— 1 oz	28	42	100	6	8	5.3	1.9	0.2	1	150	110	0.1	73	200	0.01	0.11	0.3	0
2	Camembert (3 wedges per 4-oz container)—— 1 wedge	38	52	115	8	9	5.8	2.2	.2	Trace	147	132	.1	71	350	.01	.19	.2	0
	Cheddar:																		
3	Cut pieces—— 1 oz	28	37	115	7	9	6.1	2.1	.2	Trace	204	145	.2	28	300	.01	.11	Trace	0
4	1 cu in	17.2	37	70	4	6	3.7	1.3	.1	Trace	124	88	.1	17	180	Trace	.06	Trace	0
5	Shredded—— 1 cup	113	37	455	28	37	24.2	8.5	.7	1	815	579	.8	111	1,200	.03	.42	.1	0
	Cottage (curd not pressed down):																		
	Creamed (cottage cheese, 4% fat):																		
6	Large curd—— 1 cup	225	79	235	28	10	6.4	2.4	.2	6	135	297	.3	190	370	.05	.37	.3	Trace
7	Small curd—— 1 cup	210	79	220	26	9	6.0	2.2	.2	6	126	277	.3	177	340	.04	.34	.3	Trace
8	Low fat (2%)—— 1 cup	226	79	205	31	4	2.8	1.0	.1	8	155	340	.4	217	160	.05	.42	.3	Trace
9	Low fat (1%)—— 1 cup	226	82	165	28	2	1.5	.5	.1	6	138	302	.3	193	80	.05	.37	.3	Trace
10	Uncreamed (cottage cheese dry curd, less than 1/2% fat)—— 1 cup	145	80	125	25	1	.4	.1	Trace	3	46	151	.3	47	40	.04	.21	.2	0
11	Cream—— 1 oz	28	54	100	2	10	6.2	2.4	.2	1	23	30	.3	34	400	Trace	.06	Trace	0
	Mozzarella, made with—																		
12	Whole milk—— 1 oz	28	48	90	6	7	4.4	1.7	.2	1	163	117	.1	21	260	Trace	.08	Trace	0
13	Part skim milk—— 1 oz	28	49	80	8	5	3.1	1.2	.1	1	207	149	.1	27	180	.01	.10	Trace	0
	Parmesan, grated:																		
14	Cup, not pressed down—— 1 cup	100	18	455	42	30	19.1	7.7	.3	4	1,376	807	1.0	107	700	.05	.39	.3	0
15	Tablespoon—— 1 tbsp	5	18	25	2	2	1.0	.4	Trace	Trace	69	40	Trace	5	40	Trace	.02	Trace	0
16	Ounce—— 1 oz	28	18	130	12	9	5.4	2.2	.2	1	390	229	.3	30	200	Trace	.11	.1	0
17	Provolone—— 1 oz	28	41	100	7	8	4.8	1.7	.1	1	214	141	.1	39	230	.01	.09	Trace	0
	Ricotta, made with—																		
18	Whole milk—— 1 cup	246	72	428	28	32	20.4	7.1	.7	7	509	389	.9	257	1,210	.03	.48	.3	0
19	Part skim milk—— 1 cup	246	74	340	28	19	12.1	4.7	.5	13	669	449	1.1	308	1,060	.05	.46	.2	0
20	Romano—— 1 oz	28	31	110	9	8	—	—	—	1	302	215	—	—	—	—	.11	Trace	0
21	Swiss—— 1 oz	28	37	105	8	8	5.0	1.7	.2	1	272	171	Trace	31	240	.01	.10	Trace	0
	Pasteurized process cheese:																		
22	American—— 1 oz	28	39	105	6	9	5.6	2.1	.2	Trace	174	211	.1	46	340	.01	.10	Trace	0
23	Swiss—— 1 oz	28	42	95	7	7	4.5	1.7	.1	1	219	216	.2	61	230	Trace	.08	Trace	0
24	Pasteurized process cheese food, American—— 1 oz	28	43	95	6	7	4.4	1.7	.1	2	163	130	.2	79	260	.01	.13	Trace	0
25	Pasteurized process cheese spread, American—— 1 oz	28	48	82	5	6	3.8	1.5	.1	2	159	202	.1	69	220	.01	.12	Trace	0
	Cream, sweet:																		
26	Half-and-half (cream and milk)—— 1 cup	242	81	315	7	28	17.3	7.0	.6	10	254	230	.2	314	260	.08	.36	.2	2
27	1 tbsp	15	81	20	Trace	2	1.1	.4	Trace	1	16	14	Trace	19	20	.01	.02	Trace	Trace
28	Light, coffee, or table—— 1 cup	240	74	470	6	46	28.8	11.7	1.0	9	231	192	.1	292	1,730	.08	.36	.1	2
29	1 tbsp	15	74	30	Trace	3	1.8	.7	.1	1	14	12	Trace	18	110	Trace	.02	Trace	Trace

(A)	(B)	Grams	(C)	(D)	(E)	(F)	(G)	(H)	(I)	(J)	(K)	(L)	(M)	(N)	(O)	(P)	(Q)	(R)	(S)
	Whipping, unwhipped (volume about double when whipped):																		
30	Light — 1 cup	239	64	700	5	74	46.2	18.3	1.5	7	166	146	0.1	231	2,690	0.06	0.30	0.1	1
31	1 tbsp	15	64	45	Trace	5	2.9	1.1	.1	Trace	10	9	Trace	15	170	Trace	.02	Trace	Trace
32	Heavy — 1 cup	238	58	820	5	88	54.8	22.2	2.0	7	154	149	.1	179	3,500	.05	.26	.1	1
33	1 tbsp	15	58	80	Trace	6	3.5	1.4	.1	Trace	10	9	Trace	11	220	Trace	.02	Trace	Trace
34	Whipped topping, (pressurized) — 1 cup	60	61	155	2	13	8.3	3.4	.3	7	61	54	Trace	88	550	.02	.04	Trace	0
35	1 tbsp	3	61	10	Trace	1	.4	.2	Trace	Trace	3	3	Trace	4	30	Trace	Trace	Trace	0
36	Cream, sour — 1 cup	230	71	495	7	48	30.0	12.1	1.1	10	268	195	.1	331	1,820	.08	.34	.2	2
37	1 tbsp	12	71	25	Trace	3	1.6	.6	.1	1	14	10	Trace	17	90	Trace	.02	Trace	Trace
	Cream products, imitation (made with vegetable fat):																		
	Sweet:																		
	Creamers:																		
38	Liquid (frozen) — 1 cup	245	77	335	2	24	22.8	.3	Trace	28	23	157	.1	467	[1]220	0	0	0	0
39	1 tbsp	15	77	20	Trace	1	1.4	Trace	0	2	1	10	Trace	29	[1]10	0	0	0	0
40	Powdered — 1 cup	94	2	515	5	33	30.6	.9	Trace	52	21	397	Trace	763	[1]190	0	[1].16	0	0
41	1 tsp	2	2	10	Trace	1	.7	Trace	0	1	Trace	8	Trace	16	[1]Trace	0	[1]Trace	0	0
	Whipped topping:																		
42	Frozen — 1 cup	75	50	240	1	19	16.3	1.0	.2	17	5	6	.1	14	[1]650	0	0	0	0
43	1 tbsp	4	50	15	Trace	1	.9	.1	Trace	1	Trace	Trace	Trace	1	[1]30	0	0	0	0
44	Powdered, made with whole milk — 1 cup	80	67	150	3	10	8.5	.6	.1	13	72	69	Trace	121	[1]290	.02	.09	Trace	1
45	1 tbsp	4	67	10	Trace	1	.4	Trace	Trace	1	4	3	Trace	6	[1]110	Trace	Trace	Trace	Trace
46	Pressurized — 1 cup	70	60	185	1	16	13.2	1.4	.2	11	4	13	Trace	13	[1]330	0	0	0	0
47	1 tbsp	4	60	10	Trace	1	.8	Trace	Trace	1	1	1	Trace	1	[1]20	0	0	0	0
48	Sour dressing (imitation sour cream) made with nonfat dry milk — 1 cup	235	75	415	8	39	31.2	4.4	1.1	11	266	205	.1	380	[1]20	.09	.38	.2	2
49	1 tbsp	12	75	20	1	2	1.6	.2	.1	2	14	10	Trace	19	[1]Trace	.01	.02	Trace	Trace
	Ice cream. See Milk desserts, frozen (items 75-80).																		
	Ice milk. See Milk desserts, frozen (items 81-83).																		
	Milk:																		
	Fluid:																		
50	Whole (3.3% fat) — 1 cup	244	88	150	8	8	5.1	2.1	.2	11	291	228	.1	370	[2]310	.09	.40	.2	2
	Lowfat (2%):																		
	No milk solids added:																		
51	1 cup	244	89	120	8	5	2.9	1.2	.1	12	297	232	.1	377	500	.10	.40	.2	2
	Milk solids added:																		
52	Label claim less than 10 g of protein per cup — 1 cup	245	89	125	9	5	2.9	1.2	.1	12	313	245	.1	397	500	.10	.42	.2	2
53	Label claim 10 or more grams of protein per cup (protein fortified) — 1 cup	246	88	135	10	5	3.0	1.2	.1	14	352	276	.1	447	500	.11	.48	.2	3
	Lowfat (1%):																		
	No milk solids added:																		
54	1 cup	244	90	100	8	3	1.6	.7	.1	12	300	235	.1	381	500	.10	.41	.2	2
	Milk solids added:																		
55	Label claim less than 10 g of protein per cup — 1 cup	245	90	105	9	2	1.5	.6	.1	12	313	245	.1	397	500	.10	.42	.2	2
56	Label claim 10 or more grams of protein per cup (protein fortified) — 1 cup	246	89	120	10	3	1.8	.7	.1	14	349	273	.1	444	500	.11	.47	.2	3
	Nonfat (skim):																		
57	No milk solids added — 1 cup	245	91	85	8	Trace	.3	.1	Trace	12	302	247	.1	406	500	.09	.37	.2	2

[1] Vitamin A value is largely from beta-carotene used for coloring. Riboflavin value for items 40-41 apply to products with added riboflavin.

[2] Applies to product without added vitamin A. With added vitamin A, value is 500 International Units (I.U.).

(Dashes (—) denote lack of reliable data for a constituent believed to be present in measurable amount)

NUTRIENTS IN INDICATED QUANTITY

Item No. (A)	Foods, approximate measures, units, and weight (edible part unless footnotes indicate otherwise) (B)	Grams	Water (C) Per cent	Food energy (D) Cal ories	Pro tein (E) grams	Fat (F) grams	Fatty Acids Satu rated (total) (G) grams	Unsaturated Oleic (H) grams	Unsaturated Lino leic (I) grams	Carbo hydrate (J) grams	Calcium (K) Milli grams	Phos phorus (L) Milli grams	Iron (M) Milli grams	Potas sium (N) Milli grams	Vitamin A value (O) Inter national units	Thiamin (P) Milli grams	Ribo flavin (Q) Milli grams	Niacin (R) Milli grams	Ascorbic acid (S) Milli grams
	DAIRY PRODUCTS (CHEESE, CREAM, IMITATION CREAM, MILK; RELATED PRODUCTS)—Con.																		
	Milk—Continued																		
	Fluid—Continued																		
	Nonfat (skim)—Continued																		
	Milk solids added:																		
58	Label claim less than 10 g of protein per cup. 1 cup	245	90	90	9	1	0.4	Trace	0.1	12	315	255	0.1	416	500	0.10	0.43	0.2	2
59	Label claim 10 or more grams of protein per cup (protein fortified). 1 cup	246	89	100	10	1	.4	.1	Trace	14	352	275	.1	446	500	.11	.48	.2	3
60	Buttermilk 1 cup	245	90	100	8	2	1.3	.5	Trace	12	285	219	.1	371	80	.08	.38	.1	2
	Canned:																		
	Evaporated, unsweetened:																		
61	Whole milk 1 cup	252	74	340	17	19	11.6	5.3	0.4	25	657	510	.5	764	610	.12	.80	.5	5
62	Skim milk 1 cup	255	79	200	19	1	.3	.1	Trace	29	738	497	.7	845	1,000	.11	.79	.4	3
63	Sweetened, condensed 1 cup	306	27	980	24	27	16.8	6.7	.7	166	868	775	.6	1,136	1,000	.28	1.27	.6	8
	Dried:																		
64	Buttermilk 1 cup	120	3	465	41	7	4.3	1.7	.2	59	1,421	1,119	.4	1,910	260	.47	1.90	1.1	7
	Nonfat instant:																		
65	Envelope, net wt., 3.2 oz. 1 envelope	91	4	325	32	1	.4	.1	Trace	47	1,120	896	.3	1,552	2,160	.38	1.59	.8	5
66	Cup. 1 cup	68	4	245	24	Trace	.3	.1	Trace	35	837	670	.2	1,160	1,610	.28	1.19	.6	4
	Milk beverages:																		
	Chocolate milk (commercial):																		
67	Regular 1 cup	250	82	210	8	8	5.3	2.2	.2	26	280	251	.6	417	300	.09	.41	.3	2
68	Lowfat (2%) 1 cup	250	84	180	8	5	3.1	1.3	.1	26	284	254	.6	422	500	.10	.42	.3	2
69	Lowfat (1%) 1 cup	250	85	160	8	3	1.5	.7	.1	26	287	257	.6	426	500	.10	.40	.2	2
70	Eggnog (commercial) 1 cup	254	74	340	10	19	11.3	5.0	.6	34	330	278	.5	420	890	.09	.48	.3	4
	Malted milk, home-prepared with 1 cup of whole milk and 2 to 3 heaping tsp of malted milk powder (about 3/4 oz):																		
71	Chocolate 1 cup of milk plus 3/4 oz of powder.	265	81	235	9	9	5.5	—	—	29	304	265	.5	500	330	.14	.43	.7	2
72	Natural 1 cup of milk plus 3/4 oz of powder.	265	81	235	11	10	6.0	—	—	27	347	307	.3	529	380	.20	.54	1.3	2
	Shakes, thick:																		
73	Chocolate, container, net wt., 10.6 oz. 1 container	300	72	355	9	8	5.0	2.0	.2	63	396	378	.9	672	260	.14	.67	.4	0
74	Vanilla, container, net wt., 11 oz. 1 container	313	74	350	12	9	5.9	2.4	.2	56	457	361	.3	572	360	.09	.61	.5	0
	Milk desserts, frozen:																		
	Ice cream:																		
	Regular (about 11% fat):																		
75	Hardened 1/2 gal	1,064	61	2,155	38	115	71.3	28.8	2.6	254	1,406	1,075	1.0	2,052	4,340	.42	2.63	1.1	6
76	1 cup	133	61	270	5	14	8.9	3.6	.3	32	176	134	.1	257	540	.05	.33	.1	1
77	3-fl oz container	50	61	100	2	5	3.4	1.4	.1	12	66	51	Trace	96	200	.02	.12	.1	Trace
78	Soft serve (frozen custard) 1 cup	173	60	375	7	23	13.5	5.9	.6	38	236	199	.4	338	790	.08	.45	.2	1
79	Rich (about 16% fat), hardened. 1/2 gal	1,188	59	2,805	33	190	118.3	47.8	4.3	256	1,213	927	.8	1,771	7,200	.36	2.27	.9	5
80	1 cup	148	59	350	4	24	14.7	6.0	.5	32	151	115	.1	221	900	.04	.28	.1	1
	Ice milk:																		
81	Hardened (about 4.3% fat) 1/2 gal	1,048	69	1,470	41	45	28.1	11.3	1.0	232	1,409	1,035	1.5	2,117	1,710	.61	2.78	.9	6
82	1 cup	131	69	185	5	6	3.5	1.4	.1	29	176	129	.1	265	210	.08	.35	.1	1

(A)	(B)		wt (g)	(C)	(D)	(E)	(F)	(G)	(H)	(I)	(J)	(K)	(L)	(M)	(N)	(O)	(P)	(Q)	(R)	(S)
83	Soft serve (about 2.6% fat)	1 cup	175	70	225	8	5	2.9	1.2	0.7	38	274	202	0.3	412	180	0.12	0.54	0.2	1
84	Sherbet (about 2% fat)	1/2 gal	1,542	66	2,160	17	31	19.0	7.7	.7	469	827	594	2.5	1,585	1,480	.26	.71	.2	31
85		1 cup	193	66	270	2	4	2.4	1.0	.1	59	103	74	.3	198	190	.03	.09	.1	4
	Milk desserts, other:																			
86	Custard, baked	1 cup	265	77	305	14	15	6.8	5.4	.7	29	297	310	1.1	387	930	.11	.50	.3	1
	Puddings:																			
	From home recipe:																			
	Starch base:																			
87	Chocolate	1 cup	260	66	385	8	12	7.6	3.3	.3	67	250	255	1.3	445	390	.05	.36	.3	1
88	Vanilla (blancmange)	1 cup	255	76	285	9	10	6.2	2.5	.2	41	298	232	Trace	352	410	.08	.41	.3	2
89	Tapioca cream	1 cup	165	72	220	8	8	4.1	2.5	.5	28	173	180	.7	223	480	.07	.30	.2	2
	From mix (chocolate) and milk:																			
90	Regular (cooked)	1 cup	260	70	320	9	8	4.3	2.6	.2	59	265	247	.8	354	340	.05	.39	.3	2
91	Instant	1 cup	260	69	325	8	7	3.6	2.2	.3	63	374	237	1.3	335	340	.08	.39	.3	2
	Yogurt:																			
	With added milk solids:																			
	Made with lowfat milk:																			
92	Fruit-flavored[9]	1 container, net wt., 8 oz	227	75	230	10	3	1.8	.6	.1	42	343	269	.2	439	[10]120	.08	.40	.2	1
93	Plain	1 container, net wt., 8 oz	227	85	145	12	4	2.3	.8	.1	16	415	326	.2	531	[10]150	.10	.49	.3	2
94	Made with nonfat milk	1 container, net wt., 8 oz	227	85	125	13	Trace	.3	.1	Trace	17	452	355	.2	579	[10]20	.11	.53	.3	2
	Without added milk solids:																			
95	Made with whole milk	1 container, net wt., 8 oz	227	88	140	8	7	4.8	1.7	.1	11	274	215	.1	351	280	.07	.32	.2	1
	EGGS																			
	Eggs, large (24 oz per dozen):																			
	Raw:																			
96	Whole, without shell	1 egg	50	75	80	6	6	1.7	2.0	.6	1	28	90	1.0	65	260	.04	.15	Trace	0
97	White	1 white	33	88	15	3	Trace	0	0	0	Trace	4	4	Trace	45	0	Trace	.09	Trace	0
98	Yolk	1 yolk	17	49	65	3	6	1.7	2.1	.6	Trace	26	86	.9	15	310	.04	.07	Trace	0
	Cooked:																			
99	Fried in butter	1 egg	46	72	85	5	6	2.4	2.2	.6	1	26	80	.9	58	290	.03	.13	Trace	0
100	Hard-cooked, shell removed	1 egg	50	75	80	6	6	1.7	2.0	.6	1	28	90	1.0	65	260	.04	.14	Trace	0
101	Poached	1 egg	50	74	80	6	6	1.7	2.0	.6	1	28	90	1.0	65	260	.04	.13	Trace	0
102	Scrambled (milk added) in butter. Also omelet	1 egg	64	76	95	6	7	2.8	2.3	.6	1	47	97	.9	85	310	.04	.16	Trace	0
	FATS, OILS; RELATED PRODUCTS																			
	Butter:																			
	Regular (1 brick or 4 sticks per lb):																			
103	Stick (1/2 cup)	1 stick	113	16	815	1	92	57.3	23.1	2.1	Trace	27	26	.2	29	[11]3,470	.01	.04	Trace	0
104	Tablespoon (about 1/8 stick)	1 tbsp	14	16	100	Trace	12	7.2	2.9	.3	Trace	3	3	Trace	4	[11]430	Trace	Trace	Trace	0
105	Pat (1 in square, 1/3 in high; 90 per lb)	1 pat	5	16	35	Trace	4	2.5	1.0	.1	Trace	1	1	Trace	1	[11]150	Trace	Trace	Trace	0
	Whipped (6 sticks or two 8-oz containers per lb):																			
106	Stick (1/2 cup)	1 stick	76	16	540	1	61	38.2	15.4	1.4	Trace	18	17	.1	20	[11]2,310	Trace	.03	Trace	0
107	Tablespoon (about 1/8 stick)	1 tbsp	9	16	65	Trace	8	4.7	1.9	.2	Trace	2	2	Trace	2	[11]290	Trace	Trace	Trace	0
108	Pat (1 1/4 in square, 1/3 in high; 120 per lb)	1 pat	4	16	25	Trace	3	1.9	.8	.1	Trace	1	1	Trace	1	[11]120	0	Trace	Trace	0

[3] Applies to product without vitamin A added.
[4] Applies to product with added vitamin A. Without added vitamin A, value is 20 International Units (I.U.).
[5] Yields 1 qt of fluid milk when reconstituted according to package directions.
[7] Weight applies to product with label claim of 1 1/3 cups equal 3.2 oz.
[8] Applies to products made from thick shake mixes and that do not contain added ice cream. Products made from milk shake mixes are higher in fat and usually contain added ice cream.
[9] Content of fat, vitamin A, and carbohydrate varies. Consult the label when precise values are needed for special diets.
[10] Applies to product made with milk containing no added vitamin A.
[11] Based on year-round average.

(Dashes (—) denote lack of reliable data for a constituent believed to be present in measurable amount)

NUTRIENTS IN INDICATED QUANTITY

Item No. (A)	Foods, approximate measure, units, and weight (edible part unless footnotes indicate otherwise) (B)	Grams	Water (C) Per cent	Food energy (D) Calories	Protein (E) Grams	Fat (F) Grams	Fatty Acids Saturated (total) (G) Grams	Oleic (H) Grams	Linoleic (I) Grams	Carbohydrate (J) Grams	Calcium (K) Milligrams	Phosphorus (L) Milligrams	Iron (M) Milligrams	Potassium (N) Milligrams	Vitamin A value (O) International units	Thiamin (P) Milligrams	Riboflavin (Q) Milligrams	Niacin (R) Milligrams	Ascorbic acid (S) Milligrams
	FATS, OILS; RELATED PRODUCTS—Con.																		
109	Fats, cooking (vegetable shortening). 1 cup	200	0	1,770	0	200	48.8	88.2	48.4	0	0	0	0	0	—	0	0	0	0
110	1 tbsp	13	0	110	0	13	3.2	5.7	3.1	0	0	0	0	0	0	0	0	0	0
111	Lard 1 cup	205	0	1,850	0	205	81.0	83.8	20.5	0	0	0	0	0	0	0	0	0	0
112	1 tbsp	13	0	115	0	13	5.1	5.3	1.3	0	0	0	0	0	0	0	0	0	0
	Margarine: Regular (1 brick or 4 sticks per lb):																		
113	Stick (1/2 cup) 1 stick	113	16	815	1	92	16.7	42.9	24.9	Trace	27	26	.2	29	[12]3,750	.01	.04	Trace	0
114	Tablespoon (about 1/8 stick) 1 tbsp	14	16	100	Trace	12	2.1	5.3	3.1	Trace	3	3	Trace	4	[12]470	Trace	Trace	Trace	0
115	Pat (1 in square, 1/3 in high; 90 per lb). 1 pat	5	16	35	Trace	4	.7	1.9	1.1	Trace	1	1	Trace	1	[12]170	Trace	Trace	Trace	0
116	Soft, two 8-oz containers per lb. 1 container	227	16	1,635	1	184	32.5	71.5	65.4	Trace	53	52	.4	59	[12]7,500	.01	.08	.1	0
117	1 tbsp	14	16	100	Trace	12	2.0	4.5	4.1	Trace	3	3	Trace	4	[12]470	Trace	Trace	Trace	0
	Whipped (6 sticks per lb):																		
118	Stick (1/2 cup) 1 stick	76	16	545	Trace	61	11.2	28.7	16.7	Trace	18	17	.1	20	[12]2,500	Trace	.03	Trace	0
119	Tablespoon (about 1/8 stick). 1 tbsp	9	16	70	Trace	8	1.4	3.6	2.1	Trace	2	2	Trace	2	[12]310	Trace	Trace	Trace	0
	Oils, salad or cooking:																		
120	Corn 1 cup	218	0	1,925	0	218	27.7	53.6	125.1	0	0	0	0	0	—	0	0	0	0
121	1 tbsp	14	0	120	0	14	1.7	3.3	7.8	0	0	0	0	0	—	0	0	0	0
122	Olive 1 cup	216	0	1,910	0	216	30.7	154.4	17.7	0	0	0	0	0	—	0	0	0	0
123	1 tbsp	14	0	120	0	14	1.9	9.7	1.1	0	0	0	0	0	—	0	0	0	0
124	Peanut 1 cup	216	0	1,910	0	216	37.4	98.5	67.0	0	0	0	0	0	—	0	0	0	0
125	1 tbsp	14	0	120	0	14	2.3	6.2	4.2	0	0	0	0	0	—	0	0	0	0
126	Safflower 1 cup	218	0	1,925	0	218	20.5	25.9	159.8	0	0	0	0	0	—	0	0	0	0
127	1 tbsp	14	0	120	0	14	1.3	1.6	10.0	0	0	0	0	0	—	0	0	0	0
128	Soybean oil, hydrogenated (partially hardened). 1 cup	218	0	1,925	0	218	31.8	93.1	75.6	0	0	0	0	0	—	0	0	0	0
129	1 tbsp	14	0	120	0	14	2.0	5.8	4.7	0	0	0	0	0	—	0	0	0	0
130	Soybean-cottonseed oil blend, hydrogenated. 1 cup	218	0	1,925	0	218	38.2	63.0	99.6	0	0	0	0	0	—	0	0	0	0
131	1 tbsp	14	0	120	0	14	2.4	3.9	6.2	0	0	0	0	0	—	0	0	0	0
	Salad dressings: Commercial: Blue cheese:																		
132	Regular 1 tbsp	15	32	75	1	8	1.6	1.7	3.8	1	12	11	Trace	6	30	Trace	.02	Trace	Trace
133	Low calorie (5 Cal per tsp) 1 tbsp	16	84	10	Trace	1	.5	.3	Trace	1	10	8	Trace	5	30	Trace	.01	Trace	Trace
	French:																		
134	Regular 1 tbsp	16	39	65	Trace	6	1.1	1.3	3.2	3	2	2	.1	13	—	Trace	—	—	—
135	Low calorie (5 Cal per tsp) 1 tbsp	16	77	15	Trace	1	.1	.1	.4	2	2	2	.1	13	—	Trace	—	—	—
	Italian:																		
136	Regular 1 tbsp	15	28	85	Trace	9	1.6	1.9	4.7	1	2	1	Trace	2	Trace	Trace	Trace	Trace	—
137	Low calorie (2 Cal per tsp) 1 tbsp	15	90	10	Trace	1	.1	.1	.4	Trace	2	1	Trace	2	Trace	Trace	Trace	Trace	—
138	Mayonnaise 1 tbsp	14	15	100	Trace	11	2.0	2.4	5.6	Trace	3	4	.1	5	40	Trace	.01	Trace	—
	Mayonnaise type:																		
139	Regular 1 tbsp	15	41	65	Trace	6	1.1	1.4	3.2	2	2	4	Trace	1	30	Trace	Trace	Trace	—
140	Low calorie (8 Cal per tsp) 1 tbsp	16	81	20	Trace	2	.4	.4	1.0	2	3	1	Trace	1	40	Trace	Trace	Trace	—
141	Tartar sauce, regular 1 tbsp	14	34	75	Trace	8	1.5	1.8	4.1	1	3	4	.1	11	30	Trace	Trace	Trace	Trace
	Thousand Island:																		
142	Regular 1 tbsp	16	32	80	Trace	8	1.4	1.7	4.0	2	2	3	.1	18	50	Trace	Trace	Trace	Trace
143	Low calorie (10 Cal per tsp) 1 tbsp	15	68	25	Trace	2	.4	.4	1.0	2	2	3	.1	17	50	Trace	Trace	Trace	Trace
144	From home recipe: Cooked type[13] 1 tbsp	16	68	25	1	2	.5	.6	.3	2	14	15	.1	19	80	.01	.03	Trace	Trace

FISH, SHELLFISH, MEAT, POULTRY: RELATED PRODUCTS

(A)	(B)	(g)	(C)	(D)	(E)	(F)	(G)	(H)	(I)	(J)	(K)	(L)	(M)	(N)	(O)	(P)	(Q)	(R)	(S)
	Fish and shellfish:																		
145	Bluefish, baked with butter or margarine[13], 3 oz	85	68	135	22	4	—	—	—	0	25	244	0.6	—	40	0.09	0.08	1.6	—
	Clams:																		
146	Raw, meat only, 3 oz	85	82	65	11	1	—	—	—	2	59	138	5.2	154	90	.08	.15	1.1	8
147	Canned, solids and liquid, 3 oz	85	86	45	7	1	0.2	Trace	Trace	2	47	116	3.5	119	—	—	.09	.9	—
148	Crabmeat (white or king), canned, not pressed down, 1 cup	135	77	135	24	3	.6	0.4	0.1	1	61	246	1.1	149	—	.11	.11	2.6	—
149	Fish sticks, breaded, cooked, frozen (stick, 4 by 1 by 1/2 in), 1 fish stick or 1 oz	28	66	50	5	3	—	—	—	2	3	47	.1	—	0	.01	.02	.5	—
150	Haddock, breaded, fried[14], 3 oz	85	66	140	17	5	1.4	2.2	1.2	5	34	210	1.0	296	—	.03	.06	2.7	—
151	Ocean perch, breaded, fried[14], 1 fillet	85	59	195	16	11	2.7	4.4	2.3	6	28	192	1.1	242	—	.10	.10	1.6	—
152	Oysters, raw, meat only (13–19 medium Selects), 1 cup	240	85	160	20	4	1.3	.2	.1	8	226	343	13.2	290	740	.34	.43	6.0	2
153	Salmon, pink, canned, solids and liquid, 3 oz	85	71	120	17	5	.9	.8	.1	0	167[15]	243	.7	307	60	.03	.16	6.8	—
154	Sardines, Atlantic, canned in oil, drained solids, 3 oz	85	62	175	20	9	3.0	2.5	.5	0	372	424	2.5	502	190	.02	.17	4.6	—
155	Scallops, frozen, breaded, fried, reheated, 6 scallops	90	60	175	16	8	—	—	—	9	—	—	—	—	—	—	—	—	—
156	Shad, baked with butter or margarine, bacon[13], 3 oz	85	64	170	20	10	—	—	—	0	20	266	.5	320	30	.11	.22	7.3	—
	Shrimp:																		
157	Canned meat, 3 oz	85	70	100	21	1	.1	.1	Trace	1	98	224	2.6	104	50	.01	.03	1.5	—
158	French fried[16], 3 oz	85	57	190	17	9	2.3	3.7	2.0	9	61	162	1.7	195	—	.03	.07	2.3	—
159	Tuna, canned in oil, drained solids, 3 oz	85	61	170	24	7	1.7	1.7	.7	0	7	199	1.6	—	70	.04	.10	10.1	2
160	Tuna salad[17], 1 cup	205	70	350	30	22	4.3	6.3	6.7	7	41	291	2.7	—	590	.08	.23	10.3	2
	Meat and meat products:																		
161	Bacon, (20 slices per lb, raw), broiled or fried, crisp, 2 slices	15	8	85	4	8	2.5	3.7	.7	Trace	2	34	.5	35	0	.08	.05	.8	—
	Beef, cooked:																		
	Cuts braised, simmered or pot roasted:																		
162	Lean and fat (piece, 2 1/2 by 2 1/2 by 3/4 in), 3 oz	85	53	245	23	16	6.8	6.5	.4	0	10	114	2.9	184	30	.04	.18	3.6	—
163	Lean only from item 162[18], 2.5 oz	72	62	140	22	5	2.1	1.8	.2	0	10	108	2.7	176	10	.04	.17	3.3	—
	Ground beef, broiled:																		
164	Lean with 10% fat, 3 oz or patty 3 by 5/8 in	85	60	185	23	10	4.0	3.9	.3	0	10	196	3.0	261	20	.08	.20	5.1	—
165	Lean with 21% fat, 2.9 oz or patty 3 by 5/8 in	82	54	235	20	17	7.0	6.7	.4	0	9	159	2.6	221	30	.07	.17	4.4	—
	Roast, oven cooked, no liquid added:																		
	Relatively fat, such as rib:																		
166	Lean and fat (2 pieces, 4 1/8 by 2 1/4 by 1/4 in), 3 oz	85	40	375	17	33	14.0	13.6	.8	0	8	158	2.2	189	70	.05	.13	3.1	—
167	Lean only from item 166[18], 1.8 oz	51	57	125	14	7	3.0	2.5	.3	0	6	131	1.8	161	10	.04	.11	2.6	—
	Relatively lean, such as heel of round:																		
168	Lean and fat (2 pieces, 4 1/8 by 2 1/4 by 1/4 in), 3 oz	85	62	165	25	7	2.8	2.7	.2	0	11	208	3.2	279	10	.06	.19	4.5	—

[12] Based on average vitamin A content of fortified margarine. Federal specifications for fortified margarine require a minimum of 15,000 International Units (I.U.) of vitamin A per pound.

[13] Fatty acid values apply to product made with regular-type margarine.

[14] Dipped in egg, milk or water, and breadcrumbs; fried in vegetable shortening.

[15] If bones are discarded, value for calcium will be greatly reduced.

[16] Dipped in egg, breadcrumbs, and flour or batter.

[17] Prepared with tuna, celery, salad dressing (mayonnaise type), pickle, onion, and egg.

[18] Outer layer of fat on the cut was removed to within approximately 1/2 in of the lean. Deposits of fat within the cut were not removed.

(Dashes (—) denote lack of reliable data for a constituent believed to be present in measurable amount)

Item No. (A)	Foods, approximate measures, units, and weight (edible part unless footnotes indicate otherwise) (B)	Weight (Grams)	Water (C) Percent	Food energy (D) Calories	Protein (E) Grams	Fat (F) Grams	Saturated (total) (G) Grams	Oleic (H) Grams	Linoleic (I) Grams	Carbohydrate (J) Grams	Calcium (K) Milligrams	Phosphorus (L) Milligrams	Iron (M) Milligrams	Potassium (N) Milligrams	Vitamin A value (O) International units	Thiamin (P) Milligrams	Riboflavin (Q) Milligrams	Niacin (R) Milligrams	Ascorbic acid (S) Milligrams
	FISH, SHELLFISH, MEAT, POULTRY: RELATED PRODUCTS—Con.																		
	Meat and meat products—Continued																		
	Beef,[1] cooked—Continued																		
	Roast, oven cooked, no liquid added—Continued																		
	Relatively lean such as heel of round—Continued																		
169	Lean only from item 168, 2.8 oz	78	65	125	24	3	1.2	1.0	0.1	0	10	199	3.0	268	Trace	0.06	0.18	4.3	—
	Steak:																		
	Relatively fat-sirloin, broiled:																		
170	Lean and fat (piece, 2 1/2 by 2 1/2 by 3/4 in), 3 oz	85	44	330	20	27	11.3	11.1	.6	0	9	162	2.5	220	50	.05	.15	4.0	—
171	Lean only from item 170, 2.0 oz	56	59	115	18	4	1.8	1.6	.2	0	7	146	2.2	202	10	.05	.14	3.6	—
	Relatively lean-round, braised:																		
172	Lean and fat (piece, 4 1/8 by 2 1/4 by 1/2 in), 3 oz	85	55	220	24	13	5.5	5.2	.4	0	10	213	3.0	272	20	.07	.19	4.8	—
173	Lean only from item 172, 2.4 oz	68	61	130	21	4	1.7	1.5	.2	0	9	182	2.5	238	10	.05	.16	4.1	—
	Beef, canned:																		
174	Corned beef, 3 oz	85	59	185	22	10	4.9	4.5	.2	0	17	90	3.7	—	—	.01	.20	2.9	—
175	Corned beef hash, 1 cup	220	67	400	19	25	11.9	10.9	.5	24	29	147	4.4	440	—	.02	.20	4.6	—
176	Beef, dried, chipped, 2 1/2-oz jar	71	48	145	24	4	2.1	2.0	.1	0	14	287	3.6	142	—	.05	.23	2.7	0
177	Beef and vegetable stew, 1 cup	245	82	220	16	11	4.9	4.5	.2	15	29	184	2.9	613	2,400	.15	.17	4.7	17
178	Beef potpie (home recipe), baked[19] (piece, 1/3 of 9-in diam. pie), 1 piece	210	55	515	21	30	7.9	12.8	6.7	39	29	149	3.8	334	1,720	.30	.30	5.5	6
179	Chili con carne with beans, canned, 1 cup	255	72	340	19	16	7.5	6.8	.3	31	82	321	4.3	594	150	.08	.18	3.3	—
180	Chop suey with beef and pork (home recipe), 1 cup	250	75	300	26	17	8.5	6.2	.7	13	60	248	4.8	425	600	.28	.38	5.0	33
181	Heart, beef, lean, braised, 3 oz	85	61	160	27	5	1.5	1.1	.6	1	5	154	5.0	197	20	.21	1.04	6.5	1
	Lamb, cooked:																		
	Chop, rib (cut 3 per lb with bone), broiled:																		
182	Lean and fat, 3.1 oz	89	43	360	18	32	14.8	12.1	1.2	0	8	139	1.0	200	—	.11	.19	4.1	—
183	Lean only from item 182, 2 oz	57	60	120	16	6	2.5	2.1	.2	0	6	121	1.1	174	—	.09	.15	3.4	—
	Leg, roasted:																		
184	Lean and fat (2 pieces, 4 1/8 by 2 1/4 by 1/4 in), 3 oz	85	54	235	22	16	7.3	6.0	.6	0	9	177	1.4	241	—	.13	.23	4.7	—
185	Lean only from item 184, 2.5 oz	71	62	130	20	5	2.1	1.8	.2	0	9	169	1.4	227	—	.12	.21	4.4	—
	Shoulder, roasted:																		
186	Lean and fat (3 pieces, 2 1/2 by 2 1/2 by 1/4 in), 3 oz	85	50	285	18	23	10.8	8.8	.9	0	9	146	1.0	206	—	.11	.20	4.0	—
187	Lean only from item 186, 2.3 oz	64	61	130	17	6	3.6	2.3	.2	0	8	140	1.0	193	—	.10	.18	3.7	—
188	Liver, beef, fried[20] (slice, 6 1/2 by 2 3/8 by 3/8 in), 3 oz	85	56	195	22	9	2.5	3.5	.9	5	9	405	7.5	323	[21]45,390	.22	3.56	14.0	23
	Pork, cured, cooked:																		
189	Ham, light cure, lean and fat, roasted (2 pieces, 4 1/8 by 2 1/4 by 1/4 in)[22], 3 oz	85	54	245	18	19	6.8	7.9	1.7	0	8	146	2.2	199	0	.40	.15	3.1	—
	Luncheon meat:																		
190	Boiled ham, slice (8 per 8-oz pkg.), 1 oz	28	59	65	5	5	1.7	2.0	.4	0	3	47	.8	—	0	.12	.04	.7	—
191	Canned, spiced or unspiced: Slice, approx. 3 by 2 by 1/2 in, 1 slice	60	55	175	9	15	5.4	6.7	1.0	1	5	65	1.3	133	0	.19	.13	1.8	—

(A)	(B)	(C)	(D)	(E)	(F)	(G)	(H)	(I)	(J)	(K)	(L)	(M)	(N)	(O)	(P)	(Q)	(R)	(S)
	Pork, fresh,[18] cooked:																	
	Chop, loin (cut 3 per lb with bone), broiled:																	
192	Lean and fat---- 2.7 oz	78	305	19	25	8.9	10.4	2.2	0	9	209	2.7	216	0	0.75	0.22	4.5	—
193	Lean only from item 192---- 2 oz	56	150	17	.9	3.1	3.6	.8	0	7	181	2.2	192	0	.63	.18	3.8	—
	Roast, oven cooked, no liquid added:																	
194	Lean and fat (piece, 2 1/2 by 2 1/2 by 3/4 in). 3 oz	85	310	21	24	8.7	10.2	2.2	0	9	218	2.7	233	0	.78	.22	4.8	—
195	Lean only from item 194---- 2.4 oz	68	175	20	10	3.5	4.1	.8	0	9	211	2.6	224	0	.73	.21	4.4	—
	Shoulder cut, simmered:																	
196	Lean and fat (3 pieces, 2 1/2 by 2 1/2 by 1/4 in). 3 oz	85	320	20	26	9.3	10.9	2.3	0	9	118	2.6	158	0	.46	.21	4.1	—
197	Lean only from item 196---- 2.2 oz	63	135	18	6	2.2	2.6	.6	0	8	111	2.3	146	0	.42	.19	3.7	—
	Sausages (see also Luncheon meat: (items 190-191)):																	
198	Bologna, slice (8 per 8-oz pkg.). 1 slice	28	85	3	8	3.0	3.4	.5	Trace	2	36	.5	65	—	.05	.06	.7	—
199	Braunschweiger, slice (6 per 6-oz pkg.). 1 slice	28	90	4	8	2.6	3.4	.8	1	3	69	1.7	—	1,850	.05	.41	2.3	—
200	Brown and serve (10-11 per 8-oz pkg.), browned. 1 link	17	70	3	6	2.3	2.8	.7	Trace	—	—	—	—	0	—	—	—	—
201	Deviled ham, canned---- 1 tbsp	13	45	2	4	1.5	1.8	.4	0	—	12	.3	—	0	.02	.01	.2	—
202	Frankfurter (8 per 1-lb pkg.), cooked (reheated)---- 1 frankfurter	56	170	7	15	5.6	6.5	1.2	1	3	57	.8	—	—	.08	.11	1.4	—
203	Meat, potted (beef, chicken, turkey), canned. 1 tbsp	13	30	2	2	—	—	—	0	—	—	—	—	—	Trace	.03	.2	—
204	Pork link (16 per 1-lb pkg.), cooked. 1 link	13	60	2	6	2.1	2.4	.5	Trace	1	21	.3	35	0	.10	.04	.5	—
	Salami:																	
205	Dry type, slice (12 per 4-oz pkg.). 1 slice	10	45	2	4	1.6	1.6	.1	Trace	1	28	.4	—	—	.04	.03	.5	—
206	Cooked type, slice (8 per 8-oz pkg.). 1 slice	28	90	5	7	3.1	3.0	.2	Trace	3	57	.7	—	—	.07	.07	1.2	—
207	Vienna sausage (7 per 4-oz can). 1 sausage	16	40	2	3	1.2	1.4	.2	Trace	1	24	.3	—	—	.01	.02	.4	—
	Veal, medium fat, cooked, bone removed:																	
208	Cutlet (4 1/8 by 2 1/4 by 1/2 in), braised or broiled. 3 oz	85	185	23	9	4.0	3.4	.4	0	9	196	2.7	258	—	.06	.21	4.6	—
209	Rib (2 pieces, 4 1/8 by 2 1/4 by 1/4 in), roasted. 3 oz	85	230	23	14	6.1	5.1	.6	0	10	211	2.9	259	—	.11	.26	6.6	—
	Poultry and poultry products:																	
	Chicken, cooked:																	
210	Breast, fried,[23] bones removed, 1/2 breast (3.3 oz with bones). 2.8 oz	79	160	26	5	1.4	1.8	1.1	1	9	218	1.3	—	70	.04	.17	11.6	—
211	Drumstick, fried,[23] bones removed (2 oz with bones). 1.3 oz	38	90	12	4	1.1	1.3	.9	Trace	6	89	.9	—	50	.03	.15	2.7	—
212	Half broiler, broiled, bones removed (10.4 oz with bones). 6.2 oz	176	240	42	7	2.2	2.5	1.3	0	16	355	3.0	483	160	.09	.34	15.5	—
213	Chicken, canned, boneless---- 3 oz	85	170	18	10	3.2	3.8	2.0	0	18	210	1.3	117	200	.03	.11	3.7	3
214	Chicken a la king, cooked (home recipe)---- 1 cup	245	470	27	34	12.7	14.3	3.3	12	127	358	2.5	404	1,130	.10	.42	5.4	12
215	Chicken and noodles, cooked (home recipe). 1 cup	240	365	22	18	5.9	7.1	3.5	26	26	247	2.2	149	430	.05	.17	4.3	Trace

[18] Outer layer of fat on the cut was removed to within approximately 1/2 in. of the lean. Deposits of fat within the cut were not removed.
[19] Crust made with vegetable shortening and enriched flour.
[20] Value varies widely.
[21] Regular-type margarine used.
[22] About one-fourth of the outer layer of fat on the cut was removed. Deposits of fat within the cut were not removed.
[23] Vegetable shortening used.

(Dashes (—) denote lack of reliable data for a constituent believed to be present in measurable amount)

								Fatty Acids												
									Unsaturated											
Item No.	Foods, approximate measures, units, and weight (edible part unless footnotes indicate otherwise)		Water	Food energy	Protein	Fat	Saturated (total)	Oleic	Linoleic	Carbohydrate	Calcium	Phosphorus	Iron	Potassium	Vitamin A value	Thiamin	Riboflavin	Niacin	Ascorbic acid
(A)	(B)	Grams	(C) Percent	(D) Calories	(E) Grams	(F) Grams	(G) Grams	(H) Grams	(I) Grams	(I) Grams	(K) Milligrams	(L) Milligrams	(M) Milligrams	(N) Milligrams	(O) International units	(P) Milligrams	(Q) Milligrams	(R) Milligrams	(S) Milligrams
	FISH, SHELLFISH, MEAT, POULTRY: RELATED PRODUCTS—Con.																		
	Poultry and poultry products—Continued																		
	Chicken chow mein:																		
216	Canned	250	89	95	7	Trace				18	45	35	1.3	418	150	0.05	0.10	1.0	13
217	From home recipe	250	78	255	31	10	2.4	3.4	3.1	10	58	293	2.5	473	280	.08	.23	4.3	10
218	Chicken potpie (home recipe), baked,19 piece (1/3 or 9-in diam.18 pie).	232	57	545	23	31	11.3	10.9	5.6	42	70	232	3.0	343	3,090	.34	.31	5.5	5
	Turkey, roasted, flesh without skin:																		
219	Dark meat, piece, 2 1/2 by 1 5/8 by 1/4 in.	85	61	175	26	7	2.1	1.5	1.5	0	—	—	2.0	338	—	.03	.20	3.6	—
220	Light meat, piece, 4 by 2 by 1/4 in.	85	62	150	28	3	.9	.6	.7	0	—	—	1.0	349	—	.04	.12	9.4	—
	Light and dark meat:																		
221	Chopped or diced	140	61	265	44	9	2.5	1.7	1.8	0	11	351	2.5	514	—	.07	.25	10.8	—
222	Pieces (1 slice white meat, 4 by 2 by 1/4 in with 2 slices dark meat, 2 1/2 by 1 5/8 by 1/4 in).	85	61	160	27	5	1.5	1.0	1.1	0	7	213	1.5	312	—	.04	.15	6.5	—
	FRUITS AND FRUIT PRODUCTS																		
	Apples, raw, unpeeled, without cores:																		
223	2 3/4-in diam. (about 3 per lb with cores).	138	84	80	Trace	1				20	10	14	.4	152	120	.04	.03	.1	6
224	3 1/4 in diam. (about 2 per lb with cores).	212	84	125	Trace	1				31	15	21	.6	233	190	.06	.04	.2	8
225	Applejuice, bottled or canned2ᵃ	248	88	120	Trace	Trace				30	15	22	1.5	250	.	.02	.05	.2	2²5
	Applesauce, canned:																		
226	Sweetened	255	76	230	1	Trace				61	10	13	1.3	166	100	.05	.03	.1	2³5
227	Unsweetened	244	89	100	Trace	Trace				26	10	12	1.2	190	100	.05	.02	.1	2³5
	Apricots:																		
228	Raw, without pits (about 12 per lb with pits).	107	85	55	1	Trace				14	18	25	.5	301	2,890	.03	.04	.6	11
229	Canned in heavy syrup (halves and syrup).	258	77	220	2	Trace				57	28	39	.8	604	4,490	.05	.05	1.0	10
	Dried:																		
230	Uncooked (28 large or 37 medium halves per cup).	130	25	340	7	1				86	87	140	7.2	1,273	14,170	.01	.21	4.3	16
231	Cooked, unsweetened, fruit and liquid.	250	76	215	4	1				54	55	88	4.5	795	7,500	.01	.13	2.5	8
232	Apricot nectar, canned	251	85	145	1	Trace				37	23	30	.5	379	2,380	.03	.03	.5	2⁴36
	Avocados, raw, whole, without skins and seeds:																		
233	California, mid- and late-winter (with skin and seed, 3 1/8-in diam.; wt. 10 oz).	216	74	370	5	37	5.5	22.0	3.7	13	22	91	1.3	1,303	630	.24	.43	3.5	30
234	Florida, late summer and fall (with skin and seed, 3 5/8-in diam.; wt. 1 lb).	304	78	390	4	33	6.7	15.7	5.3	27	30	128	1.8	1,836	880	.33	.61	4.9	43
235	Banana without peel (about 2.6 per lb with peel).	119	76	100	1	Trace				26	10	31	.8	440	230	.06	.07	.8	12
236	Banana flakes	6	3	20	Trace	Trace				5	2	6	.2	92	50	.01	.01	.2	Trace

(A)	(B)	(C)	(D)	(E)	(F)	(G)	(H)	(I)	(J)	(K)	(L)	(M)	(N)	(O)	(P)	(Q)	(R)	(S)
237	Blackberries, raw——— 1 cup———	144	85	85	2	1	—	—	—	19	46	27	1.3	245	290	0.04	0.06	0.6	30
238	Blueberries, raw——— 1 cup———	145	83	90	1	1	—	—	—	22	22	19	1.5	117	150	.04	.09	.7	20
	Cantaloup. See Muskmelons (item 271).																		
	Cherries:																		
239	Sour (tart), red, pitted, canned, water pack. 1 cup———	244	88	105	2	Trace	—	—	—	26	37	32	.7	317	1,660	.07	.05	.5	12
240	Sweet, raw, without pits and stems. 10 cherries———	68	80	45	1	Trace	—	—	—	12	15	13	.3	129	70	.03	.04	.3	7
241	Cranberry juice cocktail, bottled, sweetened. 1 cup———	253	83	165	Trace	Trace	—	—	—	42	13	8	.8	25	Trace	.03	.03	.1	[27]81
242	Cranberry sauce, sweetened, canned, strained. 1 cup———	277	62	405	Trace	1	—	—	—	104	17	11	.6	83	60	.03	.03	.1	6
	Dates:																		
243	Whole, without pits——— 10 dates———	80	23	220	2	Trace	—	—	—	58	47	50	2.4	518	40	.07	.08	1.8	0
244	Chopped——— 1 cup———	178	23	490	4	1	—	—	—	130	105	112	5.3	1,153	90	.16	.18	3.9	0
245	Fruit cocktail, canned, in heavy sirup. 1 cup———	255	80	195	1	Trace	—	—	—	50	23	31	1.0	411	360	.05	.03	1.0	5
	Grapefruit:																		
	Raw, medium, 3 3/4-in diam. (about 1 lb 1 oz):																		
246	Pink or red[28] 1/2 grapefruit with peel[28]	241	89	50	1	Trace	—	—	—	13	20	20	.5	166	540	.05	.02	.2	44
247	White[28] 1/2 grapefruit with peel[28]	241	89	45	1	Trace	—	—	—	12	19	19	.5	159	10	.05	.02	.2	44
248	Canned, sections with sirup 1 cup———	254	81	180	2	Trace	—	—	—	45	33	36	.8	343	30	.08	.05	.5	76
	Grapefruit juice:																		
249	Raw, pink, red, or white 1 cup———	246	90	95	1	Trace	—	—	—	23	22	37	.5	399	([29])	.10	.05	.5	93
	Canned, white:																		
250	Unsweetened——— 1 cup———	247	89	100	1	Trace	—	—	—	24	20	35	1.0	400	20	.07	.05	.5	84
251	Sweetened——— 1 cup———	250	86	135	1	Trace	—	—	—	32	20	35	1.0	405	30	.08	.05	.5	78
	Frozen, concentrate, unsweetened:																		
252	Undiluted, 6-fl oz can——— 1 can———	207	62	300	4	1	—	—	—	72	70	124	.8	1,250	60	.29	.12	1.4	286
253	Diluted with 3 parts water by volume. 1 cup———	247	89	100	1	Trace	—	—	—	24	25	42	.2	420	20	.10	.04	.5	96
254	Dehydrated crystals, prepared with water (1 lb yields about 1 gal). 1 cup———	247	90	100	1	Trace	—	—	—	24	22	40	.2	412	20	.10	.05	.5	91
	Grapes, European type (adherent skin), raw:																		
255	Thompson Seedless——— 10 grapes———	50	81	35	Trace	Trace	—	—	—	9	6	10	.2	87	50	.03	.02	.2	2
256	Tokay and Emperor, seeded types 10 grapes[30]	60	81	40	Trace	Trace	—	—	—	10	7	11	.2	99	60	.03	.02	.2	2
	Grapejuice:																		
257	Canned or bottled——— 1 cup———	253	83	165	1	Trace	—	—	—	42	28	30	.8	293	—	.10	.05	.5	[25]Trace
	Frozen concentrate, sweetened:																		
258	Undiluted, 6-fl oz can——— 1 can———	216	53	395	1	Trace	—	—	—	100	22	32	.9	255	40	.13	.22	1.5	[31]32
259	Diluted with 3 parts water by volume. 1 cup———	250	86	135	1	Trace	—	—	—	33	8	10	.3	85	10	.05	.08	.5	[31]10
260	Grape drink, canned——— 1 cup———	250	86	135	Trace	Trace	—	—	—	35	8	10	.3	88	[32]10	[32].03	[32].03	.3	([32])
261	Lemon, raw, size 165, without peel and seeds (about 4 per lb with peels and seeds). 1 lemon———	74	90	20	1	Trace	—	—	—	6	19	12	.4	102	10	.03	.01	.1	39
	Lemon juice:																		
262	Raw——— 1 cup———	244	91	60	1	Trace	—	—	—	20	17	24	.5	344	50	.07	.02	.2	112
263	Canned, or bottled, unsweetened 1 cup———	244	92	55	1	Trace	—	—	—	19	17	24	.5	344	50	.07	.02	.2	102
264	Frozen, single strength, unsweetened, 6-fl oz can. 1 can———	183	92	40	1	Trace	—	—	—	13	13	16	.5	258	40	.05	.02	.2	81
	Lemonade concentrate, frozen:																		
265	Undiluted, 6-fl oz can——— 1 can———	219	49	425	Trace	Trace	—	—	—	112	9	13	.4	153	40	.05	.06	.7	66
266	Diluted with 4 1/3 parts water by volume. 1 cup———	248	89	105	Trace	Trace	—	—	—	28	2	3	.1	40	10	.01	.02	.2	17

[13]Crust made with vegetable shortening and enriched flour.

[24]Also applies to pasteurized apple cider.

[25]Applies to product without added ascorbic acid. For value of product with added ascorbic acid, refer to label.

[26]Based on product with label claim of 45% of U.S. RDA in 6 fl oz.

[27]Based on product with label claim of 100% of U.S. RDA in 6 fl oz.

[28]Weight includes peel and membranes between sections. Without these parts, the weight of the edible portion is 123 g for item 246 and 118 g for item 247.

[29]For white-fleshed varieties, value is about 20 International Units (I.U.) per cup; for red-fleshed varieties, 1,080 I.U.

[30]Weight includes seeds. Without seeds, weight of the edible portion is 57 g.

[31]Applies to product without added ascorbic acid. With added ascorbic acid, based on claim that 6 fl oz of reconstituted juice contain 45% or 50% of the U.S. RDA, value in milligrams is 108 or 120 for a 6-fl oz can (item 258), 36 or 40 for 1 cup of diluted juice (item 259).

[32]Applies to product with added thiamin and riboflavin but without added ascorbic acid, values in milligrams would be 0.60 for thiamin, 0.80 for riboflavin, and trace for ascorbic acid. For products with only ascorbic acid added, value varies with the brand. Consult the label.

(Dashes (—) denote lack of reliable data for a constituent believed to be present in measurable amount)

							Fatty Acids												
								Unsaturated											
Item No.	Foods, approximate measures, units, and weight (edible part unless footnotes indicate otherwise)		Water	Food energy	Pro-tein	Fat	Satu-rated (total)	Oleic	Lino-leic	Carbo-hydrate	Calcium	Phos-phorus	Iron	Potas-sium	Vitamin A value	Thiamin	Ribo-flavin	Thia-min	Ascorbic acid
(A)	(B)		(C)	(D)	(E)	(F)	(G)	(H)	(I)	(I)	(K)	(L)	(M)	(N)	(O)	(P)	(Q)	(R)	(S)
		Grams	Per-cent	Cal-ories	Grams	Grams	Grams	Grams	Grams	Grams	Milli-grams	Milli-grams	Milli-grams	Milli-grams	Inter-national units	Milli-grams	Milli-grams	Milli-grams	Milli-grams
	FRUITS AND FRUIT PRODUCTS—Con.																		
	Limeade concentrate, frozen:																		
267	Undiluted, 6-fl oz can	218	50	410	Trace	Trace	---	---	---	108	11	13	0.2	129	Trace	0.02	0.02	0.2	26
268	Diluted with 4 1/3 parts water by volume.	247	89	100	Trace	Trace	---	---	---	27	3	3	Trace	32	Trace	Trace	Trace	Trace	6
	Limejuice:																		
269	Raw	246	90	65	1	Trace	---	---	---	22	22	27	.5	256	20	.05	.02	.2	79
270	Canned, unsweetened	246	90	65	1	Trace	---	---	---	22	22	27	.5	256	20	.05	.02	.2	52
	Muskmelons, raw, with rind, with-out seed cavity:																		
271	Cantaloup, orange-fleshed (with rind and seed cavity, 5-in diam., 2 1/3 lb). 1/2 melon with rind[33]	477	91	80	2	Trace	---	---	---	20	38	44	1.1	682	9,240	.11	.08	1.6	90
272	Honeydew (with rind and seed cavity, 6 1/2-in diam., 5 1/4 lb). 1/10 melon with rind[33]	226	91	50	1	Trace	---	---	---	11	21	24	.6	374	60	.06	.04	.9	34
	Oranges, all commercial varieties, raw:																		
273	Whole, 2 5/8-in diam., without peel and seeds (about 2 1/2 per lb with peel and seeds). 1 orange	131	86	65	1	Trace	---	---	---	16	54	26	.5	263	260	.13	.05	.5	66
274	Sections without membranes	180	86	90	2	Trace	---	---	---	22	74	36	.7	360	360	.18	.07	.7	90
	Orange juice:																		
275	Raw, all variet s	248	88	110	2	Trace	---	---	---	26	27	42	.5	496	500	.22	.07	1.0	124
276	Canned, unsweetened	249	87	120	2	Trace	---	---	---	28	25	45	1.0	496	500	.17	.05	.7	100
	Frozen concentrate:																		
277	Undiluted, 6-fl oz can	213	55	360	5	Trace	---	---	---	87	75	126	.9	1,500	1,620	.68	.11	2.8	360
278	Diluted with 3 parts water by volume.	249	87	120	2	Trace	---	---	---	29	25	42	.2	503	540	.23	.03	.9	120
279	Dehydrated crystals, prepared with water (1 lb yields about 1 gal). 1 cup	248	88	115	1	Trace	---	---	---	27	25	40	.5	518	500	.20	.07	1.0	109
	Orange and grapefruit juice:																		
	Frozen concentrate:																		
280	Undiluted, 6-fl oz can	210	59	330	4	1	---	---	---	78	61	99	.8	1,308	800	.48	.06	2.3	302
281	Diluted with 3 parts water by volume.	248	88	110	1	Trace	---	---	---	26	20	32	.2	439	270	.15	.02	.7	102
282	Papayas, raw, 1/2-in cubes	140	89	55	1	Trace	---	---	---	14	28	22	.4	328	2,450	.06	.06	.4	78
	Peaches:																		
	Raw:																		
283	Whole, 2 1/2-in diam., peeled, pitted (about 4 per lb with peels and pits). 1 peach	100	89	40	1	Trace	---	---	---	10	9	19	.5	202	[33]1,330	.02	.05	1.0	7
284	Sliced	170	89	65	1	Trace	---	---	---	16	15	32	.9	343	[33]2,260	.03	.09	1.7	12
	Canned, yellow-fleshed, solids and liquid (halves or slices):																		
285	Sirup pack	256	79	200	1	Trace	---	---	---	51	10	31	.8	333	1,100	.03	.05	1.5	8
286	Water pack	244	91	75	1	Trace	---	---	---	20	10	32	.7	334	1,100	.02	.07	1.5	7
	Dried:																		
287	Uncooked	160	25	420	5	1	---	---	---	109	77	187	9.6	1,520	6,240	.02	.30	8.5	29
288	Cooked, unsweetened, halves and juice.	250	77	205	3	1	---	---	---	54	38	93	4.8	743	3,050	.01	.15	3.8	5

(A)	(B)	(C)	(D)	(E)	(F)	(G)	(H)	(I)	(J)	(K)	(L)	(M)	(N)	(O)	(P)	(Q)	(R)	(S)
289 290	Frozen, sliced, sweetened: 10-oz container —— 1 container Cup ——————— 1 cup	77 77	250 220	1 1	Trace Trace	— —	— —	— —	64 57	11 10	37 33	1.4 1.3	352 310	1,850 1,630	0.03 .03	0.11 .10	2.0 1.8	[35]116 [35]103
291	Pears: Raw, with skin, cored: Bartlett, 2 1/2-in diam. (about 2 1/2 per lb with cores and stems). 1 pear	83	100	1	1	—	—	—	25	13	18	.5	213	30	.03	.07	.2	7
292	Bosc, 2 1/2-in diam. (about 3 per lb with cores and stems). 1 pear	83	85	1	1	—	—	—	22	11	16	.4	83	30	.03	.06	.1	6
293	D'Anjou, 3-in diam. (about 2 per lb with cores and stems). 1 pear	83	120	1	1	—	—	—	31	16	22	.6	260	40	.04	.08	.2	8
294	Canned, solids and liquid, sirup pack, heavy (halves or slices). 1 cup	80	195	1	1	—	—	—	50	13	18	.5	214	10	.03	.05	.3	3
295	Pineapple: Raw, diced. 1 cup	85	80	1	Trace	—	—	—	21	26	12	.8	226	110	.14	.05	.3	26
296	Canned, heavy sirup pack, solids and liquid: Crushed, chunks, tidbits. 1 cup	80	190	1	Trace	—	—	—	49	28	13	.8	245	130	.20	.05	.5	18
297	Slices and liquid: Large. 1 slice; 2 1/4 tbsp liquid.	80	80	Trace	Trace	—	—	—	20	12	5	.3	101	50	.08	.02	.2	7
298	Medium. 1 slice; 1 1/4 tbsp liquid.	80	45	Trace	Trace	—	—	—	11	6	3	.2	56	30	.05	.01	.1	4
299	Pineapple juice, unsweetened, canned. 1 cup	86	140	1	Trace	—	—	—	34	38	23	.8	373	130	.13	.05	.5	[27]80
300	Plums: Raw, without pits: Japanese and hybrid (2 1/8-in diam., about 6 1/2 per lb with pits). 1 plum	87	30	Trace	Trace	—	—	—	8	8	12	.3	112	160	.02	.02	.3	4
301	Prune-type (1 1/2-in diam., about 15 per lb with pits). 1 plum	79	20	Trace	Trace	—	—	—	6	3	5	.1	48	80	.01	.01	.1	1
302 303	Canned, heavy sirup pack (Italian prunes), with pits and liquid: Cup ——————— 1 cup[36] Portion ——— 3 plums; 2 3/4 tbsp liquid.[36]	77 77	215 110	1 1	Trace Trace	— —	— —	— —	56 29	23 12	26 13	2.3 1.2	367 189	3,130 1,610	.05 .03	.05 .03	1.0 .5	5 3
304	Prunes, dried, "softenized," with pits: Uncooked. 4 extra large or 5 large prunes.[35]	28	110	1	Trace	—	—	—	29	22	34	1.7	298	690	.04	.07	.7	1
305	Cooked, unsweetened, all sizes, fruit and liquid. 1 cup[35]	66	255	2	1	—	—	—	67	51	79	3.8	695	1,590	.07	.15	1.5	2
306	Prune juice, canned or bottled. 1 cup	80	195	1	Trace	—	—	—	49	36	51	1.8	602	—	.03	.03	1.0	5
307 308	Raisins, seedless: Cup, not pressed down —— 1 cup Packet, 1/2 oz (1 1/2 tbsp) — 1 packet	18 18	420 40	4 Trace	Trace Trace	— —	— —	— —	112 11	90 9	146 14	5.1 .5	1,106 107	30 Trace	.16 .02	.12 .01	.7 .1	1 Trace
309 310	Raspberries, red: Raw, capped, whole —— 1 cup Frozen, sweetened, 10-oz container — 1 container	84 74	70 280	1 2	1 1	— —	— —	— —	17 70	27 37	27 48	1.1 1.7	207 284	160 200	.04 .06	.11 .17	1.1 1.7	31 60
311 312	Rhubarb, cooked, added sugar: From raw ———— 1 cup From frozen, sweetened — 1 cup	63 63	380 385	1 1	Trace 1	— —	— —	— —	97 93	211 211	41 32	1.6 1.9	548 475	220 190	.05 .05	.14 .11	.8 .5	16 16

[27] Based on product with label claim of 100% of U.S. RDA in 6 fl oz.
[33] Weight includes rind. Without rind, the weight of the edible portion is 272 g for item 271 and 149 g for item 272.
[34] Represents yellow-fleshed varieties. For white-fleshed varieties, value is 50 International Units (I.U.) for 1 peach, 90 I.U. for 1 cup of slices.
[35] Value represents products with added ascorbic acid. For products without added ascorbic acid, value in milligrams is 116 for a 10-oz container, 103 for 1 cup.
[36] Weight includes pits. After removal of the pits, the weight of the edible portion is 258 g for item 302, 133 g for item 304, and 213 g for item 305.

(Dashes (—) denote lack of reliable data for a constituent believed to be present in measurable amount)

NUTRIENTS IN INDICATED QUANTITY

Item No. (A)	Foods, approximate measures, units, and weight (edible part unless footnotes indicate otherwise) (B)	Grams	Water (C) Per cent	Food energy (D) Calories	Protein (E) Grams	Fat (F) Grams	Fatty Acids Saturated (total) (G) Grams	Unsaturated Oleic (H) Grams	Linoleic (I) Grams	Carbohydrate (J) Grams	Calcium (K) Milligrams	Phosphorus (L) Milligrams	Iron (M) Milligrams	Potassium (N) Milligrams	Vitamin A value (O) International units	Thiamin (P) Milligrams	Riboflavin (Q) Milligrams	Niacin (R) Milligrams	Ascorbic acid (S) Milligrams
	FRUITS AND FRUIT PRODUCTS—Con.																		
313	Strawberries: Raw, whole berries, capped --- 1 cup	149	90	55	1	1	—	—	—	13	31	31	1.5	244	90	0.04	0.10	0.9	88
	Frozen, sweetened:																		
314	Sliced, 10-oz container --- 1 container	284	71	310	1	1	—	—	—	79	40	48	2.0	318	90	.06	.17	1.4	151
315	Whole, 1-lb container (about 1 3/4 cups) --- 1 container	454	76	415	2	1	—	—	—	107	59	73	2.7	472	140	.09	.27	2.3	249
316	Tangerine, raw, 2 3/8-in diam., size 176, about 4 per lb with peels and seeds) --- 1 tangerine	86	87	40	1	Trace	—	—	—	10	34	15	.3	108	360	.05	.02	.1	27
317	Tangerine juice, canned, sweetened --- 1 cup	249	87	125	1	Trace	—	—	—	30	44	35	.5	440	1,040	.15	.05	.2	54
318	Watermelon, raw, 4 by 8 in wedge with rind and seeds (1/16 of 32 2/3-lb melon, 10 by 16 in).[37] --- 1 wedge with rind and seeds[37]	926	93	110	2	1	—	—	—	27	30	43	2.1	426	2,510	.13	.13	.9	30
	GRAIN PRODUCTS																		
	Bagel, 3-in diam.:																		
319	Egg --- 1 bagel	55	32	165	6	2	0.5	0.9	0.8	28	9	43	1.2	41	30	.14	.10	1.2	0
320	Water --- 1 bagel	55	29	165	6	1	.2	.4	.6	30	8	41	1.2	42	0	.15	.11	1.4	0
321	Barley, pearled, light, uncooked --- 1 cup	200	11	700	16	2	.3	.2	.8	158	32	378	4.0	320	0	.24	.10	6.2	0
	Biscuits, baking powder, 2-in diam. (enriched flour, vegetable shortening):																		
322	From home recipe --- 1 biscuit	28	27	105	2	5	1.2	2.0	1.2	13	34	49	.4	33	Trace	.08	.08	.7	Trace
323	From mix --- 1 biscuit	28	29	90	2	3	.6	1.1	.7	15	19	65	.6	32	Trace	.09	.08	.8	Trace
324	Breadcrumbs (enriched):[38] Dry, grated --- 1 cup	100	7	390	13	5	1.0	1.6	1.4	73	122	141	3.6	152	Trace	.35	.35	4.8	Trace
	Soft. See White bread (items 349-350).																		
	Breads:																		
325	Boston brown bread, canned, slice, 3 1/4 by 1/2 in.[38] --- 1 slice	45	45	95	2	1	.1	.2	.2	21	41	72	.9	131	0	.06	.04	.7	0
	Cracked-wheat bread (3/4 enriched wheat flour, 1/4 cracked wheat):[38]																		
326	Loaf, 1 lb --- 1 loaf	454	35	1,195	39	10	2.2	3.0	3.9	236	399	581	9.5	608	Trace	1.52	1.13	14.4	Trace
327	Slice (18 per loaf) --- 1 slice	25	35	65	2	1	.1	.2	.2	13	22	32	.5	34	Trace	.08	.06	.8	Trace
328	French or vienna bread, enriched:[38] Loaf, 1 lb --- 1 loaf	454	31	1,315	41	14	3.2	4.7	4.6	251	195	386	10.0	408	Trace	1.80	1.10	15.0	Trace
	Slice:																		
329	French (5 by 2 1/2 by 1 in) --- 1 slice	35	31	100	3	1	.4	.4	.4	19	15	30	.8	32	Trace	.14	.08	1.2	Trace
330	Vienna (4 3/4 by 4 by 1/2 in) --- 1 slice	25	31	75	2	1	.2	.3	.3	14	11	21	.6	23	Trace	.10	.06	.8	Trace
	Italian bread, enriched:																		
331	Loaf, 1 lb --- 1 loaf	454	32	1,250	41	4	.6	.3	1.5	256	77	349	10.0	336	0	1.80	1.10	15.0	0
332	Slice, 4 1/2 by 3 1/4 by 3/4 in --- 1 slice	30	32	85	3	Trace	Trace	Trace	.1	17	5	23	.7	22	0	.12	.07	1.0	0
	Raisin bread, enriched:[38]																		
333	Loaf, 1 lb --- 1 loaf	454	35	1,190	30	13	3.0	4.7	3.9	243	322	395	10.0	1,057	Trace	1.70	1.07	10.7	Trace
334	Slice (18 per loaf) --- 1 slice	25	35	65	2	1	.2	.3	.2	13	18	22	.6	58	Trace	.09	.06	.6	Trace

(A)	(B)	(C)	(D)	(E)	(F)	(G)	(H)	(I)	(J)	(K)	(L)	(M)	(N)	(O)	(P)	(Q)	(R)	(S)	(T)
	Rye Bread:																		
	American, light (2/3 enriched wheat flour, 1/3 rye flour):																		
335	Loaf, 1 lb — 1 loaf	454	36	1,100	41	5	0.7	0.5	2.2	236	340	667	9.1	658	0	1.35	0.98	12.9	0
336	Slice (4 3/4 by 3 3/4 by 7/16 in) — 1 slice	25	36	60	2	Trace	Trace	Trace	.1	13	19	37	.5	36	0	.07	.05	.7	0
	Pumpernickel (2/3 rye flour, 1/3 enriched wheat flour):																		
337	Loaf, 1 lb — 1 loaf	454	34	1,115	41	5	.5	.7	2.4	241	381	1,039	11.8	2,059	0	1.30	.93	8.5	0
338	Slice (5 by 4 by 3/8 in)[38] — 1 slice	32	34	80	3	Trace	Trace	.1	.2	17	27	73	.8	145	0	.09	.07	.6	0
	White bread, enriched:[38]																		
	Soft-crumb type:																		
339	Loaf, 1 lb — 1 loaf	454	36	1,225	39	15	3.4	5.3	4.6	229	381	440	11.3	476	Trace	1.80	1.10	15.0	Trace
340	Slice (18 per loaf) — 1 slice	25	36	70	2	1	.3	.3	.3	13	21	24	.6	26	Trace	.10	.06	.8	Trace
341	Slice, toasted — 1 slice	22	25	70	2	1	.3	.2	.2	13	21	24	.6	26	Trace	.08	.06	.8	Trace
342	Slice (22 per loaf) — 1 slice	20	36	55	2	1	.2	.2	.2	10	17	19	.5	21	Trace	.08	.05	.7	Trace
343	Slice, toasted — 1 slice	17	25	55	2	1	.2	.2	.2	10	17	19	.5	21	Trace	.06	.05	.7	Trace
344	Loaf, 1 1/2 lb — 1 loaf	680	36	1,835	59	22	5.2	7.9	6.9	343	571	660	17.0	714	Trace	2.70	1.65	22.5	Trace
345	Slice (24 per loaf) — 1 slice	28	36	75	2	1	.2	.3	.3	14	24	27	.7	29	Trace	.11	.07	.9	Trace
346	Slice, toasted — 1 slice	24	25	75	2	1	.2	.3	.3	14	24	27	.7	29	Trace	.09	.07	.9	Trace
347	Slice (28 per loaf) — 1 slice	24	36	65	2	1	.2	.2	.2	12	20	23	.6	25	Trace	.10	.06	.8	Trace
348	Slice, toasted — 1 slice	21	25	65	2	1	.2	.2	.2	12	20	23	.6	25	Trace	.08	.06	.8	Trace
349	Cubes — 1 cup	30	36	80	2	1	.2	.3	.3	15	25	29	.8	32	Trace	.12	.07	1.0	Trace
350	Crumbs — 1 cup	45	36	120	4	1	.3	.5	.5	23	38	44	1.1	47	Trace	.18	.11	1.5	Trace
	Firm-crumb type:																		
351	Loaf, 1 lb — 1 loaf	454	35	1,245	41	17	3.9	5.9	5.2	228	435	463	11.3	549	Trace	1.80	1.10	15.0	Trace
352	Slice (20 per loaf) — 1 slice	23	35	65	2	1	.2	.3	.3	12	22	23	.6	28	Trace	.09	.06	.8	Trace
353	Slice, toasted — 1 slice	20	24	65	2	1	.2	.3	.3	12	22	23	.6	28	Trace	.07	.06	.8	Trace
354	Loaf, 2 lb — 1 loaf	907	35	2,495	82	34	7.7	11.8	10.4	455	871	925	22.7	1,097	Trace	3.60	2.20	30.0	Trace
355	Slice (34 per loaf) — 1 slice	27	35	75	2	1	.2	.3	.3	14	26	28	.7	33	Trace	.11	.06	.9	Trace
356	Slice, toasted — 1 slice	23	24	75	2	1	.2	.3	.3	14	26	28	.7	33	Trace	.09	.06	.9	Trace
	Whole-wheat bread:[38]																		
	Soft-crumb type:[38]																		
357	Loaf, 1 lb — 1 loaf	454	36	1,095	41	12	2.2	2.9	4.2	224	381	1,152	13.6	1,161	Trace	1.37	.45	12.7	Trace
358	Slice (16 per loaf) — 1 slice	28	36	65	3	1	.1	.2	.2	14	24	71	.8	72	Trace	.09	.03	.8	Trace
359	Slice, toasted — 1 slice	24	24	65	3	1	.1	.2	.2	14	24	71	.8	72	Trace	.07	.03	.8	Trace
	Firm-crumb type:[38]																		
360	Loaf, 1 lb — 1 loaf	454	36	1,100	48	14	2.5	3.3	4.9	216	449	1,034	13.6	1,238	Trace	1.17	.54	12.7	Trace
361	Slice (18 per loaf) — 1 slice	25	36	60	3	1	.1	.2	.3	12	25	57	.8	68	Trace	.06	.03	.7	Trace
362	Slice, toasted — 1 slice	21	24	60	3	1	.1	.2	.3	12	25	57	.8	68	Trace	.05	.03	.7	Trace
	Breakfast cereals:																		
	Hot type, cooked:																		
	Corn (hominy) grits, degermed:																		
363	Enriched — 1 cup	245	87	125	3	Trace	Trace	Trace	.1	27	2	25	.7	27	Trace[40]	.10	.07	1.0	0
364	Unenriched — 1 cup	245	87	125	3	Trace	Trace	Trace	.1	27	2	25	.2	27	Trace[40]	.05	.02	.5	0
365	Farina, quick-cooking, enriched — 1 cup	245	89	105	3	Trace	Trace	Trace	.1	22	147	113[41]	[42]	25	0	.12	.07	1.0	0
366	Oatmeal or rolled oats — 1 cup	240	87	130	5	2	—	—	—	23	22	137	1.4	146	0	.19	.05	.2	0
367	Wheat, rolled — 1 cup	240	80	180	5	1	—	—	—	41	19	182	1.7	202	0	.17	.07	2.2	0
368	Wheat, whole-meal — 1 cup	245	88	110	4	1	—	—	—	23	17	127	1.2	118	0	.15	.05	1.5	0
	Ready-to-eat:																		
369	Bran flakes (40% bran), added sugar, salt, iron, vitamins — 1 cup	35	3	105	4	1	Trace	—	—	28	19	125	15.6	137	1,650	.41	.49	4.1	12
370	Bran flakes with raisins, added sugar, salt, iron, vitamins — 1 cup	50	7	145	4	1	—	—	—	40	28	146	16.9	154	2,350	.58	.71	5.8	18

[37] Weight includes rind and seeds. Without rind and seeds, weight of the edible portion is 426 g.
[38] Made with vegetable shortening.
[39] Applies to product made with white cornmeal. With yellow cornmeal, value is 30 International Units (I.U.).
[40] Applies to white varieties. For yellow varieties, value is 150 International Units (I.U.).
[41] Applies to products that do not contain di-sodium phosphate. If di-sodium phosphate is an ingredient, value is 162 mg.
[42] Value may range from less than 1 mg to about 8 mg depending on the brand. Consult the label.

(Dashes (—) denote lack of reliable data for a constituent believed to be present in measurable amount)

| | | | | | | | Fatty Acids | | | | | | | | | | | | |
| | | | | | | | Saturated | Unsaturated | | | | | | | | | | | |
Item No. (A)	Foods, approximate measures, units, and weight (edible part unless footnotes indicate otherwise) (B)	Grams	Water (C) Per-cent	Food energy (D) Cal-ories	Pro-tein (E) Grams	Fat (F) Grams	(total) (G) Grams	Oleic (H) Grams	Lino-leic (I) Grams	Carbo-hydrate (J) Grams	Calcium (K) Milli-grams	Phos-phorus (L) Milli-grams	Iron (M) Milli-grams	Potas-sium (N) Milli-grams	Vitamin A value (O) International units	Thiamin (P) Milli-grams	Ribo-flavin (Q) Milli-grams	Niacin (R) Milli-grams	Ascorbic acid (S) Milli-grams
	GRAIN PRODUCTS—Con.																		
	Breakfast cereals—Continued																		
	Ready-to-eat—Continued																		
	Corn flakes:																		
371	Plain, added sugar, salt, iron, vitamins. 1 cup	25	4	95	2	Trace	—	—	—	21	(23)	9	0.6	30	1,180	0.29	0.35	2.9	9
372	Sugar-coated, added salt, iron, vitamins. 1 cup	40	2	155	2	Trace	—	—	—	37	1	10	1.0	27	1,880	.46	.56	4.6	14
373	Corn, puffed, plain, added sugar, salt, iron, vita-mins. 1 cup	20	4	80	2	1	—	—	—	16	4	18	2.3	—	940	.23	.28	2.3	7
374	Corn, shredded, added sugar, salt, iron, thiamin, niacin. 1 cup	25	3	95	2	Trace	—	—	—	22	1	10	.6	—	0	.11	.05	.5	0
375	Oats, puffed, added sugar, salt, minerals, vitamins. 1 cup	25	3	100	3	1	—	—	—	19	44	102	2.9	—	1,180	.29	.35	2.9	9
	Rice, puffed:																		
376	Plain, added iron, thiamin, niacin. 1 cup	15	4	60	1	Trace	—	—	—	13	3	14	.3	15	0	.07	.01	.7	0
377	Presweetened, added salt, iron, vitamins. 1 cup	28	3	115	1	0	—	—	—	26	3	14	[41]1.1	43	1,250	.38	.43	5.0	[45]15
378	Wheat flakes, added sugar, salt, iron, vitamins. 1 cup	30	4	105	3	Trace	—	—	—	24	12	83	(44)	81	1,410	.35	.42	3.5	11
	Wheat, puffed:																		
379	Plain, added iron, thiamin, niacin. 1 cup	15	3	55	2	Trace	—	—	—	12	4	48	.6	51	0	.08	.03	1.2	0
380	Presweetened, added salt, iron, vitamins. 1 cup	38	3	140	3	Trace	—	—	—	33	7	[4]52	[41]1.6	63	1,680	.50	.57	6.7	[45]20
381	Wheat, shredded, plain. 1 oblong biscuit or 1/2 cup spoon-size biscuits	25	7	90	2	1	—	—	—	20	11	97	.9	87	0	.06	.03	1.1	0
382	Wheat germ, without salt and sugar, toasted. 1 tbsp	6	4	25	2	1	—	—	—	3	3	70	.5	57	10	.11	.05	.3	1
383	Buckwheat flour, light, sifted. 1 cup	98	12	340	6	1	0.2	0.4	0.4	78	11	86	1.0	314	0	.08	.04	.4	0
384	Bulgur, canned, seasoned. 1 cup	135	56	245	8	4	—	—	—	44	27	263	1.9	151	0	.08	.05	4.1	0
	Cake icings. See Sugars and Sweets (items 532-536).																		
	Cakes made from cake mixes with enriched flour:[16]																		
	Angelfood:																		
385	Whole cake (9 3/4-in diam. tube cake). 1 cake	635	34	1,645	36	1	—	—	—	377	603	756	2.5	381	0	.37	.95	3.6	0
386	Piece, 1/12 of cake. 1 piece	53	34	135	3	Trace	—	—	—	32	50	63	.2	32	0	.03	.08	.3	0
	Coffeecake:																		
387	Whole cake (7 3/4 by 5 5/8 by 1 1/4 in). 1 cake	430	30	1,385	27	41	11.7	16.3	8.8	225	262	748	6.9	469	690	.82	.91	7.7	1
388	Piece, 1/6 of cake. 1 piece	72	30	230	5	7	2.0	2.7	1.5	38	44	125	1.2	78	120	.14	.15	1.3	Trace
	Cupcakes, made with egg, milk, 2 1/2-in diam.:																		
389	Without icing. 1 cupcake	25	26	90	1	3	.8	1.2	.7	14	40	59	.3	21	40	.05	.05	.4	Trace
390	With chocolate icing. 1 cupcake	36	22	130	2	5	2.0	1.6	.6	21	47	71	.4	42	60	.05	.06	.4	Trace
	Devil's food with chocolate icing:																		
391	Whole, 2 layer cake (8- or 9-in diam.). 1 cake	1,107	24	3,755	49	136	50.0	44.9	17.0	645	653	1,162	16.6	1,439	1,660	1.06	1.65	10.1	1
392	Piece, 1/16 of cake. 1 piece	69	24	235	3	8	3.1	2.8	1.1	40	41	72	1.0	90	100	.07	.10	.6	Trace
393	Cupcake, 2 1/2-in diam. 1 cupcake	35	24	120	2	4	1.6	1.4	.5	20	21	37	.5	46	50	.03	.05	.3	Trace

(A)	(B)		(C)	(D)	(E)	(F)	(G)	(H)	(I)	(J)	(K)	(L)	(M)	(N)	(O)	(P)	(Q)	(R)	(S)
	Gingerbread:																		
394	Whole cake (8-in square)	1 cake	570	1,575	18	39	9.7	16.6	10.0	291	513	570	8.6	1,562	Trace	0.84	1.00	7.4	Trace
395	Piece, 1/9 of cake	1 piece	63	175	2	4	1.1	1.8	1.1	32	57	63	.9	173	Trace	.09	.11	.8	Trace
	White, 2 layer with chocolate icing:																		
396	Whole cake (8- or 9-in diam.)	1 cake	1,140	4,000	44	122	48.2	46.4	20.0	716	1,129	2,041	11.4	1,322	680	1.50	1.77	12.5	2
397	Piece, 1/16 of cake	1 piece	71	250	3	8	3.0	2.9	1.2	45	70	127	.7	82	40	.09	.11	.8	Trace
	Yellow, 2 layer with chocolate icing:																		
398	Whole cake (8- or 9-in diam.)	1 cake	1,108	3,735	45	125	47.8	47.8	20.3	638	1,008	2,017	12.2	1,208	1,550	1.24	1.67	10.6	2
399	Piece, 1/16 of cake	1 piece	69	235	3	8	3.0	3.0	1.3	40	63	126	.8	75	100	.08	.10	.7	Trace
	Cakes made from home recipes using enriched flour:[47]																		
	Boston cream pie with custard filling:[47]																		
400	Whole cake (8-in diam.)	1 cake	825	2,490	41	78	23.0	30.1	15.2	412	553	833	8.2	[48]734	1,730	1.04	1.27	9.6	2
401	Piece, 1/12 of cake	1 piece	69	210	3	6	1.9	2.5	1.3	34	46	70	.7	[48]61	140	.09	.11	.8	Trace
	Fruitcake, dark:																		
402	Loaf, 1-lb (7 1/2 by 2 by 1 1/2 in).	1 loaf	454	1,720	22	69	14.4	33.5	14.8	271	327	513	11.8	2,250	540	.72	.73	4.9	2
403	Slice, 1/30 of loaf	1 slice	15	55	1	2	.5	1.1	.5	9	11	17	.4	74	20	.02	.02	.2	Trace
	Plain, sheet cake:																		
	Without icing:																		
404	Whole cake (9-in square)	1 cake	777	2,830	35	108	29.5	44.4	23.9	434	497	793	8.5	[48]614	1,320	1.21	1.40	10.2	2
405	Piece, 1/9 of cake	1 piece	86	315	4	12	3.3	4.9	2.6	48	55	88	.9	[48]68	150	.13	.15	1.1	Trace
	With uncooked white icing:																		
406	Whole cake (9-in square)	1 cake	1,096	4,020	37	129	42.2	49.5	24.4	694	548	822	8.2	[48]669	2,190	1.22	1.47	10.2	2
407	Piece, 1/9 of cake	1 piece	121	445	4	14	4.7	5.5	2.7	77	61	91	.8	[48]74	240	.14	.16	1.1	Trace
	Pound:[49]																		
408	Loaf, 8 1/2 by 3 1/2 by 3 1/4 in.	1 loaf	565	2,725	31	170	42.9	73.1	39.6	273	107	418	7.9	345	1,410	.90	.99	7.3	0
409	Slice, 1/17 of loaf	1 slice	33	160	2	10	2.5	4.3	2.3	16	6	24	.5	20	80	.05	.06	.4	0
	Spongecake:																		
410	Whole cake (9 3/4-in diam. tube cake).	1 cake	790	2,345	60	45	13.1	15.8	5.7	427	237	885	13.4	687	3,560	1.10	1.64	7.4	Trace
411	Piece, 1/12 of cake	1 piece	66	195	5	4	1.1	1.3	.5	36	20	74	1.1	57	300	.09	.14	.6	Trace
	Cookies made with enriched flour:[50][51]																		
	Brownies with nuts:																		
	Home-prepared, 1 3/4 by 1 3/4 by 7/8 in:																		
412	From home recipe	1 brownie	20	95	1	6	1.5	3.0	1.2	10	8	30	.4	38	40	.04	.03	.2	Trace
413	From commercial recipe[52]	1 brownie	20	85	1	4	.9	1.4	1.3	13	9	27	.4	34	20	.03	.02	.2	Trace
414	Frozen, with chocolate icing,[52] 1 1/2 by 1 3/4 by 7/8 in.	1 brownie	25	105	1	5	2.0	2.2	.7	15	10	31	.4	44	50	.03	.03	.2	Trace
	Chocolate chip:																		
415	Commercial, 2 1/4-in diam., 3/8 in thick.	4 cookies	42	200	2	9	2.8	2.9	2.2	29	16	48	1.0	56	50	.10	.17	.9	Trace
416	From home recipe, 2 1/3-in diam.	4 cookies	40	205	2	12	3.5	4.5	2.9	24	14	40	.8	47	40	.06	.06	.5	Trace
417	Fig bars, square (1 5/8 by 1 5/8 by 3/8 in) or rectangular (1 1/2 by 1 3/4 by 1/2 in).	4 cookies	56	200	2	3	.8	1.2	.7	42	44	34	1.0	111	60	.04	.14	.9	Trace
418	Gingersnaps, 2-in diam., 1/4 in thick.	4 cookies	28	90	2	2	.7	1.0	.6	22	20	13	.7	129	20	.08	.06	.7	0
419	Macaroons, 2 3/4-in diam., 1/4 in thick.	2 cookies	38	180	2	9	—	—	—	25	10	32	.3	176	0	.02	.06	.2	0
420	Oatmeal with raisins, 2 5/8-in diam., 1/4 in thick.	4 cookies	52	235	3	8	2.0	3.3	2.0	38	11	53	1.4	192	30	.15	.10	1.0	Trace

[43]Value varies with the brand. Consult the label.
[44]Value varies with the brand. Consult the label.
[45]Applies to product with added ascorbic acid. Without added ascorbic acid, value is trace.
[46]Applies to product with added ascorbic acid.
[47]Excepting angelfood cake, cakes were made from mixes containing vegetable shortening; icings, with butter.
[48]Excepting spongecake, vegetable shortening used for cake portion; butter, for icing. If butter or margarine used for cake portion, vitamin A values would be higher.
[49]Applies to product made with a sodium aluminum-sulfate type baking powder. With a low-sodium type baking powder containing potassium, value would be about twice the amount shown.
[50]Equal weights of flour, sugar, eggs, and vegetable shortening.
[51]Products are commercial unless otherwise specified.
[52]Made with enriched flour and vegetable shortening except for macaroons which do not contain flour or shortening.
[53]Icing made with butter.

(Dashes (—) denote lack of reliable data for a constituent believed to be present in measurable amount)

								Fatty Acids												
Item No.	Foods, approximate measures, units, and weight (edible part unless footnotes indicate otherwise)		Water	Food energy	Protein	Fat	Saturated (total)	Unsaturated Oleic	Linoleic	Carbohydrate	Calcium	Phosphorus	Iron	Potassium	Vitamin A value	Thiamin	Riboflavin	Niacin	Ascorbic acid
(A)	(B)	Grams	(C) Percent	(D) Calories	(E) Grams	(F) Grams	(G) Grams	(H) Grams	(I) Grams	(J) Grams	(K) Milligrams	(L) Milligrams	(M) Milligrams	(N) Milligrams	(O) International units	(P) Milligrams	(Q) Milligrams	(R) Milligrams	(S) Milligrams
	GRAIN PRODUCTS—Con.																		
	Cookies made with enriched flour[50][51]—Continued																		
421	Plain, prepared from commercial chilled dough, 2 1/2-in diam., 1/4 in thick. 4 cookies	48	5	240	2	12	3.0	5.2	2.9	31	17	35	0.6	23	30	0.10	0.08	0.9	0
422	Sandwich type (chocolate or vanilla), 1 3/4-in diam., 3/8 in thick. 4 cookies	40	2	200	2	9	2.2	3.9	2.2	28	10	96	.7	15	0	.06	.10	.7	0
423	Vanilla wafers, 1 3/4-in diam., 1/4 in thick. 10 cookies	40	3	185	2	6	—	—	—	30	16	25	.6	29	50	.10	.09	.8	0
	Cornmeal:																		
424	Whole-ground, unbolted, dry form. 1 cup	122	12	435	11	5	.5	1.0	2.5	90	24	312	2.9	346	[53]620	.46	.13	2.4	0
425	Bolted (nearly whole-grain), dry form. 1 cup	122	12	440	11	4	.5	.9	2.1	91	21	272	2.2	303	[53]590	.37	.10	2.3	0
	Degermed, enriched:																		
426	Dry form. 1 cup	138	12	500	11	2	.2	.4	.9	108	8	137	4.0	166	[53]610	.61	.36	4.8	0
427	Cooked. 1 cup	240	88	120	3	Trace	Trace	.1	.2	26	2	34	1.0	38	[53]140	.14	.10	1.2	0
	Degermed, unenriched:																		
428	Dry form. 1 cup	138	12	500	11	2	.2	.4	.9	108	8	137	1.5	166	[53]610	.19	.07	1.4	0
429	Cooked. 1 cup	240	88	120	3	Trace	Trace	.1	.2	26	2	34	.5	38	[53]140	.05	.02	.2	0
	Crackers:[34]																		
430	Graham, plain, 2 1/2-in square. 2 crackers	14	6	55	1	1	.3	.5	.3	10	6	21	.5	55	0	.02	.08	.5	0
431	Rye wafers, whole-grain, 1 7/8 by 3 1/2 in. 2 wafers	13	6	45	2	Trace	—	—	—	10	7	50	.5	78	0	.04	.03	.2	0
432	Saltines, made with enriched flour. 4 crackers or 1 packet	11	4	50	1	1	.3	.5	.4	8	2	10	.5	13	0	.05	.05	.4	0
	Danish pastry (enriched flour), plain without fruit or nuts:[54]																		
433	Packaged ring, 12 oz. 1 ring	340	22	1,435	25	80	24.3	31.7	16.5	155	170	371	6.1	381	1,050	.97	1.01	8.6	Trace
434	Round piece, about 4 1/4-in diam. by 1 in. 1 pastry	65	22	275	5	15	4.7	6.1	3.2	30	33	71	1.2	73	200	.18	.19	1.7	Trace
435	Ounce. 1 oz	28	22	120	2	7	2.0	2.7	1.4	13	14	31	.5	32	90	.08	.08	.7	Trace
	Doughnuts, made with enriched flour:[55]																		
436	Cake type, plain, 2 1/2-in diam., 1 in high. 1 doughnut	25	24	100	1	5	1.2	2.0	1.1	13	10	48	.4	23	20	.05	.05	.4	Trace
437	Yeast-leavened, glazed, 3 3/4-in diam., 1 1/4 in high. 1 doughnut	50	26	205	3	11	3.3	5.8	3.3	22	16	33	.6	34	25	.10	.10	.8	0
	Macaroni, enriched, cooked (cut lengths, elbows, shells):																		
438	Firm stage (hot). 1 cup	130	64	190	7	1	—	—	—	39	14	85	1.4	103	0	.23	.13	1.8	0
	Tender stage:																		
439	Cold macaroni. 1 cup	105	73	115	4	Trace	—	—	—	24	8	53	.9	64	0	.15	.08	1.2	0
440	Hot macaroni. 1 cup	140	73	155	5	1	—	—	—	32	11	70	1.3	85	0	.20	.11	1.5	0
	Macaroni (enriched) and cheese:																		
441	Canned[55]. 1 cup	240	80	230	9	10	4.2	3.1	1.4	26	199	182	1.0	139	260	.12	.24	1.0	Trace
442	From home recipe (served hot)[56]. 1 cup	200	58	430	17	22	8.9	8.8	2.9	40	362	322	1.8	240	860	.20	.40	1.8	Trace
	Muffins made with enriched flour:[38] From home recipe:																		
443	Blueberry, 2 3/8-in diam., 1 1/2 in high. 1 muffin	40	39	110	3	4	1.1	1.4	.7	17	34	53	.6	46	90	.09	.10	.7	Trace
444	Bran. 1 muffin	40	35	105	3	4	1.2	1.4	.8	17	57	162	1.5	172	90	.07	.10	1.7	Trace
445	Corn (enriched degermed cornmeal and flour), 2 3/8-in diam., 1 1/2 in high. 1 muffin	40	33	125	3	4	1.2	1.6	.9	19	42	68	.7	54	[57]120	.10	.10	.7	Trace

(A)	(B)	(grams)	(C)	(D)	(E)	(F)	(G)	(H)	(I)	(J)	(K)	(L)	(M)	(N)	(O)	(P)	(Q)	(R)	(S)
446	Plain, 3-in diam., 1 1/2 in high. — 1 muffin	40	38	120	3	4	1.0	1.7	1.0	17	42	60	0.6	50	40	0.09	0.12	0.9	Trace
447	From mix, egg, milk: Corn, 2 3/8-in diam., 1 1/2 in high.[58] — 1 muffin	40	30	130	3	4	1.2	1.7	.9	20	96	152	.6	44	[57]100	.08	.09	.7	Trace
448	Noodles (egg noodles), enriched, cooked. — 1 cup	160	71	200	7	2	—	—	—	37	16	94	1.4	70	110	.22	.13	1.9	0
449	Noodles, chow mein, canned.[58] — 1 cup	45	1	220	6	11	—	—	—	26	—	—	—	—	—	—	—	—	—
450	Pancakes, (4-in diam.):[58] Buckwheat, made from mix (with buckwheat and enriched flours), egg and milk added. — 1 cake	27	58	55	2	2	.8	.9	.4	6	59	91	.4	66	60	.04	.05	.2	Trace
451	Plain: Made from home recipe using enriched flour. — 1 cake	27	50	60	2	2	.5	.8	.5	9	27	38	.4	33	30	.06	.07	.5	Trace
452	Made from mix with enriched flour, egg and milk added. — 1 cake	27	51	60	2	2	.7	.7	.3	9	58	70	.3	42	70	.04	.06	.2	Trace
	Pies, piecrust made with enriched flour, vegetable shortening (9-in diam.):																		
	Apple:																		
453	Whole — 1 pie	945	48	2,420	21	105	27.0	44.5	25.2	360	76	208	6.6	756	280	1.06	.79	9.3	9
454	Sector, 1/7 of pie — 1 sector	135	48	345	3	15	3.9	6.4	3.6	51	11	30	.9	108	40	.15	.11	1.3	2
	Banana cream:																		
455	Whole — 1 pie	910	54	2,010	41	85	26.7	33.2	16.2	279	601	746	7.3	1,847	2,280	.77	1.51	7.0	9
456	Sector, 1/7 of pie — 1 sector	130	54	285	6	12	3.8	4.7	2.3	40	86	107	1.0	264	330	.11	.22	1.0	1
	Blueberry:																		
457	Whole — 1 pie	945	51	2,285	23	102	24.8	43.7	25.1	330	104	217	9.5	614	280	1.03	.80	10.0	28
458	Sector, 1/7 of pie — 1 sector	135	51	325	3	15	3.5	6.2	3.6	47	15	31	1.4	88	40	.15	.11	1.4	4
	Cherry:																		
459	Whole — 1 pie	945	47	2,465	25	107	28.2	45.0	25.3	363	132	236	6.6	992	4,160	1.09	.84	9.8	Trace
460	Sector, 1/7 of pie — 1 sector	135	47	350	4	15	4.0	6.4	3.6	52	19	34	.9	142	590	.16	.12	1.4	Trace
	Custard:																		
461	Whole — 1 pie	910	58	1,985	56	101	33.9	38.5	17.5	213	874	1,028	8.2	1,247	2,090	.79	1.92	5.6	0
462	Sector, 1/7 of pie — 1 sector	130	58	285	8	14	4.8	5.5	2.5	30	125	147	1.2	178	300	.11	.27	.8	0
	Lemon meringue:																		
463	Whole — 1 pie	840	47	2,140	31	86	26.1	33.8	16.4	317	118	412	6.7	420	1,430	.61	.84	5.2	25
464	Sector, 1/7 of pie — 1 sector	120	47	305	4	12	3.7	4.8	2.3	45	17	59	1.0	60	200	.09	.12	.7	4
	Mince:																		
465	Whole — 1 pie	945	43	2,560	24	109	28.0	45.9	25.2	389	265	359	13.3	1,682	20	.96	.86	9.8	9
466	Sector, 1/7 of pie — 1 sector	135	43	365	3	16	4.0	6.6	3.6	56	38	51	1.9	240	Trace	.14	.12	1.4	1
	Peach:																		
467	Whole — 1 pie	945	48	2,410	24	101	24.8	43.7	25.1	361	95	274	8.5	1,408	6,900	1.04	.97	14.0	28
468	Sector, 1/7 of pie — 1 sector	135	48	345	3	14	3.5	6.2	3.6	52	14	39	1.2	201	990	.15	.14	2.0	4
	Pecan:																		
469	Whole — 1 pie	825	20	3,450	42	189	27.8	101.0	44.2	423	388	850	25.6	1,015	1,320	1.80	.95	6.9	Trace
470	Sector, 1/7 of pie — 1 sector	118	20	495	6	27	4.0	14.4	6.3	61	55	122	3.7	145	190	.26	.14	1.0	Trace
	Pumpkin:																		
471	Whole — 1 pie	910	59	1,920	36	102	37.4	37.5	16.6	223	464	628	7.3	1,456	22,480	.78	1.27	7.0	Trace
472	Sector, 1/7 of pie — 1 sector	130	59	275	5	15	5.4	5.4	2.4	32	66	90	1.0	208	3,210	.11	.18	1.0	Trace
473	Piecrust (home recipe) made with enriched flour and vegetable shortening, baked. — 1 pie shell, 9-in diam.	180	15	900	11	60	14.8	26.1	14.9	79	25	90	3.1	89	0	.47	.40	5.0	0
474	Piecrust mix with enriched flour and vegetable shortening, 10-oz pkg. prepared and baked. — Piecrust for 2-crust pie, 9-in diam.	320	19	1,485	20	93	22.7	39.7	23.4	141	131	272	6.1	179	0	1.07	.79	9.9	0

[48] Made with vegetable shortening.
[50] Products are commercial unless otherwise specified.
[51] Made with enriched flour and vegetable shortening except for macaroons which do not contain flour or shortening.
[52] Applies to yellow varieties; white varieties contain only a trace.
[53] Contains vegetable shortening and butter.
[54] Made with corn oil.
[55] Made with regular margarine.
[56] Applies to product made with yellow cornmeal.
[57] Applies to product made with yellow cornmeal and enriched flour.
[58] Made with enriched degermed cornmeal and enriched flour.

(Dashes (—) denote lack of reliable data for a constituent believed to be present in measurable amount)

							Fatty Acids												
Item No.	Foods, approximate measures, units, and weight (edible part unless footnotes indicate otherwise)		Water	Food energy	Pro-tein	Fat	Satu-rated (total)	Unsaturated Oleic	Lino-leic	Carbo-hydrate	Calcium	Phos-phorus	Iron	Potas-sium	Vitamin A value	Thiamin	Ribo-flavin	Niacin	Ascorbic acid
(A)	(B)		(C)	(D)	(E)	(F)	(G)	(H)	(I)	(J)	(K)	(L)	(M)	(N)	(O)	(P)	(Q)	(R)	(S)
		Grams	Per-cent	Cal-ories	Grams	Grams	Grams	Grams	Grams	Grams	Milli-grams	Milli-grams	Milli-grams	Milli-grams	Inter-national units	Milli-grams	Milli-grams	Milli-grams	Milli-grams
	GRAIN PRODUCTS—Con.																		
475	Pizza (cheese) baked, 4 3/4-in sector; 1/8 of 12-in diam. pie.[19] 1 sector	60	45	145	6	4	1.7	1.5	0.6	22	86	89	1.1	67	230	0.16	0.18	1.6	4
	Popcorn, popped:																		
476	Plain, large kernel. 1 cup	6	4	25	1	Trace	Trace	.1	.2	5	1	17	.2	—	—	—	.01	.1	0
477	With oil (coconut) and salt added, large kernel. 1 cup	9	3	40	1	2	1.5	.2	.2	5	1	19	.2	—	—	—	.01	.2	0
478	Sugar coated. 1 cup	35	4	135	2	1	.5	.2	.4	30	2	47	.5	—	—	—	.02	.4	0
	Pretzels, made with enriched flour:																		
479	Dutch, twisted, 2 3/4 by 2 5/8 in. 1 pretzel	16	5	60	2	1	—	—	—	12	4	21	.2	21	0	.05	.04	.7	0
480	Thin, twisted, 3 1/4 by 2 1/4 by 1/4 in. 10 pretzels	60	5	235	6	3	—	—	—	46	13	79	.9	78	0	.20	.15	2.5	0
481	Stick, 2 1/4 in long. 10 pretzels	3	5	10	Trace	Trace	—	—	—	2	1	4	Trace	4	0	.01	.01	.1	0
	Rice, white, enriched:																		
	Instant, ready-to-serve, hot:																		
482	1 cup	165	73	180	4	Trace	Trace	Trace	Trace	40	5	31	1.3	—	0	.21	(59)	1.7	0
	Long grain:																		
483	Raw. 1 cup	185	12	670	12	1	.2	.2	.2	149	44	174	5.4	170	0	.81	.06	6.5	0
484	Cooked, served hot. 1 cup	205	73	225	4	Trace	.1	.1	.1	50	21	57	1.8	57	0	.23	.02	2.1	0
	Parboiled:																		
485	Raw. 1 cup	185	10	685	14	1	.2	.1	.2	150	111	370	5.4	278	0	.81	.07	6.5	0
486	Cooked, served hot.[38] 1 cup	175	73	185	4	Trace	.1	.1	.1	41	33	100	1.4	75	0	.19	.02	2.1	0
	Rolls, enriched:[38]																		
	Commercial:																		
487	Brown-and-serve (12 per 12-oz pkg.), browned. 1 roll	26	27	85	2	2	.4	.7	.5	14	20	23	.5	25	Trace	.10	.06	.9	Trace
488	Cloverleaf or pan, 2 1/2-in diam., 2 in high. 1 roll	28	31	85	2	2	.4	.6	.4	15	21	24	.5	27	Trace	.11	.07	.9	Trace
489	Frankfurter and hamburger (8 per 11 1/2-oz pkg.). 1 roll	40	31	120	3	2	.5	.8	.6	21	30	34	.8	38	Trace	.16	.10	1.3	Trace
490	Hard, 3 3/4-in diam., 2 in high. 1 roll	50	25	155	5	2	.4	.6	.5	30	24	46	1.2	49	Trace	.20	.12	1.7	Trace
491	Hoagie or submarine, 11 1/2 by 3 by 2 1/2 in. 1 roll	135	31	390	12	4	.9	1.4	1.4	75	58	115	3.0	122	Trace	.54	.32	4.5	Trace
	From home recipe:																		
492	Cloverleaf, 2 1/2-in diam., 2 in high. 1 roll	35	26	120	3	3	.8	1.1	.7	20	16	36	.7	41	30	.12	.12	1.2	Trace
	Spaghetti, enriched, cooked:																		
493	Firm stage, "al dente," served hot. 1 cup	130	64	190	7	1	—	—	—	39	14	85	1.4	103	0	.23	.13	1.8	0
494	Tender stage, served hot. 1 cup	140	73	155	5	1	—	—	—	32	11	70	1.3	85	0	.20	.11	1.5	0
	Spaghetti (enriched) in tomato sauce with cheese:																		
495	From home recipe. 1 cup	250	77	260	9	9	2.0	5.4	.7	37	80	135	2.3	408	1,080	.25	.18	2.3	13
496	Canned. 1 cup	250	80	190	6	2	.5	.3	.4	39	40	88	2.8	303	930	.35	.28	4.5	10
	Spaghetti (enriched) with meat balls and tomato sauce:																		
497	From home recipe. 1 cup	248	70	330	19	12	3.3	6.3	.9	39	124	236	3.7	665	1,590	.25	.30	4.0	22
498	Canned. 1 cup	250	78	260	12	10	2.2	3.3	3.9	29	53	113	3.3	245	1,000	.15	.18	2.3	5
499	Toaster pastries. 1 pastry	50	12	200	3	6	—	—	—	36	60[54]	60[67]	1.9	60[74]	500	.16	.17	2.1	(60)
	Waffles, made with enriched flour, 7-in diam.:[38]																		
500	From home recipe. 1 waffle	75	41	210	7	7	2.3	2.8	1.4	28	85	130	1.3	109	250	.17	.23	1.4	Trace
501	From mix, egg and milk added. 1 waffle	75	42	205	7	8	2.8	2.9	1.2	27	179	257	1.0	146	170	.14	.22	.9	Trace

(A)	(B)	(g)	(C)	(D)	(E)	(F)	(G)	(H)	(I)	(J)	(K)	(L)	(M)	(N)	(O)	(P)	(Q)	(R)	(S)
	Wheat flours: All-purpose or family flour, enriched:																		
502	Sifted, spooned — 1 cup	115	12	420	12	1	0.2	0.1	0.5	88	18	100	3.3	109	0	0.74	0.46	6.1	0
503	Unsifted, spooned — 1 cup	125	12	455	13	1	.2	.1	.5	95	20	109	3.6	119	0	.80	.50	6.6	0
504	Cake or pastry flour, enriched, sifted, spooned — 1 cup	96	12	350	7	1	.1	.1	.3	76	16	70	2.8	91	0	.61	.38	5.1	0
505	Self-rising, enriched, unsifted, spooned — 1 cup	125	12	440	12	1	.2	.1	.5	93	331	583	3.6	—	0	.80	.50	6.6	0
506	Whole-wheat, from hard wheats, stirred — 1 cup	120	12	400	16	2	.4	.2	1.0	85	49	446	4.0	444	0	.66	.14	5.2	0
	LEGUMES (DRY), NUTS, SEEDS: RELATED PRODUCTS																		
	Almonds, shelled:																		
507	Chopped (about 130 almonds) — 1 cup	130	5	775	24	70	5.6	47.7	12.8	25	304	655	6.1	1,005	0	.31	1.20	4.6	Trace
508	Slivered, not pressed down (about 115 almonds) — 1 cup	115	5	690	21	62	5.0	42.2	11.3	22	269	580	5.4	889	0	.28	1.06	4.0	Trace
	Beans, dry: Common varieties as Great Northern, navy, and others: Cooked, drained:																		
509	Great Northern — 1 cup	180	69	210	14	1	—	—	—	38	90	266	4.9	749	0	.25	.13	1.3	0
510	Pea (navy) — 1 cup	190	69	225	15	1	—	—	—	40	95	281	5.1	790	0	.27	.13	1.3	0
	Canned, solids and liquid: White with:																		
511	Frankfurters (sliced) — 1 cup	255	71	365	19	18	—	—	—	32	94	303	4.8	668	330	.18	.15	3.3	Trace
512	Pork and tomato sauce — 1 cup	255	71	310	16	7	2.4	2.8	.6	48	138	235	4.6	536	330	.20	.08	1.5	5
513	Pork and sweet sauce — 1 cup	255	66	385	16	12	4.3	5.0	1.1	54	161	291	5.9	—	10	.15	.10	1.3	—
514	Red kidney — 1 cup	255	76	230	15	1	—	—	—	42	74	278	4.6	673	—	.13	.11	1.5	—
515	Lima, cooked, drained — 1 cup	190	64	260	16	1	—	—	—	49	55	293	5.9	1,163	—	.25	.11	1.3	—
516	Blackeye peas, dry, cooked (with residual cooking liquid) — 1 cup	250	80	190	13	1	—	—	—	35	43	238	3.3	573	30	.40	.10	1.0	—
517	Brazil nuts, shelled (6-8 large kernels) — 1 oz	28	5	185	4	19	4.8	6.2	7.1	3	53	196	1.0	203	Trace	.27	.03	.5	—
518	Cashew nuts, roasted in oil — 1 cup	140	5	785	24	64	12.9	36.8	10.2	41	53	522	5.3	650	140	.60	.35	2.5	—
	Coconut meat, fresh:																		
519	Piece, about 2 by 2 by 1/2 in — 1 piece	45	51	155	2	16	14.0	.9	.3	4	6	43	.8	115	0	.02	.01	.2	1
520	Shredded or grated, not pressed down — 1 cup	80	51	275	3	28	24.8	1.6	.5	8	10	76	1.4	205	0	.04	.02	.4	2
521	Filberts (hazelnuts), chopped (about 80 kernels) — 1 cup	115	6	730	14	72	5.1	55.2	7.3	19	240	388	3.9	810	—	.53	—	1.0	Trace
522	Lentils, whole, cooked — 1 cup	200	72	210	16	Trace	—	—	—	39	50	238	4.2	498	40	.14	.12	1.2	0
523	Peanuts, roasted in oil, salted (whole, halves, chopped) — 1 cup	144	2	840	37	72	13.7	33.0	20.7	27	107	577	3.0	971	—	.46	.19	24.8	0
524	Peanut butter — 1 tbsp	16	2	95	4	8	1.5	3.7	2.3	3	9	61	.3	100	—	.02	.02	2.4	0
525	Peas, split, dry, cooked — 1 cup	200	70	230	16	1	—	—	—	42	22	178	3.4	592	80	.30	.18	1.8	—
526	Pecans, chopped or pieces (about 120 large halves) — 1 cup	118	3	810	11	84	7.2	50.5	20.0	17	86	341	2.8	712	150	1.01	.15	1.1	2
527	Pumpkin and squash kernels, dry, hulled — 1 cup	140	4	775	41	65	11.8	23.5	27.5	21	71	1,602	15.7	1,386	100	.34	.27	3.4	—
528	Sunflower seeds, dry, hulled — 1 cup	145	5	810	35	69	8.2	13.7	43.2	29	174	1,214	10.3	1,334	70	2.84	.33	7.8	—
	Walnuts: Black:																		
529	Chopped or broken kernels — 1 cup	125	3	785	26	74	6.3	13.3	45.7	19	Trace	713	7.5	575	380	.28	.14	.9	—
530	Ground (finely) — 1 cup	80	3	500	16	47	4.0	8.5	29.2	12	Trace	456	4.8	368	240	.18	.09	.6	—
531	Persian or English, chopped (about 60 halves) — 1 cup	120	4	780	18	77	8.4	11.8	42.2	19	119	456	3.7	540	40	.40	.16	1.1	2

[13] Crust made with vegetable shortening and enriched flour.
[14] Made with vegetable shortening.
[15] Product may or may not be enriched with riboflavin. Consult the label.
[16] Value varies with the brand. Consult the label.

(Dashes (—) denote lack of reliable data for a constituent believed to be present in measurable amount)

NUTRIENTS IN INDICATED QUANTITY

SUGARS AND SWEETS

Item No. (A)	Foods, approximate measures, units, and weight (edible part unless footnotes indicate otherwise) (B)	Weight (Grams)	Water (C) Percent	Food energy (D) Calories	Protein (E) Grams	Fat (F) Grams	Fatty Acids Saturated (total) (G) Grams	Oleic (H) Grams	Linoleic (I) Grams	Carbohydrate (J) Grams	Calcium (K) Milligrams	Phosphorus (L) Milligrams	Iron (M) Milligrams	Potassium (N) Milligrams	Vitamin A value (O) International units	Thiamin (P) Milligrams	Riboflavin (Q) Milligrams	Niacin (R) Milligrams	Ascorbic acid (S) Milligrams
	Cake icings:																		
	Boiled, white:																		
532	Plain — 1 cup	94	18	295	1	0		0	0	75	2	2	Trace	17	0	Trace	0.03	Trace	0
533	With coconut — 1 cup	166	15	605	3	13	11.0	.9	Trace	124	10	50	0.8	277	0	0.02	.07	0.3	0
	Uncooked:																		
534	Chocolate made with milk and butter — 1 cup	275	14	1,035	9	38	23.4	11.7	1.0	185	165	305	3.3	536	580	.06	.28	.6	1
535	Creamy fudge from mix and water — 1 cup	245	15	830	7	16	5.1	6.7	3.1	183	96	218	2.7	238	Trace	.05	.20	.7	Trace
536	White — 1 cup	319	11	1,200	2	21	12.7	5.1	.5	260	48	38	Trace	57	860	Trace	.06	Trace	Trace
	Candy:																		
537	Caramels, plain or chocolate — 1 oz	28	8	115	1	3	1.6	1.1	.1	22	42	35	.4	54	Trace	.01	.05	.1	Trace
	Chocolate:																		
538	Milk, plain — 1 oz	28	1	145	2	9	5.5	3.0	.3	16	65	65	.3	109	80	.02	.10	.1	Trace
539	Semisweet, small pieces (60 per oz) — 1 cup or 6-oz pkg	170	1	860	7	61	36.2	19.8	1.7	97	51	255	4.4	553	30	.02	.14	.9	0
540	Chocolate-coated peanuts — 1 oz	28	1	160	5	12	4.0	4.7	2.1	11	33	84	.4	143	Trace	.10	.05	2.1	Trace
541	Fondant, uncoated (mints, candy corn, other) — 1 oz	28	8	105	Trace	1	.1	.3	.1	25	4	2	.3	1	0	Trace	Trace	Trace	0
542	Fudge, chocolate, plain — 1 oz	28	8	115	1	3	1.3	1.4	.6	21	22	24	.3	42	Trace	.01	.03	.1	Trace
543	Gum drops — 1 oz	28	12	100	Trace	Trace	—	—	—	25	2	Trace	.1	1	0	0	Trace	0	0
544	Hard — 1 oz	28	1	110	0	Trace	—	—	—	28	6	2	.5	1	0	0	0	Trace	0
545	Marshmallows — 1 oz	28	17	90	1	Trace	—	—	—	23	5	2	.5	2	0	0	Trace	0	0
	Chocolate-flavored beverage powders (about 4 heaping tsp per oz):																		
546	With nonfat dry milk — 1 oz	28	2	100	5	1	.5	.3	Trace	20	167	155	.5	227	10	.04	.21	.2	1
547	Without milk — 1 oz	28	1	100	1	1	.4	.2	0	25	9	48	.6	142	0	.01	.03	.1	0
548	Honey, strained or extracted — 1 tbsp	21	17	65	Trace	0	0	0	0	17	4	1	.2	11	0	Trace	.01	Trace	Trace
549	Jams and preserves — 1 tbsp	20	29	55	Trace	Trace	—	—	—	14	4	2	.2	18	Trace	Trace	.01	Trace	Trace
550	Jams and preserves — 1 packet	14	29	40	Trace	Trace	—	—	—	10	3	1	.1	12	Trace	Trace	.01	Trace	Trace
551	Jellies — 1 tbsp	18	29	50	Trace	Trace	—	—	—	13	4	1	.3	14	Trace	Trace	Trace	Trace	Trace
552	Jellies — 1 packet	14	29	40	Trace	Trace	—	—	—	10	3	1	.2	11	Trace	Trace	Trace	Trace	1
	Syrups:																		
	Chocolate-flavored sirup or topping:																		
553	Thin type — 1 fl oz or 2 tbsp	38	32	90	1	1	.5	.3	Trace	24	6	35	.6	106	Trace	.01	.03	.2	0
554	Fudge type — 1 fl oz or 2 tbsp	38	25	125	2	5	3.1	1.6	.1	20	48	60	.5	107	60	.02	.08	.2	Trace
	Molasses, cane:																		
555	Light (first extraction) — 1 tbsp	20	24	50	—	—	—	—	—	13	33	9	.9	183	—	.01	.01	Trace	—
556	Blackstrap (third extraction) — 1 tbsp	20	24	45	—	—	—	—	—	11	137	17	3.2	585	—	.02	.04	.4	—
557	Sorghum — 1 tbsp	21	23	55	—	—	—	—	—	14	35	5	2.6	—	—	—	.02	Trace	—
558	Table blends, chiefly corn, light and dark — 1 tbsp	21	24	60	0	0	0	0	0	15	9	3	.8	1	0	0	0	Trace	0
	Sugars:																		
559	Brown, pressed down — 1 cup	220	2	820	0	0	0	0	0	212	187	42	7.5	757	0	.02	.07	.4	0
	White:																		
560	Granulated — 1 cup	200	1	770	0	0	0	0	0	199	0	0	.2	6	0	0	0	0	0
561	Granulated — 1 tbsp	12	1	45	0	0	0	0	0	12	0	0	Trace	Trace	0	0	0	0	0
562	Granulated — 1 packet	6	1	23	0	0	0	0	0	6	0	0	Trace	Trace	0	0	0	0	0
563	Powdered, sifted, spooned into cup — 1 cup	100	1	385	0	0	0	0	0	100	0	0	.1	3	0	0	0	0	0

VEGETABLE AND VEGETABLE PRODUCTS

(A)	(B)	(C)	(D)	(E)	(F)	(G)	(H)	(I)	(J)	(K)	(L)	(M)	(N)	(O)	(P)	(Q)	(R)	(S)
	Asparagus, green:																	
	Cooked, drained:																	
	Cuts and tips, 1 1/2- to 2-in lengths:																	
564	From raw---------- 1 cup	94	30	3	Trace	—	—	—	5	30	73	0.9	265	1,310	0.23	0.26	2.0	38
565	From frozen------- 1 cup	93	40	6	Trace	—	—	—	6	40	115	2.2	396	1,530	.25	.23	1.8	41
	Spears, 1/2-in diam. at base:																	
566	From raw------- 4 spears	94	10	1	Trace	—	—	—	2	13	30	.4	110	540	.10	.11	.8	16
567	From frozen---- 4 spears	92	15	2	Trace	—	—	—	2	13	40	.7	143	470	.10	.08	.7	16
568	Canned, spears, 1/2-in diam. at base. 4 spears	93	15	2	Trace	—	—	—	3	15	42	1.5	133	640	.05	.08	.6	12
	Beans:																	
	Lima, immature seeds, frozen, cooked, drained:																	
569	Thick-seeded types (Fordhooks) 1 cup	74	170	10	Trace	—	—	—	32	34	153	2.9	724	390	.12	.09	1.7	29
570	Thin-seeded types (baby limas) 1 cup	69	210	13	Trace	—	—	—	40	63	227	4.7	709	400	.16	.09	2.2	22
	Snap:																	
	Green:																	
571	Cooked, drained: From raw (cuts and French style). 1 cup	92	30	2	Trace	—	—	—	7	63	46	.8	189	680	.09	.11	.6	15
	From frozen:																	
572	Cuts------------ 1 cup	92	35	2	Trace	—	—	—	8	54	43	.9	205	780	.09	.12	.5	7
573	French style---- 1 cup	92	35	2	Trace	—	—	—	8	49	39	1.2	177	690	.08	.10	.4	9
574	Canned, drained solids (cuts). 1 cup	92	30	2	Trace	—	—	—	7	61	34	2.0	128	630	.04	.07	.4	5
	Yellow or wax:																	
575	Cooked, drained: From raw (cuts and French style). 1 cup	93	30	2	Trace	—	—	—	6	63	46	.8	189	290	.09	.11	.6	16
576	From frozen (cuts)----- 1 cup	92	35	2	Trace	—	—	—	8	47	42	.9	221	140	.09	.11	.5	8
577	Canned, drained solids (cuts). 1 cup	92	30	2	Trace	—	—	—	7	61	34	2.0	128	140	.04	.07	.4	7
	Beans, mature. See Beans, dry (items 509-515) and Blackeye peas, dry (item 516).																	
	Bean sprouts (mung):																	
578	Raw------------------- 1 cup	89	35	4	Trace	—	—	—	7	20	67	1.4	234	20	.14	.14	.8	20
579	Cooked, drained------- 1 cup	91	35	4	Trace	—	—	—	7	21	60	1.1	195	30	.11	.13	.9	8
	Beets:																	
	Cooked, drained, peeled:																	
580	Whole beets, 2-in diam.---- 2 beets	91	30	1	Trace	—	—	—	7	14	23	.5	208	20	.03	.04	.3	6
581	Diced or sliced------------ 1 cup	91	55	2	Trace	—	—	—	12	24	39	.9	354	30	.05	.07	.5	10
	Canned, drained solids:																	
582	Whole beets, small-------- 1 cup	89	60	2	Trace	—	—	—	14	30	29	1.1	267	30	.02	.05	.2	5
583	Diced or sliced----------- 1 cup	89	65	2	Trace	—	—	—	15	32	31	1.2	284	30	.02	.05	.2	5
584	Beet greens, leaves and stems, cooked, drained. 1 cup	94	25	2	Trace	—	—	—	5	144	36	2.8	481	7,400	.10	.22	.4	22
	Blackeye peas, immature seeds, cooked and drained:																	
585	From raw------------- 1 cup	72	180	13	1	—	—	—	30	40	241	3.5	625	580	.50	.18	2.3	28
586	From frozen---------- 1 cup	66	220	15	1	—	—	—	40	43	286	4.8	573	290	.68	.19	2.4	15
	Broccoli, cooked, drained:																	
	From raw:																	
587	Stalk, medium size------ 1 stalk	91	45	6	1	—	—	—	8	158	112	1.4	481	4,500	.16	.36	1.4	162
588	Stalks cut into 1/2-in pieces 1 cup	91	40	5	Trace	—	—	—	7	136	96	1.2	414	3,880	.14	.31	1.2	140
	From frozen:																	
589	Stalk, 4 1/2 to 5 in long--- 1 stalk	91	10	1	Trace	—	—	—	1	12	17	.2	66	570	.02	.03	.2	22
590	Chopped----------------- 1 cup	92	50	5	1	—	—	—	9	100	104	1.3	392	4,810	.11	.22	.9	105
591	Brussels sprouts, cooked, drained: From raw, 7-8 sprouts (1 1/4- to 1 1/2-in diam.). 1 cup	88	55	7	1	—	—	—	10	50	112	1.7	423	810	.12	.22	1.2	135
592	From frozen----------- 1 cup	89	50	5	Trace	—	—	—	10	33	95	1.2	457	880	.12	.16	.9	126

(Dashes (−) denote lack of reliable data for a constituent believed to be present in measurable amount)

							Fatty Acids													
								Unsaturated												
Item No.	Foods, approximate measures, units, and weight (edible part unless footnotes indicate otherwise)		Water	Food energy	Protein	Fat	Saturated (total)	Oleic	Linoleic	Carbohydrate	Calcium	Phosphorus	Iron	Potassium	Vitamin A value	Thiamin	Riboflavin	Niacin	Ascorbic acid
(A)	(B)	Grams	(C) Per cent	(D) Calories	(E) Grams	(F) Grams	(G) Grams	(H) Grams	(I) Grams	(I) Grams	(K) Milligrams	(L) Milligrams	(M) Milligrams	(N) Milligrams	(O) International units	(P) Milligrams	(Q) Milligrams	(R) Milligrams	(S) Milligrams
	VEGETABLE AND VEGETABLE PRODUCTS—Con.																		
	Cabbage:																		
	Common varieties:																		
	Raw:																		
593	Coarsely shredded or sliced— 1 cup	70	92	15	1	Trace	—	—	—	4	34	20	0.3	163	90	0.04	0.04	0.02	33
594	Finely shredded or chopped— 1 cup	90	92	20	1	Trace	—	—	—	5	44	26	.4	210	120	.05	.05	.3	42
595	Cooked, drained— 1 cup	145	94	30	2	Trace	—	—	—	6	64	29	.4	236	190	.06	.06	.4	48
596	Red, raw, coarsely shredded or sliced. 1 cup	70	90	20	1	Trace	—	—	—	5	29	25	.6	188	30	.06	.04	.3	43
597	Savoy, raw, coarsely shredded or sliced. 1 cup	70	92	15	2	Trace	—	—	—	3	47	38	.6	188	140	.04	.06	.2	39
598	Cabbage, celery (also called pe-tsai or wongbok), raw, 1-in pieces. 1 cup	75	95	10	1	Trace	—	—	—	2	32	30	.5	190	110	.04	.03	.5	19
599	Cabbage, white mustard (also called bokchoy or pakchoy), cooked, drained. 1 cup	170	95	25	2	Trace	—	—	—	4	252	56	1.0	364	5,270	.07	.14	1.2	26
	Carrots:																		
	Raw, without crowns and tips, scraped:																		
600	Whole, 7 1/2 by 1 1/8 in, or strips, 2 1/2 to 3 in long— 1 carrot or 18 strips	72	88	30	1	Trace	—	—	—	7	27	26	.5	246	7,930	.04	.04	.4	6
601	Grated— 1 cup	110	88	45	1	Trace	—	—	—	11	41	40	.8	375	12,100	.07	.06	.7	9
602	Cooked (crosswise cuts), drained. 1 cup	155	91	50	1	Trace	—	—	—	11	51	48	.9	344	16,280	.08	.08	.8	9
	Canned:																		
603	Sliced, drained solids— 1 cup	155	91	45	1	Trace	—	—	—	10	47	34	1.1	186	23,250	.03	.05	.6	3
604	Strained or junior (baby food)— 1 oz (1 3/4 to 2 tbsp)	28	92	10	Trace	Trace	—	—	—	2	7	6	.1	51	3,690	.01	.01	.1	1
	Cauliflower:																		
605	Raw, chopped— 1 cup	115	91	31	3	Trace	—	—	—	6	29	64	1.3	339	70	.13	.12	.8	90
	Cooked, drained:																		
606	From raw (flower buds)— 1 cup	125	93	30	3	Trace	—	—	—	5	26	53	.9	258	80	.11	.10	.8	69
607	From frozen (flowerets)— 1 cup	180	94	30	3	Trace	—	—	—	6	31	68	.9	373	50	.07	.09	.7	74
	Celery, Pascal type, raw:																		
608	Stalk, large outer, 8 by 1 1/2 in, at root end. 1 stalk	40	94	5	Trace	Trace	—	—	—	2	16	11	.1	136	110	.01	.01	.1	4
609	Pieces, diced— 1 cup	120	94	20	1	Trace	—	—	—	5	47	34	.4	409	320	.04	.04	.4	11
	Collards, cooked, drained:																		
610	From raw (leaves without stems)— 1 cup	190	90	65	7	1	—	—	—	10	357	99	1.5	498	14,820	.21	.38	2.3	144
611	From frozen (chopped)— 1 cup	170	90	50	5	1	—	—	—	10	299	87	1.7	401	11,560	.10	.24	1.0	56
	Corn, sweet:																		
	Cooked, drained:																		
612	From raw, ear 5 by 1 3/4 in— 1 ear[61]	140	74	70	2	1	—	—	—	16	2	69	.5	151	[62]310	.09	.08	1.1	7
	From frozen:																		
613	Ear, 5 in long— 1 ear[61]	229	73	120	4	1	—	—	—	27	4	121	1.0	291	[62]440	.18	.10	2.1	9
614	Kernels— 1 cup	165	77	130	5	1	—	—	—	31	5	120	1.3	304	[62]580	.15	.10	2.5	8
	Canned:																		
615	Cream style— 1 cup	256	76	210	5	2	—	—	—	51	8	143	1.5	248	[62]840	.08	.13	2.6	13
	Whole kernel:																		
616	Vacuum pack— 1 cup	210	76	175	5	1	—	—	—	43	6	153	1.1	204	[62]740	.06	.13	2.3	11
617	Wet pack, drained solids— 1 cup	165	76	140	4	1	—	—	—	33	8	81	.8	160	[62]580	.05	.08	1.5	7
	Cowpeas. See Blackeye peas. (Items 585-586).																		
	Cucumber slices, 1/8 in thick (large, 2 1/8-in diam.; small, 1 3/4-in diam.):																		
618	With peel— 6 large or 8 small slices	28	95	5	Trace	Trace	—	—	—	1	7	8	.3	45	70	.01	.01	.1	3

(A)	(B)	(wt. g)	(C)	(D)	(E)	(F)	(G)	(H)	(I)	(J)	(K)	(L)	(M)	(N)	(O)	(P)	(Q)	(R)	(S)
619	Without peel——6 1/2 large or 9 small pieces.	28	96	5	Trace	Trace	—	—	—	1	5	5	0.1	45	Trace	0.01	0.01	0.1	3
620	Dandelion greens, cooked, drained——1 cup	105	90	35	2	1	—	—	—	7	147	44	1.9	244	12,290	.14	.17	—	19
621	Endive, curly (including escarole), raw, small pieces——1 cup	50	93	10	1	Trace	—	—	—	2	41	27	.9	147	1,650	.04	.07	.3	5
622	Kale, cooked, drained: From raw (leaves without stems and midribs)——1 cup	110	88	45	5	1	—	—	—	7	206	64	1.8	243	9,130	.11	.20	1.8	102
623	From frozen (leaf style)——1 cup	130	91	40	4	1	—	—	—	7	157	62	1.3	251	10,660	.08	.20	.9	49
	Lettuce, raw:																		
624	Butterhead, as Boston types: Head, 5-in diam.——1 head[63]	220	95	25	2	Trace	—	—	—	4	57	42	3.3	430	1,580	.10	.10	.5	13
625	Leaves——1 outer or 2 inner or 3 heart leaves.	15	95	Trace	Trace	Trace	—	—	—	Trace	5	4	.3	40	150	.01	.01	Trace	1
626	Crisphead, as Iceberg: Head, 6-in diam.——1 head[64]	567	96	70	5	1	—	—	—	16	108	118	2.7	943	1,780	.32	.32	1.6	32
627	Wedge, 1/4 of head——1 wedge	135	96	20	1	Trace	—	—	—	4	27	30	.7	236	450	.08	.08	.4	8
628	Pieces, chopped or shredded——1 cup	55	96	5	1	Trace	—	—	—	2	11	12	.3	96	180	.03	.03	.2	3
629	Looseleaf (bunching varieties including romaine or cos), chopped or shredded pieces——1 cup	55	94	10	1	Trace	—	—	—	2	37	14	.8	145	1,050	.03	.04	.2	10
630	Mushrooms, raw, sliced or chopped pieces——1 cup	70	90	20	2	Trace	—	—	—	3	4	81	.6	290	Trace	.07	.32	2.9	2
631	Mustard greens, without stems and midribs, cooked, drained——1 cup	140	93	30	3	1	—	—	—	6	193	45	2.5	308	8,120	.11	.20	.8	67
632	Okra pods, 3 by 5/8 in, cooked——10 pods	106	91	30	2	Trace	—	—	—	6	98	43	.5	184	520	.14	.19	1.0	21
	Onions: Mature: Raw:																		
633	Chopped——1 cup	170	89	65	3	Trace	—	—	—	15	46	61	.9	267	[65]Trace	.05	.07	.3	17
634	Sliced——1 cup	115	89	45	2	Trace	—	—	—	10	31	41	.6	181	[65]Trace	.03	.05	.2	12
635	Cooked (whole or sliced), drained——1 cup	210	92	60	3	Trace	—	—	—	14	50	61	.8	231	[65]Trace	.06	.06	.4	15
636	Young green, bulb (3/8 in diam.) and white portion of top——6 onions	30	88	15	Trace	Trace	—	—	—	3	12	12	.2	69	Trace	.02	.01	.1	8
637	Parsley, raw, chopped——1 tbsp	4	85	Trace	Trace	Trace	—	—	—	Trace	7	2	.2	25	300	Trace	.01	Trace	6
638	Parsnips, cooked (diced or 2-in lengths)——1 cup	155	82	100	2	1	—	—	—	23	70	96	.9	587	50	.11	.12	.2	16
	Peas, green: Canned:																		
639	Whole, drained solids——1 cup	170	77	150	8	1	—	—	—	29	44	129	3.2	163	1,170	.15	.10	1.4	14
640	Strained (baby food)——1 oz (1 3/4 to 2 tbsp)	28	86	15	1	Trace	—	—	—	3	3	18	.3	28	140	.02	.03	.3	3
641	Frozen, cooked, drained——1 cup	160	82	110	8	Trace	—	—	—	19	30	138	3.0	216	960	.43	.14	2.7	21
642	Peppers, hot, red, without seeds, dried (ground chili powder, added seasonings)——1 tsp	2	9	5	Trace	Trace	—	—	—	1	5	4	.3	20	1,300	Trace	.02	.2	Trace
	Peppers, sweet (about 5 per lb, whole), stem and seeds removed:																		
643	Raw——1 pod	74	93	15	1	Trace	—	—	—	4	7	16	.5	157	310	.06	.06	.4	94
644	Cooked, boiled, drained——1 pod	73	95	15	1	Trace	—	—	—	3	7	12	.4	109	310	.05	.05	.4	70
645	Potatoes, cooked: Baked, peeled after baking (about 2 per lb, raw)——1 potato	156	75	145	4	Trace	—	—	—	33	14	101	1.1	782	Trace	.15	.07	2.7	31
	Boiled (about 3 per lb, raw):																		
646	Peeled after boiling——1 potato	137	80	105	3	Trace	—	—	—	23	10	72	.8	556	Trace	.12	.05	2.0	22
647	Peeled before boiling——1 potato	135	83	90	3	Trace	—	—	—	20	8	57	.7	385	Trace	.12	.05	1.6	22
648	French-fried, strip, 2 to 3 1/2 in long: Prepared from raw——10 strips	50	45	135	2	7	1.7	1.2	3.3	18	8	56	.7	427	Trace	.07	.04	1.6	11
649	Frozen, oven heated——10 strips	50	53	110	2	4	1.1	.8	2.1	17	5	43	.9	326	Trace	.07	.01	1.3	11
650	Hashed brown, prepared from frozen——1 cup	155	56	345	3	18	4.6	3.2	9.0	45	28	78	1.9	439	Trace	.11	.03	1.6	12
	Mashed, prepared from—																		
651	Milk added——1 cup	210	83	135	4	2	.7	.4	Trace	27	50	103	.8	548	40	.17	.11	2.1	21

[61] Weight includes cob. Without cob, weight is 77 g for item 612, 126 g for item 613.
[62] Based on yellow varieties. For white varieties, value is trace.
[63] Weight includes refuse of outer leaves and core. Without these parts, weight is 163 g.
[64] Weight includes core. Without core, weight is 539 g.
[65] Value based on white-fleshed varieties. For yellow-fleshed varieties, value in International Units (I.U.) is 70 for item 633, 50 for item 634, and 80 for item 635.

(Dashes (—) denote lack of reliable data for a constituent believed to be present in measurable amount)

Item No.	Foods, approximate measures, units, and weight (edible part unless footnotes indicate otherwise)	Grams	Water (Percent)	Food energy (Calories)	Protein (Grams)	Fat (Grams)	Saturated (total) (Grams)	Oleic (Grams)	Linoleic (Grams)	Carbohydrate (Grams)	Calcium (Milligrams)	Phosphorus (Milligrams)	Iron (Milligrams)	Potassium (Milligrams)	Vitamin A value (International units)	Thiamin (Milligrams)	Riboflavin (Milligrams)	Niacin (Milligrams)	Ascorbic acid (Milligrams)
(A)	(B)		(C)	(D)	(E)	(F)	(G)	(H)	(I)	(J)	(K)	(L)	(M)	(N)	(O)	(P)	(Q)	(R)	(S)
	VEGETABLE AND VEGETABLE PRODUCTS—Con.																		
	Potatoes, cooked—Continued																		
	Mashed, prepared from raw—Continued																		
652	Milk and butter added------ 1 cup	210	80	195	4	9	5.6	2.3	0.2	26	50	101	0.8	525	360	0.17	0.11	2.1	19
653	1 cup	210	79	195	4	7	3.6	2.1	.2	30	65	99	.6	601	270	.08	.08	1.9	11
	Dehydrated flakes (without milk), water, milk, butter, and salt added.																		
654	Potato chips, 1 3/4 by 2 1/2 in oval cross section. 10 chips	20	2	115	1	8	2.1	1.4	4.0	10	8	28	.4	226	Trace	.04	.01	1.0	3
655	Potato salad, made with cooked salad dressing. 1 cup	250	76	250	7	7	2.0	2.7	1.3	41	80	160	1.5	798	350	.20	.18	2.8	28
656	Pumpkin, canned------ 1 cup	245	90	80	2	1	—	—	—	19	61	64	1.0	588	15,680	.07	.12	1.5	12
657	Radishes, raw (prepackaged) stem ends, rootlets cut off. 4 radishes	18	95	5	Trace	Trace				1	5	6	.2	58	Trace	.01	.01	.1	5
658	Sauerkraut, canned, solids and liquid. 1 cup	235	93	40	2	Trace				9	85	42	1.2	329	120	.07	.09	.5	33
	Southern peas. See Blackeye peas (items 585-586).																		
	Spinach:																		
659	Raw, chopped------ 1 cup	55	91	15	2	Trace	—	—	—	2	51	28	1.7	259	4,460	.06	.11	.3	28
	Cooked, drained:																		
660	From raw------ 1 cup	180	92	40	5	1	—	—	—	6	167	68	4.0	583	14,580	.13	.25	.9	50
	From frozen:																		
661	Chopped------ 1 cup	205	92	45	6	1	—	—	—	8	232	90	4.3	683	16,200	.14	.31	.8	39
662	Leaf------ 1 cup	190	92	45	6	1	—	—	—	7	200	84	4.8	688	15,390	.15	.27	1.0	53
663	Canned, drained solids------ 1 cup	205	91	50	6	1	—	—	—	7	242	53	5.3	513	16,400	.04	.25	.6	29
	Squash, cooked:																		
664	Summer (all varieties), diced, drained. 1 cup	210	96	30	2	Trace	—	—	—	7	53	53	.8	296	820	.11	.17	1.7	21
665	Winter (all varieties), baked, mashed. 1 cup	205	81	130	4	1	—	—	—	32	57	98	1.6	945	8,610	.10	.27	1.4	27
	Sweetpotatoes:																		
	Cooked (raw, 5 by 2 in; about 2 1/2 per lb):																		
666	Baked in skin, peeled------ 1 potato	114	64	160	2	1	—	—	—	37	46	66	1.0	342	9,230	.10	.08	.8	25
667	Boiled in skin, peeled------ 1 potato	151	71	170	3	1	—	—	—	40	48	71	1.1	367	11,940	.14	.09	.9	26
668	Candied, 2 1/2 by 2-in piece-- 1 piece	105	60	175	1	3	2.0	.8	.1	36	39	45	.9	200	6,620	.06	.04	.4	11
	Canned:																		
669	Solid pack (mashed)------ 1 cup	255	72	275	5	1	—	—	—	63	64	105	2.0	510	19,890	.13	.10	1.5	36
670	Vacuum pack, piece 2 3/4 by 1 in. 1 piece	40	72	45	1	Trace	—	—	—	10	10	16	.3	80	3,120	.02	.02	.2	6
	Tomatoes:																		
671	Raw, 2 3/5-in diam. (3 per 12 oz pkg.). 1 tomato[6]	135	94	25	1	Trace				6	16	33	.6	300	1,110	.07	.05	.9	[6,7]28
672	Canned, solids and liquid----- 1 cup	241	94	50	2	Trace				10	[6]14	46	1.2	523	2,170	.12	.07	1.7	41
673	Tomato catsup------ 1 cup	273	69	290	5	1				69	60	137	2.2	991	3,820	.25	.19	4.4	41
674	1 tbsp	15	69	15	Trace	Trace				4	3	8	.1	54	210	.01	.01	.2	2
	Tomato juice, canned:																		
675	Cup------ 1 cup	243	94	45	2	Trace				10	17	44	2.2	552	1,940	.12	.07	1.9	39
676	Glass (6 fl oz)------ 1 glass	182	94	35	2	Trace				8	13	33	1.6	413	1,460	.09	.05	1.5	29
677	Turnips, cooked, diced------ 1 cup	155	94	35	1	Trace				8	54	37	.6	291	Trace	.06	.08	.5	34
	Turnip greens, cooked, drained:																		
678	From raw (leaves and stems)--- 1 cup	145	94	30	3	Trace				5	252	49	1.5	—	8,270	.15	.33	.7	68
679	From frozen (chopped)------ 1 cup	165	93	40	4	Trace				6	195	64	2.6	246	11,390	.08	.15	.7	31
680	Vegetables, mixed, frozen, cooked- 1 cup	182	83	115	6	1				24	46	115	2.4	348	9,010	.22	.13	2.0	15

MISCELLANEOUS ITEMS

(A)	(B)	(C)	(D)	(E)	(F)	(G)	(H)	(I)	(J)	(K)	(L)	(M)	(N)	(O)	(P)	(Q)	(R)	(S)
	Baking powders for home use:																	
	Sodium aluminum sulfate:																	
681	With monocalcium phosphate monohydrate — 1 tsp — 3.0	2	5	Trace	Trace	0	0	0	1	58	87	—	5	0	0	0	0	0
682	With monocalcium phosphate monohydrate, calcium sulfate — 1 tsp — 2.9	1	5	Trace	Trace	0	0	0	1	183	45	—	—	0	0	0	0	0
	Barbecue sauce:																	
683	Straight phosphate — 1 tsp — 3.8	2	5	Trace	Trace	0.0	0.0	0.0	1	239	359	—	6	0	0	0	0	0
684	Low sodium — 1 tsp — 4.3	2	5	Trace	Trace	0.0	0.0	0.0	2	207	314	—	471	0	0	0	0	0
685	Barbecue sauce — 1 cup — 250	81	230	4	17	2.2	4.3	10.0	20	53	50	2.0	435	900	.03	.03	.8	13
686	**Beverages, alcoholic:** Beer — 12 fl oz — 360	92	150	1	0			0	14	18	108	Trace	90	—	.01	.11	2.2	—
	Gin, rum, vodka, whisky:																	
687	80-proof — 1 1/2-fl oz jigger — 42	67	95	—	—	0.0	0.0	0.0	Trace	—	—	—	—	—	—	—	—	—
688	86-proof — 1 1/2-fl oz jigger — 42	64	105	—	—			0.0	Trace	—	—	—	1	—	—	—	—	—
689	90-proof — 1 1/2-fl oz jigger — 42	62	110	—	—			0.0	Trace	—	—	—	1	—	—	—	—	—
	Wines:																	
690	Dessert — 3 1/2-fl oz glass — 103	77	140	Trace	0	0	0	0	8	8	—	—	77	—	.01	.02	.2	—
691	Table — 3 1/2-fl oz glass — 102	86	85	Trace	0	0	0	0	4	9	10	.4	94	—	Trace	.01	.1	—
	Beverages, carbonated, sweetened, nonalcoholic:																	
692	Carbonated water — 12 fl oz — 366	92	115	0	0	0.0	0.0	0.0	29	—	—	—	—	0	0	0	0	0
693	Cola type — 12 fl oz — 369	90	145	0	0	0.0	0.0	0.0	37	—	—	—	—	0	0	0	0	0
694	Fruit-flavored sodas and Tom Collins mixer — 12 fl oz — 372	88	170	0	0	0.0	0.0	0.0	45	—	—	—	—	0	0	0	0	0
695	Ginger ale — 12 fl oz — 366	92	115	0	0	0.0	0.0	0.0	29	—	—	—	0	0	0	0	0	0
696	Root beer — 12 fl oz — 370	90	150	0	0	0.0	0.0	0.0	39	—	—	—	0	0	0	0	0	0
	Chili powder. See Peppers, hot, red (item 642).																	
	Chocolate:																	
697	Bitter or baking. Semisweet, see Candy, chocolate (item 539). — 1 oz — 28	2	145	3	15	8.9	4.9	.4	8	22	109	1.9	235	20	.01	.07	.4	0
698	Gelatin, dry — 1 7-g envelope — 7	13	25	6	Trace	0.0	0.0	0.0	0	—	—	—	—	—	—	—	—	—
699	Gelatin dessert prepared with gelatin dessert powder and water — 1 cup — 240	84	140	4	0	0.0	0.0	0.0	34	—	—	—	—	—	—	—	—	—
700	Mustard, prepared, yellow — 1 tsp or individual serving pouch or cup — 5	80	5	Trace	Trace			Trace	Trace	4	4	.1	7	—	—	—	—	—
	Olives, pickled, canned:																	
701	Green — 4 medium or 3 extra large or 2 giant.[69] — 16	78	15	Trace	2	.2	1.2	.1	Trace	8	2	.2	7	40	—	—	—	—
702	Ripe, Mission — 3 small or 2 large[69] — 10	73	15	Trace	2	.2	1.2	.1	Trace	9	1	.1	2	10	Trace	Trace	—	—
	Pickles, cucumber:																	
703	Dill, medium, whole, 3 3/4 in long, 1 1/4-in diam — 1 pickle — 65	93	5	Trace	Trace				1	17	14	.7	130	70	Trace	.01	Trace	4
704	Fresh-pack, slices 1 1/2-in diam., 1/4 in thick — 2 slices — 15	79	10	Trace	Trace				3	5	4	.3	20	20	Trace	Trace	Trace	1
705	Sweet, gherkin, small, whole, about 2 1/2 in long, 3/4-in diam — 1 pickle — 15	61	20	Trace	Trace				5	2	2	.2	—	10	Trace	Trace	Trace	1
706	Relish, finely chopped, sweet — 1 tbsp — 15	63	20	Trace	Trace				5	3	2	.1	—	—	—	—	—	—
	Popcorn. See items 476-478.																	
707	Popsicle, 3-fl oz size — 1 popsicle — 95	80	70	0	0	0	0	0	18	0	—	Trace	—	0	0	0	0	0

[66] Weight includes cores and stem ends. Without these parts, weight is 123 g.
[67] Based on year-round average. For tomatoes marketed from November through May, value is about 12 mg; from June through October, 32 mg.
[68] Applies to product without calcium salts added. Value for products with calcium salts added may be as much as 63 mg for whole tomatoes, 241 mg for cut forms.
[69] Weight includes pits. Without pits, weight is 13 g for item 701, 9 g for item 702.

(Dashes (—) denote lack of reliable data for a constituent believed to be present in measurable amount)

NUTRIENTS IN INDICATED QUANTITY

Item No. (A)	Foods, approximate measures, units, and weight (edible part unless footnotes indicate otherwise) (B)	Grams	Water (C) Percent	Food energy (D) Calories	Protein (E) Grams	Fat (F) Grams	Fatty Acids — Saturated (total) (G) Grams	Unsaturated Oleic (H) Grams	Linoleic (I) Grams	Carbohydrate (J) Grams	Calcium (K) Milligrams	Phosphorus (L) Milligrams	Iron (M) Milligrams	Potassium (N) Milligrams	Vitamin A value (O) International units	Thiamin (P) Milligrams	Riboflavin (Q) Milligrams	Niacin (R) Milligrams	Ascorbic acid (S) Milligrams
	MISCELLANEOUS ITEMS—Con.																		
	Soups:																		
	Canned, condensed:																		
	Prepared with equal volume of milk:																		
708	Cream of chicken———— 1 cup	245	85	180	7	10	4.2	3.6	1.3	15	172	152	0.5	260	610	0.05	0.27	0.7	2
709	Cream of mushroom——— 1 cup	245	83	215	7	14	5.4	2.9	4.6	16	191	169	.5	279	250	.05	.34	.7	1
710	Tomato———————— 1 cup	250	84	175	7	7	3.4	1.7	1.0	23	168	155	.8	418	1,200	.10	.25	1.3	15
	Prepared with equal volume of water:																		
711	Bean with pork——————— 1 cup	250	84	170	8	6	1.2	1.8	2.4	22	63	128	2.3	395	650	.13	.08	1.0	3
712	Beef broth, bouillon, consomme. 1 cup	240	96	30	5	0	0	0	0	3	Trace	31	.5	130	Trace	Trace	.02	1.2	—
713	Beef noodle——————— 1 cup	240	93	65	4	3	.6	.7	.8	7	7	48	1.0	77	50	.05	.07	1.0	Trace
714	Clam chowder, Manhattan type (with tomatoes, without milk). 1 cup	245	92	80	2	3	.5	.4	1.3	12	34	47	1.0	184	880	.02	.02	1.0	—
715	Cream of chicken——————— 1 cup	240	92	95	3	6	1.6	2.3	1.1	8	24	34	.5	79	410	.02	.05	.5	Trace
716	Cream of mushroom——— 1 cup	240	90	135	2	10	2.6	1.7	4.5	10	41	50	.5	98	70	.02	.12	.7	Trace
717	Minestrone——————— 1 cup	245	90	105	5	3	.7	.9	1.3	14	37	59	1.0	314	2,350	.07	.05	1.0	—
718	Split pea——————— 1 cup	245	85	145	9	3	1.1	1.2	.4	21	29	149	1.5	270	440	.25	.15	1.5	—
719	Tomato——————— 1 cup	245	91	90	2	3	.5	.5	1.0	16	15	34	.7	230	1,000	.05	.05	1.2	12
720	Vegetable beef——————— 1 cup	245	92	80	5	2	—	—	—	10	12	49	.7	162	2,700	.05	.05	1.0	—
721	Vegetarian——————— 1 cup	245	92	80	2	2	—	—	—	13	20	39	1.0	172	2,940	.05	.05	1.0	—
	Dehydrated:																		
722	Bouillon cube, 1/2 in——— 1 cube	4	4	5	1	Trace	—	—	—	Trace	—	—	—	4	—	—	—	—	—
	Mixes:																		
	Unprepared:																		
723	Onion——————— 1 1/2-oz pkg	43	3	150	6	5	1.1	2.3	1.0	23	42	49	.6	238	30	.05	.03	.3	6
	Prepared with water:																		
724	Chicken noodle——— 1 cup	240	95	55	2	1	—	—	—	8	7	19	.2	19	50	.07	.05	.5	Trace
725	Onion——————— 1 cup	240	96	35	1	1	—	—	—	6	10	12	.2	58	Trace	Trace	Trace	Trace	2
726	Tomato vegetable with noodles. 1 cup	240	93	65	2	1	—	—	—	12	7	19	.2	29	480	.05	.02	.5	5
727	Vinegar, cider——————— 1 tbsp	15	94	Trace	Trace	0	0	0	—	1	1	1	.1	15	—	—	—	—	—
728	White sauce, medium, with enriched flour. 1 cup	250	73	405	10	31	19.3	7.8	.8	22	288	233	.5	348	1,150	.12	.43	.7	2
	Yeast:																		
729	Baker's, dry, active——— 1 pkg	7	5	20	3	Trace	—	—	—	3	3	90	1.1	140	Trace	.16	.38	2.6	Trace
730	Brewer's, dry——————— 1 tbsp	8	5	25	3	Trace	—	—	—	3	[7]17	140	1.4	152	Trace	1.25	.34	3.0	Trace

[7]Value may vary from 6 to 60 mg.

Source: *Nutritive Values of Foods,* United States Department of Agriculture, Home and Garden Bulletin No. 72.

BIBLIOGRAPHY

American Dietetic Association Foundation Cookbook. Chicago, IL, The American Dietetic Association Foundation, 1985.

An Eating Plan for Healthy Americans. Dallas, TEX, The American Heart Association, 1985.

Anderson, J: Food Allergy and Food Intolerance. *Contemporary Nutrition,* vol. 9, no. 9, Minneapolis, MN, General Mills Nutrition Dept., 1984.

Axler, BH: *Foodservice: A Managerial Aproach.* ?Supply City? NIFI and D.C. Health and Co., 1979.

Blackburn G: Fad-Reducing Diets: Separating Fads From Facts. *Contemporary Nutrition,* vol. 8, no. 7, Minneapolis, MN, General Mills Nutrition Dept., 1983.

Block Z: *It's All On The Label.* Boston, MA, Little, Brown & Company, 1981.

Bray, G: Obesity: A Blueprint for Progress. *Contemporary Nutrition,* vol. 12, no. 7, Minneapolis, MN, General Mills Nutrition Dept., 1987.

Breen, JJ and Sanderson, WD: *How to Start A Successful Restaurant: An Entrepreneur's Guide.* New York, NY, Lebhar-Friedman Books Chain Store Publishing Corp., 1981.

Brody, JE: *Jane Brody's Nutrition Book.* New York, NY, W.W. Norton and Company, 1981.

Carlson, BL: Meeting Consumer Demands—The Basis for Successful Marketing of Nutrition in Foodservices. *International Journal of Hospitality Management, vol. 5, no. 4, pp. 163–169, 1986.*

Carlson, BL: Preparing the Hospitality Student to Meet Nutrition Concerns in Today's Restaurants. 1986 Proceedings of the CHRIE Conference. ?Supply City & Publisher? pp. 161–166, 1986.

Carson, C: Coping with the Dietary-Fat Issue: A Plan of Action. *Dairy Foods,* vol. 88, p. 11, 1987.

Chait, A: Dietary Management of Diabetes Melitus. *Contemporary Nutrition,* vol. 9, no. 2, Minneapolis, MN, General Mills Nutrition Dept., 1984.

Cholesterol Counts. *U.S. Dept. of Health and Human Services,* National Institute of Health Publication No. 85–2699, October 1985.

Christian, JL and Greger, JL: *Nutrition for Living.* Menlo Park, CA, The Benjamin/Cummings Publishing Co., Inc. 1985.

Claiborne C: *Craig Claiborne's Gourmet Diet.* New York, NY, New York Times Books, 1980.

Clydesdale, FM: Dietary Iron—Chemistry and Bioavailability, vol. 10, no. 4, *Contemporary Nutrition,* Minneapolis, MN, General Mills Nutrition Dept., 1985.

Consumer Nutrition Concerns and Restaurant Choices, vol. 1, Washington, DC, 1986.

Consumers Redefine Their Additive Attitudes. *Food Engineering International,* vol. 12, p. 32, 1987.

Coppess, MH: Dietary Schizophrenia: Is America Really Counting Calories? *The NRA News,* vol. 6, pp. 10–11, 1986.

Dahringer, Le and Johnson, D: The Federal Trade Commission Redefinition of Deception and Public Policy Implications: Let The Buyer Beware. *The Journal of Consumer Affairs,* vol. 18, pp. 326–342, 1984.

Dietary Guidelines for Healthy American Adults: A Statement for Physicians and Health Professionals by the Nutrition Committee. Dallas, TEX, *The American Heart Association,* 1986.

Dietary Intervention: Main Factor in Reducing Blood Cholesterol Levels. *The American Dietetic Association Courier,* vol. 26, pp. 1–3, 1987.

Drew, K: The Work and Education of Chefs. *International Journal of Hospitality Management,* vol. 6, pp. 52–55, 1987.

Dunn, MD: *Fundamentals of Nutrition.* New York, NY, Van Nostrand Reinhold, 1983.

Dzeizak, J: Microwavable Foods—Industry's Response to Consumer Demands for Convenience. *Food Technology,* vol. 41, pp. 51–62, 1987.

Elder M: The Future of Foodservice Consumer Tastes. *Restaurant Business,* vol. 86, pp. 147–163, 1987.

Exchange Lists for Meal Planning. Chicago, IL, American Dietetic and American Diabetic Associations, 1986.

Facts About Blood Cholesterol. *The National Heart, Lung and Blood Institute/U.S. Dept. of Health and Human Services,* N.I.H. Publication No. 85–2696, 1985.

FDA Consumer, U.S. Dept. of HEW, Washington, D.C.,

    A Compendium on Fats, March, 1983.

    A New Weapon in the Battle Against Heart Disease, Nov., 1987.

Clot-Busting Drugs to 'Turn Off' Heart Attacks, Feb., 1987.

Diners' Club: The Four Varieties of Restaurant-Goers, March, 1987.

Dining Out with a Healthy Appetite, March, 1987.

Nutrition and the Athlete, May, 1987.

Planning a Diet for a Healthy Heart, March, 1987.

Please Pass That Woman Some More Calcium and Iron, September, 1984.

Selling Nutrition: Should Food Packages Carry Health Messages? Nov. 1987.

What About Nutrients and Fast Foods? May, 1983.

Fessel, C: Gastronomy 2000: A New Gastrosophy. *The Consultant.* vol. 20, pp. 43–47, 1987.

Fitness Focus at Food Firms. *Environmental Nutrition Newsletter,* vol. 8, p. 4, 1985.

Fluoridation—A Matter of Choice. *University of California Berkeley Wellness Letter,* Des Moines, IA, Health Letter Associates, 1985.

Forrest, LG: *Training for the Hospitality Industry.* New York, NY, The Educational Institute of the AH&MA, 1982.

Franz, MJ: *Exchanges for All Occasions.* Minneapolis, MN, International Diabetes Center, 1983.

Franz, J: *Fast Food Facts.* Minneapolis, MN, International Diabetes Center, 1985.

Gallup Organization, Inc: *Changes in Consumer Eating Habits.* ?Supply City? National Restaurant Association, 1986.

Greenwald, P: Dietary Fiber and Colon Cancer. *Contemporary Nutrition,* vol. 11, no. 1, Minneapolis, MN, General Mills Nutrition Dept., 1986.

Gussow, JD and Thomas PR: *The Nutrition Debate: Sorting Out Some Answers.* Palo Alto, CA, Bull Publishing Company, 1986.

Hamilton, EM and Whitney EN: *Understanding Nutrition,* ed. 3. St. Paul, MN, West Publishing, 1984.

Hamilton, EM, Whitney EN, and Sizer FS: *Nutrition Concepts and Controversies,* ed. 3. St. Paul, MN, West Publishing, 1985.

392

Hannigan K: Vegetable Protein Use Shifts Gears. *Food Engineering,* vol. 59, pp. 155–162, 1987.

Harlander S: Biotechnology in the Food Processing Industry. *Contemporary Nutrition,* vol. XI, no. 3, Minneapolis, MN, General Mills Nutrition Dept., 1986.

Hayes, DK and Hoffman L: Menu Analysis: A Better Way. *The Cornell Hotel and Restaurant Administration Quarterly,* vol. 25, no. 4, 1985.

Heaney, R: Calcium Bioavailability. *Contemporary Nutrition,* vol. 11, no. 8, Minneapolis, MN, General Mills Nutrition Dept., 1986.

Herbert V: Health Claims in Food Labeling and Advertising. *Nutrition Today,* vol. 22, pp. 25–30, 1987.

The Institute of Food Technologists' Expert Panel on Food Safety and Nutrition: Sweeteners: Nutritive and Non-Nutritive. *Contemporary Nutrition,* vol. 12, no. 9, Minneapolis, MN, General Mills Nutrition Dept., 1987.

Jarvis, T: Vitamin Use and Abuse. *Contemporary Nutrition,* vol. 9, no. 10, Minneapolis, MN, General Mills Nutrition Dept., 1984.

Jelen P: *Introduction to Food Processing.* Reston, VA, Reston Publishing Co., Inc., 1985.

Karpaty, P: Nutrition, Taste, and Economy—A Delicate Balance. *Resort and Hotel Management,* vol. 39, pp. 23–25, 1985.

Kasavana, ML and Smith, DS: *Menu Engineering: A Practical Guide to Menu Pricing.* Okemos, MI, Hospitality Publishers, 1982.

Kelly, G: Getting the Nutrition Word Out. *NRA News, National Restaurant Association,* vol. 4, pp. 17–19, 1984.

Kotschevar, L: *Management by Menu,* ed. 2. Dubuque, IA, Wm. C. Brown Company, 1986.

Kotschevar, L: *Quantity Food Production—Standards, Techniques and Principles,* ed. 4. New York, NY, Van Nostrand Reinhold, 1988.

Kraus, B: *The Dictionary of Sodium, Fats, and Cholesterol.* New York, NY, Grosset & Dunlap, 1980.

Kraus B: *Calories and Carbohydrates,* ed. 5. New York, NY, Signet, 1983.

Kraus B: *1983 Sodium Guide to Brand Names and Basic Foods.* New York, NY, New American Library, 1983.

Lappe, FM: *Diet for a Small Planet.* New York, NY, Ballantine Books, Inc., 1973.

Laudadio, D and Laudadio L: The Function of Nutrition in the Hospitality Curriculum and Industry of the Future. 1982 Proceedings of the National CHRIE Conference ?Supply city & publisher? pp. 253–278.

Lecos, CW: Cutting Cholesterol? Look to the Label. *FDA Consumer,* vol. 21, pp. 8–13, 1987.

Leontos, C: Nutrition on Menu Means $$$$ in Pocket. *Nevada Hospitality,* vol. 6, ?Supply pages? 1988.

Leveille, GA, Zabik, ME, and Morgan KJ: *Nutrients in Foods.* Cambridge, MA, The Nutrition Guild, 1983.

Lewis, CJ, Campbell-Lindzey, VS, and Lewis, KJ: A Nutrition Information/Resource Center Within A University Setting. *Journal of Nutrition Education,* vol. 17, no. 1, pp. 7–10, 1985.

Lipske, SN: The Eating Out Public's Interest in Nutrition. *Position Paper and Research Summary. G.D.R.—CREST,* NRA, ?Supply city? 1984.

McNamara, DJ: The Diet-Heart Question: How Good Is the Evidence? *Contemporary Nutrition,* vol. 12, no. 4, Minneapolis, MN, General Mills Nutrition Dept., 1987.

McWilliams, M: *Food Fundamentals,* ed. 4. New York, NY, John Wiley & Sons, 1985.

Martin, B: *Quality Service: The Restaurant Manager's Bible.* New York, NY, Cornell University School of Hotel Administration, 1986.

Medved, E: *Food Preparation and Theory.* Englewood Cliffs, NJ, Prentice Hall Co., Inc., 1986.

Miller, J: *Menu Pricing and Strategy,* ed. 2. New York, NY, Van Nostrand Reinhold, 1986.

Minor, LJ: *Nutritional Standards.* Westport, CT, A.V.I. Publishing Company, Inc., 1983.

Minor LJ: *Sanitation, Safety and Environmental Standards.* Westport, CT, The AVI Publishing Company, 1983.

Morgan, KJ: The Role of Snacking in the American Diet. *Contemporary Nutrition,* vol. 7, no. 9, Minneapolis, MN, General Mills Nutriion Dept., 1982.

Morgan, WJ, Jr: *Supervision and Management of Quantity Food Preparation,* ed. 3. Berkeley, CA, McCutchan Publishing Corp., 1988.

Murphy, TA and Murphy, D: *The Wellness for Life Workbook,* ed. 3. San Diego, CA, Fitness Publications, 1984.

National Academy of Science: *Recommended Dietary Allowances,* ed. 9. Washington, DC, National Academy of Science, 1980.

National Academy of Science: The Role of Nutrition in Disease Prevention and Health Promotion and Maintenance. *Nutrition News,* vol. 48, pp. 13–16, 1985.

National Institute of Health Statement: Health Implications of Obesity. *Contemporary Nutrition,* vol. 10, no. 9, Minneapolis, MN, General Mills Nutrition Dept., 1985.

National Restaurant Association: An Historical Perspective for Foodservice: Food Product Information. *Current Issues Report,* Washington, DC, National Restaurant Association, 1986.

National Restaurant Association: *Conducting a Feasibility Study for a New Restaurant.* Washington, DC, NRA with Cini-Grissom Association, Inc., 1983.

National Restaurant Association: *Guidelines for Providing Facts to Foodservice Patrons: Ingredient and Nutrition Information.* Washington, DC, NRA, 1987.

National Restaurant Association Current Issues Report: Nutrition and Foodservice. Washington, DC, NRA, 1983.

National Restaurant Association Current Issues Report: Consumer Food Safety Concerns, Washington, DC, NRA, 1986.

Nutrition and the American Restaurant: A Report on Nutritious Food Offerings in Consumer Information Programs. Washington, DC, The Public Voice for Food and Health Policy, 1983.

O'Connor, P: Dietary Fat, Calories, and Cancer. *Contemporary Nutrition,* vol. 10, no. 7, Minneapolis, MN, General Mills Nutrition Det., July 1985.

Patrons Seek Healthier Foods: NRA Survey Suggests New Marketing Tacks. *Nation's Restaurant News,* p. 21, June 9, 1986.

Pennington, JA and Church, HN: *Food Values of Portions Commonly Used,* ed. 14. Philadelphia, PA, J.B. Lippincott, 1985.

Person, S: Dietworks Formula Yields Natural Growth. *Restaurant Business,* pp. 210–214, July 20, 1985.

Pratscher M, Lydecker T, Weinstein J, and Bertagnoli L: Tastes of America: How America Loves to Eat Out. *Restaurants and Institutions,* vol. 97, no. 26, pp. 30–84, 1987.

Pressure on Fast Food Chains to Name Ingredients. *Tufts University Diet and Nutrition Letter,* vol. 4, p. 1, 1986.

R & I 400: Menus and Markets. *Restaurants and Institutions,* vol. 97, no. 16, 1987.

Regan, C: National Restaurant Association National Conference: Presentation on Nutrition in Foodservice. Chicago, IL, May 1987.

Shetterly, C: Healthy Employees Keep Companies Well. *The Las Vegas Sun,* p. C-1, November 11, 1985.

Southgate, D: New Thoughts on Carbohydrate Digestion. *Contemporary Nutrition,* vol. 12, no. 10, Minneapolis, MN, General Mills Nutrition Dept., 1987.

Spears, NC and Vaden, AG: *Foodservice Organizations: A Managerial and Systems Approach.* New York, NY, John Wiley & Sons, 1985.

Stare, F. et al: *Atheriosclerosis.* Englewood Cliffs, CPC International (Medcom), 1974.

Stare, J and McWilliams M: *Living Nutrition,* ed. 4. New York, NY, John Wiley & Sons, 1984.

Tabacchi, H: Targeting the Health-Conscious Consumer. *The Cornell Hotel and Restaurant Administration Quarterly,* vol. 28, pp. 21–24, 1987.

The Fiber Furor. *Consumer Reports,* pp. 640–642, October 1986.

The New Science of Nutrition: Diet Wars. *U.S. News & World Report,* vol. 100, pp. 62–69, January 20, 1986.

The Optimal Diet. *The Phi Kappa Journal,* vol. 64, ?Supply page? Winter, 1984.

Toufexis, A: Dieting: The Losing Game. *Time,* pp. 54–63, January 20, 1986.

US Dept. of HHS: *Facts About Cholesterol.* Washington, DC, National Institutes of Health Publication No. 85-2696, 1985.

USDA: Composition of Foods. Washington, DC, Agricultural Handbook No. 8, Series Nos. 1-8, 1982.

USDA: Conserving Nutritional Values in Foods. Washington, DC, *Home and Garden Bulletin No. 90,* 1983.

USDA: Nutritive Value of American Foods in Common Units. Washington, DC, *Agricultural Handbook No. 456,* 1979.

USDA Publication F.D.A. 84-1109: *Information Materials for the Food and Cosmetic Industries,* Washington, DC, 1984.

USDA and USDHHS: Dietary Guidelines for Americans. Washington, DC, *Home and Garden Bulletin No. 232,* August 1985.

Wagner, J: The Bite without the Bulge. *Food Engineering International,* vol. 12, p. 7, May 1987.

Whelan, EM and Stare FJ: *The 100% Natural, Purely Organic, Cholesterol-Free, Megavitamin, Low-Carbohydrate Nutrition Hoax.* New York, NY, Antheneum, 1983.

Williams, ER and Caliendo, MA: *Nutrition: Principles, Issues and Applications.* New York, NY, McGraw-Hill Book Company, 1984.

Williams, SR: *Nutrition and Diet Therapy,* ed. 5. St. Louis, MO, Mosby College Publishing, 1985.

Index

A

Absorption, nutrient, 50
Adding weight, 131
Adipose tissue, 97, 98
Advertising, 280, 283
Alcohol, 77, 100, 111
Aldersterone, 157, 173
Alimentary canal, 48
Allergies, 275, 326
Alternative sweeteners, 73
American Cancer Society, 5
American Council on Science and
    Health, 110
American Diabetes Association, 5, 319
American Dietetic Association, 5, 33,
    318, 319
American Heart Association, 5, 11, 31,
    102, 109, 110, 248
Amine, 81
Amino acids, 46, 81, 89, 329
Anabolism, 50, 89
Anemia, 178, 322
Angina pectoris, 109
Animal product cookery, 207
Anorexia nervosa, 118, 145
Antioxidants in fat, 96
Antivitamins, 137
Appendicitis, 67
Apprenticeship training, 298
Ascorbic acid, 152
Aspartame, 73
Athlete's diet, 88
Attitudes, consumer, 225
Attitudes, knowledge and skills (AKS),
    292
Avidin, 152

B

Basal metabolic rate, 125, 128
Basic Four Food Plan, 53, 54, 86, 102,
    328
Beriberi, 144
Bile, 49
Biotin, 151
Blood, 178

Blood clotting, 142
Biological value (BV), 84
Bitot's spots, 138
Blood sugar, 68
Body composition, 121
Body fat, 97, 98
Budgets, 241
Bulimia nervosa, 118
Bulk diets, 321
Business and industry feeding, 246
B-vitamins

C

Calcium, 140
Calculating nutrient values, 51
Calorie control, 116, 251, 303, 316
Calorie, defined, 50
Calories, 50, 271
Calories, in foods, 63, 68
Calories, consumer attitudes, 226-231
Calorie needs
    from activity, 123, 125
    from hormone activity, 123
Calories, percents consumer, 7, 9
Calories, recommended amounts, 68
Caloric needs, 124
Cancer, 67, 72, 90, 93
Cancer and fiber, 321
Capital expenses, 241
Carbohydrate, 45, 46, 48, 63, 81
Carbohydrate intake recommended, 68
Carcinogens, 73
Cardiovascular disease (CVD), 92, 97,
    98, 101, 109
Caries, 71, 140
Carotene, 138
Catabolism, 50, 89
Causes of death, 116
Causes of overweight, 119
Cellulose, 67, 116
Cereal cookery, 210
Cereal council, 32
Cerebral infarction, 109
Checker, 309
Chef's training, 306, 308

Chlorine, 139, 175
Cholesterol, 4, 73, 96, 97-99, 103, 109, 139, 303
Cholesterol and fiber, 321
Cholesterol control, 111
Choline, 137
Chlorophyll, 64
Chromium, 184
Cirrhosis, 78
Citric acid cycle, 70
Clotting of blood, 142
Cobalamin (B$_{12}$), 150, 185
Cobalt, 185
Coenzymes, 137
Collagen, 152
Collecting market data, 223
Communication steps, 294
Competition, 221; 223
Complementary proteins, 82, 329
Complete proteins, 329
Complex carbohydrates, 63, 64, 66, 68, 75
Composition, body, 121
Computers, 53, 233, 254
Conjugated lipids, 97
Consumer attitudes, 225
Consumers, kinds, 225
Controlling calories, 116
Controlling dietary cholesterol, 103
Controlling dietary fat, 104
Cooking frozen meat, 209
Cooking losses (nutrient), 206
Copper, 182
"Creative cuisine" program, 248
Cretinism, 181
Customer information (see also guest information), 306
Customers and the market, 221
Cyclamate, 67, 73

D
Dairy products, handling of, 200
Data market collection, 223
Deaminization, 68
Deaths, causes of, 116
Death rates, 3, 4
Delaney amendment, 37, 73
Diabetes, 230, 319-321
Diet adequacy, 51
Dietary Goals, 7, 9, 38, 86, 101, 285
Dietary Guidelines, 68, 101, 205

Dietary patterns, 4, 5, 20
Dietary exchange method, 86, 101, 104, 272
Diet levels, 4
Diet manuals, 317
Dietitians, 317, 318
Diet fads, 27, 127
Diet prescription, 316, 317
Diet(s), 60, 230, 316
Diets, special, 316
Digestion, 47
Digestive system, 48
Disaccharides, 64, 66
Disease, food related, 3, 4
Diverticulosis, 61, 321
DNA, 151
Drip loss, 208
Drives to eat, 20
Drug interactions, 326
Dry storage, 201-202

E
Eating habits, 20
Economic needs for food, 27
Ectomorphic, 122
Electrolytes, 163
Elimination diets for allergies, 327
Elimination (fecal waste), 50
Empty calories, 72
Endomorphic, 122
Endorsements, 282-283
Energy, 46, 63
Energy nutrients, 46, 63
Enrichment (fortification), 200
Environmental Protection Agency (EPA), 33, 57
Enzymes in digestion, 48
Equal®, 73
Equipment needs for nutrition programs, 241
Ergosterol, 137, 139
Esophagus, 48
Essential amino acids, 82
Estimating caloric need, 129
Ethnic foods, 22
Ethnic restaurants, 244
Evaluating nutrition programs, 288
Exchange method, 53, 57, 75, 86, 104, 320
Exchange method in carbohydrate control, 75, 320

Extrinsic factor, 150

F
Fad diets, 27, 127
False foods, 328
Family restaurants, 246
Fastfood nutrient information, 11, 239, 246, 269, 270
Fastfood operation, 246
Fat, 9
Fat breakdown, 69
Fat food preparation control, 211-212
Fat intake recommended, 101
Fats, 45, 46, 90, 248
Fats, calories in, 93
Fat-soluble vitamins, 136
Fats, saturated, 248
Faux foods, 328
Feasibility study steps, 231-235
Federal Trade Commission (FTC), 9, 10, 33, 35, 289, 294, 302
Feedback, 288, 306, 308
Fiber, 48, 63, 66, 67, 71, 180, 200, 321, 323, 326, 328
Flavor, 212, 229
Fluorine, 159, 183
Folacin (folic acid), 150
Food allergies, 275, 326-328
Food and Drug Administration, 7, 10, 11, 33, 34, 36, 51, 73-74
FDA and menu terms, 266
Food and health, 3
Food and Nutrition Board, 51, 109, 110
Food-away-from-home consumption, 12
Food consumption percentages, 52
Food, holding of, 308
Food intolerances, 230, 275, 326
Food, need for, 2, 44
Food, portioning of, 248, 251, 308
Food, preservation of, 197-200
Food regulation, 9
Food sensitivities, 274
Food Stamp Program, 6
Foodservices and healthful foods, 5
Foodservice workforce, 292
Food storage, 193, 194, 201, 205, 307
Fortification (enrichment), 37, 181, 200
Food value tables, 53
Fraud in nutrition, 24
Fresh foods, handling of, 199
Fresh foods, produce, 203, 209

Frozen foods, handling of, 199
Frozen meat cookery, 209
Frozen storage, 201, 204
Fructose, 64-68
Fruits, 209
Functions of protein, 87

G
Gaining weight, 131
Galactose, 64-68
Glucose, 64-68, 70, 100, 324
Glycogen, 65, 67
Goiter, 20, 180
Gout, 78
Government and nutrition, 6
Governmental nutrition information, 33
GRAS, 31, 33
Grain products, 200
Grains, whole, 37
Guest information, 264-276, 306, 327-328

H
Hard water, 158
Harvard Medical School, 110, 112
Health and Human Services, 33, 35
Health-care units and nutrition, 317
Health conscious patrons, 227
Healthful foods program (see also menu(s), menu planning, recipes, training)
    causes, of failure, 292
    goals of, 192
    guidelines for, 194
    incorporation of, 231
    program examples, 217- 218, 247-249
    program roll-out, 287-289
    purposes of, 215-218, 303
Health programs and nutrition, 285
Heart disease, 67, 72, 73, 90, 92, 109, 111
Height-weight standards, 120, 123
Hemoglobin, 177
Hemophilia, 142
Hiatal hernia, 322
High blood pressure, 90, 109, 111, 170, 171, 321
High carbohydrate diet, 88
High-density lipoproteins (HDL), 111
High fiber (residue) diets, 321

Hotels and nutrition, 243
Hydrogenation, 94
Hypertension, 170, 171, 321
Hypoglycemia, 324

I
Ideal diets, 59
Ideal weight, 122
Illnesses, food related, 3, 4
Implementing nutrition programs, 264, 287-288, 302, 306
Incaparina, 83
Incomplete proteins, 82, 329
Index of nutrient density (IND), 38
Infraction, 109
Ingredient(s), 198, 211-213, 216, 226, 248, 268, 275, 307, 331
Ingredient information, 34
Inositol, 137
Instruction, 301
Insulin, 173, 184, 319-324
Intakes (food), 7, 9
Intrinsic factor (IF), 150
Iodine, 20, 180
Iron, 177
Issuing, 307

J
Job breakdown, 299

K
Keratomalacia, 138
Ketones, 78
Ketosis, 69, 100
Kidney problems, 90, 109
Kilocalorie, 50
Krebs cycle, 70

L
Labeling, 10, 34, 175
Labor cost, 241
Lactic acid, 66, 78
Lactose, 65, 66, 68, 111
Lactose intolerance, 68, 326
Laetrile (B$_{17}$), 137
Large intestine, 48
Lecithin, 98, 101
Legumes, 330
Levulose, 64
Limiting amino acids, 82
Limiting proteins, 329

Linoleic acid, 98, 173
Lipases, 99
Lipid intakes recommended, 101
Lipid metabolism, 99
Lipids, 45, 46, 90, 93
Lipoic acid, 137
Lipoproteins, 99, 111
Liver, 49, 78, 99, 100
Losses, nutrient, 192, 307
Low blood sugar, 324
Low calorie diets, 75, 320
Low density lipoproteins (LDL), 111
Low residue diet, 322
Low salt (sodium) diets, 321

M
Macrominerals, 165
Magnesium, 176
Maintaining weight, 132
Maltose, 64, 66, 68
Manganese, 183
Management and nutrition, 192, 306
Management and training, 293
Mannitol, 73
Mannose, 64, 65
Marketing, 221-222, 276-287, 306
Marketing, cooperative, 285
Marketing mix, the, 276-284
Marketing nutrition, 215
Marketing research, 218, 221
Markets, 221-225, 243, 276
Markets, healthful foods program, 215, 221-235, 238-239
Market segments, 222, 226
Market study, 223
Matlitol, 73
Meal demand times, 242
Meal development, 260
Meals-on-wheels, 7
Meat cookery, 207
Mega-nutrient diet, 27
Menu, communicating through, 264-276
Menu development, 216-218, 259
Menu format, 243, 265
Menu offerings, number, 241, 242
Menu plans and planning, 211, 226-231, 240-247, 260-263, 321, 323, 327-329
Menu(s), 239, 264-265, 303, 310, 317
Menu terms defined (FDA), 266
Mesomorphic, 122

Milk, 209
Minerals, 45, 46, 157, 161
Misinformation in nutrition, 24
Monosaccharides, 64
Monounsaturated fats and oils, 93
Motivation in learning, 296
Mouth, 48

N
National Dairy Council, 32
National Livestock and Meat Board, 32
National Restaurant Association,
    customer markets, 226-230
National Restaurant Association, view
    on regulation, 10, 15
National School Lunch Program, 6
Natural foods, 21, 28
Needs, nutritional, 21, 22, 23
Needs of patrons, 221, 225, 239
Net protein utilization (NPU), 84
Niacin, 146
Nitrogen blance, 89
Non-nutritive sweeteners, 73
Nutrient density, 38, 68, 84
Nutrient losses, 307
Nutrient loss, prevention of, 192,
    193-211
Nutrient needs, 50, 303
Nutrient preservation, 182, 307
Nutrients, 45, 193, 211-213, 318
Nutrient absorption in the body, 56
Nutrient information (see also guest
    information), 11, 19, 33, 255, 265,
    270, 271
Nutrition in hotel foodservices, 243
Nutritional labeling, 4, 10, 34, 200-201
Nutrition management, 317
Nutrition (menu) terms defined, 266
Nutrition programs, 215
Nutrition responsibility, 12-16
Nutrition, selling, 264
Nutrition values computerized, 254

O
Obesity, 90, 111
Oils, 90, 93
On-the-job-training (OJT), 297
Optimal diet, the, 59
Organic foods, 28
Osteomalacia, 140
Osteoporosis, 165

Overweight, 72, 101, 119

P
Panaceas for weight loss, 127
Pantothentic acid, 151
Patron information, 306
Patron needs, 221, 225
Patrons, kinds, 225
Pegamic acid (B_{15}), 137
Pellagra, 146
Personal foods needs, 23
Personal selling, 280
PERT, 219, 238, 287
Phospholipids, 98
Phosphorus, 140, 168
Photosynthesis, 64
Phytic acid, 37
Place, in marketing, 276, 283
Planning nutrition programs (see also
    menus, recipes, training), 218-220,
    231-235, 238, 287-289
Plant products, 209
Plaque (arterial), 109
Plaque in tooth decay, 71
Point-of-sale selling, 281
Polysaccharides, 65, 66
Polyunsaturated fats and oils, 93, 101
Postal Service, 33
Potassium, 169
Precursors of vitamins, 137
Premising, 219
Preparation, 205-206, 308
Prepreparation and nutrient losses, 205
Prescribed diets, 316, 317
Price, in marketing, 276, 284
Produce, 203, 209
Product in marketing, 276, 307
Production, 307
Product knowledge, 309-312
Products, 88
Programmed training, 298
Programs, nutrition, 215
Promotions in marketing, 276, 280, 306
Proof in alcohol, 77
Protein, 81
Protein, cost of, 87
Protein efficiency ratio (PER), 84
Protein intolerance, 88
Protein needs, 86
Proteins, 45, 46
Protein, used for energy, 69

Protein value (USRDA), 34
Protein value (PV), 84
Provitamins, 137
Psychological needs for food, 21
Physiological needs for food, 21
Publicity in marketing, 281
Public Health Service, 33, 36
Purchasing, 197, 201, 211-212, 307
Pure Food, Drug and Cosmetic Act, 36, 37
Pyridoxine, 147

R
Receiving, 307
Recipe(s), 212, 239, 248, 249-260, 266, 330
Recipe development, 198, 249-252
Recipe evaluation, 257
Recipe nutrient analysis, 53, 252-257
Recipe testing, 257
Recipe selection, 239-240, 249, 303
Recipes, computer analyzed, 53, 254
Recommended alcoholic intake, 77, 78
Recommended carbohydrate intake, 67, 68, 72, 75
Recommended Dietary Allowances, 51, 53, 59, 86, 245
Recommended fat intake, 101
Recommended protein intake, 86
Reducing diet, 27, 320
Reducing weight, 128
Refrigerated storage, 201, 202
Reliable nutritional information, 26
Religious needs for food, 23
Research, marketing, 221
Residue-control diets, 321-322
Responsibility for nutrition, 12-16
Restaurants, 244
Retinol, 138
Riboflavin (B₂), 146
Ribonucleic acid (RNA), 149, 151
Rickets, 140
Roughage, 67

S
Saccharides, 63
Saccharine, 73
Salt, 170
Salt restriction, 111
Sampling (in marketing), 281
Sampling (in employee training), 310

Saturated fats, 93, 111, 112, 248
Scurvy, 152
Seasoning, 212, 213, 318, 323
Segments, market, 222, 226
Select Committee on Nutrition and Human Needs, 7, 9
Selenium, 184
Selling nutrition, 264, 277
Senility, 109
Selling, personal, 280, 306, 309
Service, 278, 279, 312
Service personnel training, 308, 309-312
Simple carbohydrates, 64, 48, 71
Simple lipids, 97
Simple sugars, 73
Small intestine, 48, 49
Specific dynamic action (SDA), 125
Social needs for foods, 22
Sodium, 170, 213, 307
Sodium in water, 160
Sodium-restricted diets, 321
Sodium restriction, 111, 213, 273, 321
Soft water, 158
Softening water, 160
Sorbitol, 73
Sources of minerals, 168
Special requests, 260-261, 275-276, 309
Staffing for nutrition programs, 241
Standardized recipes, 250
Standards, food, 33, 35
Standards, nutritional, 59
Standards of Identity, 23, 35
Standards of weight, 20
Starch, 63-64, 66-67
Stibesterol, 37
Stomach, 48
Storage, 307
Storage, food, 193, 194, 201-205, 307
Strokes (cardiovascular), 90, 92, 109, 111
Sucrose, 64-66, 68, 73
Sugar, 64, 68, 71, 111
Sugar alcohols, 73, 74
Suggestive selling, 280
Sulfur, 170
Sweating, 173
Sweeteners, use of, 71

T
Tables of food value, 53

Target markets, 223
Taste testing, 257
Teaching nutrition, 295
Temperature, 193-210, 308
Testing recipes, 257
Tests for fatty tissue, 122
Texture, food, 318
Thiamine (B_1), 70, 143
Thrombosis, 109
Thyroid, 124, 127, 180
Time of meal demand, 242
Title VII elderly feeding program, 7
Tocopherol, 141
Tooth decay, 71, 140
Trace minerals, 177, 185
Traditional eating patterns, 226
Trainees, 296, 302
Trainers, 295
Training, 265, 292-314
Training formats, 297-299
Training needs, 294, 299
Training objectives, 292
Training topics, 302-312
Triglycerides, 93, 99, 111

U
U.S. dietary goals, 35
Ulcers, diets and, 322-323
Unreliable nutrition information, 26
Unsaturated fats, 93, 111
USDA, 2, 3, 35, 71
US Dietary Goals, 35
US Public Health Service, 109
US RDA, 34, 53
US Senate Select Committee on
    Nutrition and Human Needs, 7, 9

V
Value perception, 284
Vegan diets, 328
Vegans, 151, 328
Vegetables, 209
Vegetarian, 328-331

Very low density lipoproteins (VLDP),
    111
Veto factor, 217, 226
Vestibule training, 298
Villi, 49
Vitamin A, 138
Vitamin B_1, 143
Vitamin B_2, 146
Vitamin B_6, 147
Vitamin B_{12}, 150
Vitamin C, 152
Vitamin D, 139
Vitamin E, 141
Vitamin K, 142
Vitamins, 45, 46, 136

W
Waitstaff training, 309
Water, 43, 47, 157
Water, need for, 158
Water softening, 160
Water-soluble vitamins, 136, 143
Whole grains, 37
Weight-conscious consumers, 227
Weight control, 116
Weight gain, 131
Weight loss, 128, 320
Weight maintenance, 132
Weight loss panaceas, 126
Weight reduction diet, 27, 124, 128,
    129, 130
Weight standards, 120
White House conference on food,
    nutrition and health, 7
Worker training, 241

X
Xerophthalmia, 138
Xylitol, 73

Z
Zen diet, 27
Zinc, 182